Age, Time, and Fertility

Applications of Exploratory Data Analysis

MARY B. BRECKENRIDGE
Department of Family Medicine
Rutgers Medical School
University of Medicine and Dentistry of New Jersey
Piscataway, New Jersey

With an Appendix by John W. Tukey
Princeton University, Princeton, New Jersey
and Bell Laboratories, Murray Hill, New Jersey

1983

ACADEMIC PRESS

A Subsidiary of Harcourt Brace Jovanovich, Publishers
New York   London
Paris   San Diego   San Francisco   São Paulo   Sydney   Tokyo   Toronto

ACADEMIC PRESS, INC.
111 Fifth Avenue, New York, New York 10003

United Kingdom Edition published by
ACADEMIC PRESS, INC. (LONDON) LTD.
24/28 Oval Road, London NW1 7DX

Library of Congress Cataloging in Publication Data

Breckenridge, Mary B.
   Age, time, and fertility.

   (Studies in population)
   Includes bibliographical references and index.
   1. Fertility, Human--Sweden--Mathematical models.
2. Sweden--Population--Mathematical models.
3. Fertility, Human--Mathematical models.   I. Title.
II. Title: Exploratory data analysis.   III. Series.
HB1027.B73   1983   304.6'32'09485   82-24474
ISBN 0-12-128750-5

PRINTED IN THE UNITED STATES OF AMERICA

83 84 85 86   9 8 7 6 5 4 3 2 1

TO BRUCE, A SUSTAINING CONSTANT AMONG THE VARIABLES

Contents

List of Figures and Tables

Figures

Fig. 8.2.   EHR time parameters α_i^*, β_i^*, and γ_i^* and total rates of fertility
$5T_i$ for selected countries: time sequences of age-specific over-
all fertility distributions expressed as weighted sums of the A_j^*,
B_j^*, and C_j^* age standards for the $X202$ sequence.

Tables

Preface

This study models change in the age pattern of fertility. It responds to a specific need in making fertility comparisons across time and place—the need for a summary measure of change that conveys more information about the dynamics of change than can total fertility rates alone. The modeling process is based on Tukey's exploratory data analysis (EDA) methods. This approach has proved very effective in other fields for detecting underlying patterns, even in flawed data. Demography has only begun to take advantage of the strengths of this approach in the description of complex data sets.

Even with the increasing availability of data on individual fertility intentions and behavior, measures of the aggregate consequences of individual behaviors continue to have a central place in demographic analysis for several good reasons:

1. to identify population trends and transitions;
2. to provide general standards against which to measure the behavior of subpopulations;
3. to permit the comparison of current patterns with historical patterns and patterns in those populations for which more detailed information is not available;
4. to summarize fertility behavior for use in population projections and in models that relate demographic change to social and economic change.

Measures of total fertility alone cannot fully serve these purposes because very different age patterns of fertility can result in the same total fertility rate.

Previous efforts to model the age pattern of fertility have encountered two difficulties: either they have not described well a sufficiently wide range of fertility schedules or they have not provided stable, interpretable descriptions of fertility change across time for actual populations. The success reported here in modeling overall and marital fertility in long time sequences is the result of the data guiding and flexibility of the EDA approach in combination with robust–resistant methods of parameter estimation. As applied in this book, the process also introduces two-stage modeling—a further innovation for demographic modeling. The first stage concentrates on the detection of the patterns that underlie a data time sequence, bringing as much as possible of the systematic variability into a small number of parameters. The model thus grows out of the data, rather than being imposed on the data. The second stage standardizes the form of the fitted parameters. That is, from the many algebraically equivalent expressions of the parameters, a demographically guided standard form of the fitted descriptions is selected for the identification of trends and transitions and brief departures from trend and for the comparison of one fertility time sequence with another. Appendix A by John W. Tukey places this approach within a broader view of modeling.

Modeling is carried out for two centuries of Swedish age-specific overall fertility rates and seven decades of marital fertility rates in both cross-sectional and cohort perspectives. The general applicability of these findings is then illustrated with fertility sequences for the 25 counties of Sweden, a six-decade sequence of U.S. fertility data, and recent data for other countries. Although the primary contribution of this work is to the modeling of demographic change in time sequence rather than to the study of Swedish history, it provides some new insights into Swedish marriage and fertility experience across two centuries and makes informative new use of 85 years of eighteenth- and nineteenth-century data that have been subjected to little previous analysis. The methodology and substantive findings will thus be of interest to several audiences: demographers, not only those working on fertility, but also those working with a variety of other data; historical demographers, especially those concerned with the problems of analyzing incomplete and error-ridden data; and European social and economic historians.

This book is organized with two groups of readers in mind: those who are specifically interested in the measures of fertility change developed and those who are primarily interested in the methods as they can be equally well applied to other types of demographic data—not only to other expressions of fertility experience such as age-parity-specific rates but also to mortality, morbidity, migration, labor force participation, and health care utilization. The chapters form two sections. The first section (Chapters II–V) provides an introduction to the philosophy and tools of EDA and to the data analyzed. It then examines in detail the process of developing and standardizing the closely fitting, few-parameter descriptions of demographic change in time sequence. The second section (Chapters VI–VIII) examines the results and applications of fertility modeling and establishes relations between change in the age pattern of fertility and change in the level of fertility. Cross-referencing permits the reader to move easily between outcome and process and among related results. Only a basic knowledge of demography and statistics is required to follow the material presented. The fundamental material on fertility modeling and re-presentation of fits in a standard form was first reported in my dissertation at Princeton University and a paper in the Technical Report Series of the Department of Statistics. A number of additional examples and refinements are presented for the first time in this book.

Acknowledgments

Many people have contributed to the evolution of this work through discussions, technical advice, review, and helpful criticism. The work owes its initiation to a challenge from Ansley Coale that I find a way to identify in aggregate data, even flawed historical data, evidence of departures from fertility pattern trends that are related to unusual circumstances—wars, severe crop failures, emigration, and economic distress. This study builds on Coale's pioneering work on modeling aggregate experience in demographically understandable terms. A timely encounter with the philosophy and tools of exploratory data analysis led me to consider old questions in productive new ways. I am particularly indebted to John W. Tukey for his advice, his encouragement in pursuing this work, and his helpful comments on an earlier draft of the manuscript. The work has also benefited from my exposure to Norman Ryder's longitudinal view of demographic phenomena, with emphasis on cohort experience and period–cohort interrelations. I appreciate his careful review of portions of an earlier draft of the manuscript and his cogent comments. The utility of bringing this work together in a single volume was first pointed out by Barbara Anderson, who has also provided perceptive criticism and encouragement at a number of stages of the research. The Department of Family Medicine has fostered both my completion of the work on this book and my application of exploratory methods in research on morbidity and health care utilization.

In the preparation of the manuscript, Ruth Easley filled many technical roles with unusual skill, ingenuity, and spirit. It is a pleasure to acknowledge her contributions over the many months from first to final draft. The staff of Academic Press deserve special thanks for the cooperative spirit and judgment that have characterized their production effort.

Age, Time, and Fertility
Applications of Exploratory Data Analysis

I

Introduction

The continuing search for more refined ways of expressing demographic fact or change in a small number of meaningful parameters grows out of the need to simplify comparisons across time and place. A summary measure, selected with care, can also yield new insight on the association of demographic change with social and economic change.

Whatever variable is of interest—fertility, mortality, migration, labor force participation—no single measure can be expected to serve all purposes. The rewards of looking at data in a number of different ways, and then again in new ways, have been repeatedly demonstrated. The problems of dealing with incomplete and error-ridden data continue to be a challenge for new methodologies.

In his assessment of trends in technology that impinge on demographic research, Winsborough (1978) emphasizes not only advances in computing, data processing, and retrieval systems but also the development of new methods of model construction, data analysis, and parameter estimation. He refers to the new methods in terms of new analytic styles for handling the increasing volume and complexity of demographic data. He also points out the Tukey and Mosteller–Tukey work on exploratory data analysis (EDA) as a style whose importance for demography has yet to be assayed. The use of the Tukey and Mosteller EDA approach in the following chapters, with a combination of flawed and very high quality data, demonstrates the value of this flexible, data-guided approach in meeting a specific need in demographic analysis—the need for a stable, interpretable description of change in the age pattern of fertility across time.

The goals that were met by these exploratory analyses were:

1. to extract the patterns underlying long time sequences of age-specific fertility,

2. to express these patterns in a small number of parameters that reveal
    not only differences in pattern but also the dynamics of change in a
    demographically understandable form, and
3. to describe trends and transitions sufficiently well that departures
    from trend can be examined in relation to singular events—wars,
    periods of economic distress, years of high emigration—that would
    be expected to have large, although temporary, effects on fertility.

Previous efforts to model the age pattern of fertility have not succeeded
in providing such descriptions of actual population experience. One approach to fertility modeling has sought to express the net maternity function in terms of specific statistical distributions, such as a log normal
curve, a beta function, or a Gompertz function. Keyfitz (1977) observes
that his tests of several proposed distributions "offer little room for satis-
faction," and Brass (1974), as well as Keyfitz, emphasizes that most
simple distributions fall far short of describing a wide range of fertility
schedules accurately.

Another approach has used empirical generalizations as fixed standards.[1] This second approach (the basis of the Coale (1971) model of
marital fertility, the Coale–McNeil (1972) marriage model, and the Coale–
Trussell (1974) model fertility schedules) incorporates the empirically derived patterns into a model and then systematically varies the patterns to
apply to populations that did not contribute to the formation of the standards. The patterns have usually been given plausible, demographically
meaningful interpretations. This approach has been far more successful in
fitting a wide range of fertility experience than have attempts to model
fertility by means of simple functional forms, but it still has encountered
numerous problems. For example, Trussell (1974) has commented on
efforts to develop a coherent time-sequence description of overall fertility
for Sweden and the United States by fitting reported schedules with
Coale–Trussell model schedules. He describes the result for both countries as, "Unfortunately . . . disappointing, since the parameters are not
very stable even in periods when we know that actual nuptiality or fertility conditions were not changing rapidly."

Whereas previous efforts have tested how age-specific fertility data fit
externally derived patterns, the EDA approach permits the model of
changing fertility patterns to grow out of the time-sequence data. The two
centuries of single-year, age-specific fertility data available for Sweden,
including 1775–1860 data that have been subjected to little previous analysis, provide an unusual opportunity for such time-sequence analysis. The
first measures of the success of the EDA procedures are the closely fitting
descriptions developed for the cross-sectional and cohort data sequences
and the coherent picture of demographic change expressed in the fitted

parameters. A further measure of success is the demonstrated applicability of the derived age standards to the description of time-sequence data from other countries, including the United States.

The separation of this book into a "process" section (Chapters II–V) and an "outcome" section (Chapters VI–VIII) recognizes the interests of several different groups of readers. The "process" chapters include sufficient detail so that the reader can visualize the application of the methods to other bodies of demographic data.[2] The "outcome" chapters group the results and applications for the use of demographers and historians whose immediate interest is in the substantive measures rather than the details of methodology.

The process–outcome separation is, of course, an artificial one. In EDA, examination of the results at each step guides the following steps of exploration. The explorations reported here have not proceeded along a broad, straight path with simultaneous analyses of overall and marital fertility from both cross-sectional and cohort perspectives. Building on the initial observation by McNeil and Tukey (1975) that twentieth-century United States fertility distributions could be well described in several forms by empirical higher rank (EHR) analysis, one of the tools of EDA, the exploration process has been one of multiple forays into age-specific fertility data. The method was first applied to the general case of cross-sectional overall fertility rates by 5-year age groups, then at another angle to the cohort perspective on these rates, and then at another depth to the marital fertility component of overall fertility. Finally, the study of overall fertility was extended to longer time sequences, single-year-of-age rates, and more complex descriptions of patterns. Each new foray has depended on the guidance and equipment acquired in the previous steps of exploration. The early work developed close fits in two age parameters and two time parameters for overall and marital fertility in cross-sectional and cohort sequences of the Swedish data (Breckenridge, 1976). These results led to extensive testing of more complex models for improvements in fit to a selected cross-sectional overall fertility sequence (Orav, 1977). At the same time, further exploratory steps made other contributions to effective description by: (1) identifying useful standard forms of the closely fitted parameters, which both simplified the descriptions and made cross-sequence comparisons valid; and (2) establishing the value of translating the time parameters to a standard level of fertility in order to uncover an additional type of transition in fertility patterns (Breckenridge, 1978). These results, in turn, have been extended in several directions, and some of this work is reported here for the first time.

Whether the reader's immediate interest is in the substantive results or the details of the methodology, an "iterative" reading of the book may be the most useful—moving back and forth between process and outcome. The first series of stops might be the summary in Chapter II as an introduction to the EDA approach and to the data analyzed, followed by Tables 4.1 and 4.2 in Chapter IV to note the closeness of fits, and then the summary in Chapter V on standard-form re-presentation of fits. The reader might then scan Chapter VII on marital fertility outcomes and their relation both to overall fertility outcomes and to results by other methods of analyzing fertility. Alternatively, the reader might choose to scan Chapter VI on the outcomes for cohort overall fertility in relation to cross-sectional overall fertility.

A return to the consideration of process would then emphasize the two aspects of developing descriptions or models of demographic data, as discussed by Tukey in Appendix A. The first concern is "to make our fit to the diversity of the real world as good as possible, subject to holding the number of parameters to a minimum." Only then does the second concern enter consideration—which structure of the empirically best-fitting models best serves the purposes of a specific investigation of demographic data.

Chapter II provides an overall view of the philosophy and some of the tools of EDA, including a simple illustration of stepwise dissection of data, the role of residuals in exploration, and the use of graphic summaries to identify data patterns. This chapter also provides an overall view of the fertility experience recorded for Sweden across two centuries—information that will help guide the modeling of age-specific fertility change by EDA methods in the subsequent chapters.

Chapter III outlines choices to be made in an exploratory analysis of any data set, describes generally useful analytic procedures, and discusses the choices made in achieving very close fits to both the cross-sectional and the cohort time sequences of overall and marital fertility. The choices include: which form of the data to use in analysis of the selected sequences, how to linearize the data by re-expression before fitting, what degree of resistance to "outliers" to use in the fitting procedure, and which ways to examine residuals for size and, more importantly, structure in estimating goodness of fit. Development of increasingly complete descriptions of the regularities underlying the diverse age distributions of fertility in the sequences starts at the three-parameter model of the classical analysis of variance and tests higher-rank fits, using the robust–resistant iteratively weighted fitting procedures that comprise EHR analysis (McNeil and Tukey, 1975). For each sequence, a well-fitting description with two age parameters and two time parameters is then carried forward to Chapters IV and V. For one overall fertility sequence—a cross-sectional sequence that includes the most recent data available—a description with three age parameters and three time parameters is also carried forward to illustrate several advantages that result, under some circumstances, from pulling into a fitted description even a small amount of pattern left in the residuals.

Chapter IV tests how well the fitting process has met the first goal in the description of fertility change—expressing the diversity of the real world in a small number of parameters. The closeness of fit achieved for all sequences is illustrated with summary measures of residual size, tests of residuals for remaining pattern, typical reported and fitted schedules, and presentation of "worst fits" for each sequence. A distinctive type of structure left in cohort residuals is identified with period effects on cohort fertility patterns.

Chapter V applies a very useful concept for modeling: the empirically best-fitting model need not be, and often should not be, the form in which the fitted parameters are examined and interpreted. Knowledge of demographic processes is used to guide the selection of a standard form for the parameters of all of the sequences, the procedures for re-presentation are outlined, and the function of each of the standard-form parameters in describing fertility patterns is tested. The resulting standard forms simplify the descriptions, aid interpretation of change, and make cross-sequence comparisons of parameters appropriate in the chapters that follow.

Chapters VI and VII focus on trends and transitions in Swedish fertility experience and on identification of the nature of brief departures from trend. Chapter VIII relates standards derived from Swedish data to fertility experience in other countries and to hypothetical experience expressed in other researchers' model fertility schedules.

Beginning with the single-year-of-age cohort sequence, which encompasses the major transition from moderately high to below-replacement-level fertility, Chapter VI directs attention to relations between cohort and cross-sectional overall fertility patterns across time. For sequences by 5-year age groups these relations are traced from the earliest periods of less accurate data to the most recent changes of pattern. The chapter also considers the relations of subpopulation experience—in this case for each of the 25 Swedish counties—to the aggregate experience expressed in the data for the country as a whole. The translation of fitted parameters and fertility distributions to a standard level of fertility helps tease out additional information about the nature of fertility change, including evidence of change in the age pattern of entry into childbearing. Departures from trend in fertility patterns are considered in relation to periods of emigration, war, and economic distress. Examination of even small residuals in conjunction with fitted parameters proves to be an important tool for interpretation, just as it was for fitting.

The information about overall fertility change and the gains in methodology from Chapter VI are then carried into Chapter VII for consideration of marital fertility change and its relation to overall fertility change in both cross-sectional and cohort perspectives. Here the focus, although it includes the traditional concern with evidence of parity-dependent control, is a broader one, examining evidence also of other types of transition in marital fertility patterns, for both all legitimate births and births occurring 9 months or more after marriage. The further dissection of time parameters to look at change in the age pattern of childbearing apart from change in the level of fertility leads to a method of estimating missing data and correcting some suspected inaccuracies. Chapter VII provides the methodological basis for a detailed analysis of the variable border between marital and nonmarital childbearing.

The standard-form age parameters that underlie two centuries of Swedish fertility experience are applied to preliminary cross-population comparisons in Chapter VIII. These parameters prove to give an equally close-fitting and coherent description of a time sequence of U.S. overall fertility experience up to the mid-1970s. They also prove to underlie a variety of Coale–Trussell model fertility schedules selected to be quite unlike any fertility distributions ever observed in Sweden. Short time sequences of overall fertility for 15 countries and selected overall and marital fertility schedules for approximately 50 countries, with fertility ranging from high to below-replacement-level, are expressed in terms of the standard-form age parameters derived from Swedish data to provide the first step in the systematic development of cross-population descriptions of difference and change in aggregate fertility patterns. The large number of close fits confirms the generality of the derived standards, even at this preliminary stage. Joint consideration of fitted parameters and residuals traces the emergence of new age patterns of childbearing in countries with high degrees of regulation of fertility. It also points to types of modification of parameters that should be expected to accommodate well these recently developing patterns.

The exploratory analyses presented here do not provide a "finished" model of time-sequence change in fertility patterns, but they do yield informative and provocative steps in the continuing search for useful, more refined ways of looking at the full diversity of fertility patterns in changing social milieux. The success in developing a sound, demographically interpretable description of a long and varied fertility history, including data of lesser accuracy, and the success in describing closely a variety of fertility patterns from other countries encourage a full exploratory analysis across populations, including the most recent variations in aggregate fertility patterns.

Notes to Chapter I

1. The trend away from predetermined forms and toward empirically derived forms is not unique to fertility modeling. The modeling of mortality has proceeded in the same direction. For examples, see the Coale–Demeny (1966) groups of model life tables, the Brass (1975) logit life tables incorporating variations on an empirical standard pattern, and the Ewbank, Gomez de Leon, and Stoto (1983) four-parameter system of model life tables.

2. Indeed, the applicability of the EDA approach to a wide variety of demographic data is becoming increasingly apparent. An early example with an exploratory emphasis is D'Souza's (1974) study of interbirth intervals. Other examples include modeling of mortality (Ewbank *et. al.*, 1983) and length of hospital postoperative stay (Stoto, 1983b), tests of population projections (Stoto, 1983a), and longitudinal study of ambulatory care utilization by the elderly (Breckenridge, in progress).

II

Preparing for an Exploratory
Analysis: Data and
Analytic Approach

Introduction

The use of Swedish fertility data in an exploratory analysis is a natural strategy for developing a time-sequence model of age patterns of fertility. No other country provides as long a single-year sequence of age-specific overall fertility rates—data of very high quality since 1860, supplemented by 85 years of little-analyzed pre-1860 data of lower quality. Exploratory data analysis (EDA), with emphasis on data guiding and flexibility, provides a powerful means of detecting the patterns that underlie these data across both age and time, in both cross-sectional and cohort perspectives, and of simultaneously identifying the effects of singular events or faulty data. Although the decision to examine Swedish data has precedent, the detailed application of EDA to related time sequences of demographic data is new.

Both the length and quality of their demographic records have led to frequent use of Sweden's data to demonstrate new analytic approaches and to test new models. For example, some of the earliest evidence presented by Ryder (1951, 1955) for the importance of the cohort perspective in understanding demographic change was based on Swedish fertility, mortality, and marriage data. Also, Lee's (1975, 1977) tests of spectral analysis as a means of relating fertility, mortality, and nuptiality change are partially based on Swedish data. Extensive records of other kinds— economic, social, climatological, medical—have permitted the examina-

8

tion of relations between demographic change and other types of change. Examples of this include Thomas's (1941) detailed study of the social and economic aspects of Swedish population movements, Hyrenius's (1946) consideration of the relation between birth rates and economic activity in Sweden from 1920 to 1944, and Friedlander's (1969) and Mosher's (1980) use of Swedish migration and fertility data to test Davis's (1963) multiphasic demographic response theory. Swedish data have been the basis of external standards incorporated in new models, such as the Coale–McNeil model of first marriage frequencies (Coale, 1971; Coale and McNeil, 1972). They have also provided the basis for extending or modifying previously derived models: examples include Ewbank's (1974) tests of Coale–McNeil marriage model variations in the description of both female and male marriage entry patterns for a sequence of Swedish birth cohorts and Page's (1977) incorporation of marriage duration effects on marital fertility patterns in an analog of the Coale (1971) marital fertility model.

Because Swedish fertility and its relation to other factors have been analyzed by a variety of quite different methods, a background exists against which the results of an exploratory analysis of Swedish age-specific fertility patterns can be examined. As we prepare to apply exploratory analysis methods to the development of a time-sequence model of age patterns of fertility, we consider first the characteristics of the data to be analyzed and then the philosophy and tools of the EDA approach that make it particularly appropriate to the task.

Data in Time Sequence—Two Centuries of Swedish Fertility Rates

For time-sequence modeling of fertility, Swedish data have a number of desirable characteristics in addition to the length and quality of data. These include considerable diversity in both the age distribution of births and the level of fertility, prominent changes in the age pattern of marriage, which should be reflected in fertility patterns, and well-documented occurrences of singular events (wars, periods of high emigration, periodic severe crop failures) that would be expected to affect temporarily the level and/or age distribution of births. For the purpose of demonstrating the effectiveness of EDA methods, the merits of the data also include the fact that they are not for an "ideal" population. The rates to be analyzed reflect most of the factors that tend to confound aggregate fertility models: significant levels of illegitimate fertility and premarital pregnancy legitimated by marriage before the birth of the child; recent increases in the rates of divorce and remarriage; and, in early data, probable errors of common types, including incorrect population totals, omission of births, misplacement of births in time, and misplacement of women by age.

The availability of overall fertility schedules by 5-year age groups (15–19 to 45–49) and single calendar years for a period of two centuries is a particular advantage. These schedules contain useful demographic information not captured in 10-year or 5-year averages, even when systematic change over time is gradual. Some of the information becomes accessible because closer approximations of cohort experience can be constructed from single-year cross-sectional schedules than from 5-year averages. Either in cross section or by cohort, the large number of data points is effectively used in the EDA approach to extract the underlying patterns, even in the presence of brief departures from trend. The availability of single-year-of-age overall fertility schedules for ages 13–50, beginning with the birth cohort of 1870, provides additional strength to the analyses covering the latter part of the time sequence. A brief discussion of the sources of data and the quality of the eighteenth- and nineteenth-century data will precede an overview of fertility change across two centuries.

Data Sources[1]

Overall Fertility   Based on parish register information systematically collected by the Statistical Commission of Sweden, yearly data on the number of confinements by age of mother in 5-year age groups (15–19, 20–24, . . . , 45–49) are available from 1775. Year-end census data on the population by sex and age in 5-year age groups are available for every fifth year beginning in 1775, with estimates for the intervening years. On degree of accuracy, the data fall into pre-1860 and post-1860 periods, divided by the founding of the Central Bureau of Statistics in Sweden and the resulting reorganization of procedures for collecting and recording population statistics. The confinement and population data for single years from 1775 to 1875, after adjustment for obvious omissions, were published by the Central Bureau of Statistics in 1878 in the single appendix often referred to as "Grunddragen."

Overall, the "Grunddragen" data on the number of confinements are thought to be relatively accurate, particularly after a tightening of reporting requirements in 1801 (Hofsten and Lundstrom, 1976). However, they are considered to contain some common types of errors: misplacement in time when the date of baptism rather than the date of birth is recorded; omission when the birth did not occur in the parish where the mother was registered; and misplacement by mother's age because of the practice of reporting the age as that at a near birthday. This last error persisted until 1895, when recording of the mother's birth date became a requirement. The error has greatest importance for fertility rates by 5-year age groups when women soon to be 20 are reported as aged 20 or women soon to be 25 are reported as aged 25. Particularly for the cities, the population data from the parish registers before 1860 are considered to be less reliable than the confinement data, in regard to both total numbers and age distributions.

The data from "Grunddragen" were the basis of Sundbärg's major reconstitution of Swedish population statistics by age and sex for quinquennial periods from 1750 to 1860. When Sundbärg carried out this work in the decades around 1900, he made only minor adjustments to the total population figures, confining revisions to the census data before 1810 and introducing no change exceeding 2 percent of the total population. He then proceeded on a stepwise adjustment of the structure of this fixed total, first for sex, then for age and sex combined, working backward by 5-year periods from the census of 1860 and using a combination of census and registration data. As Hofsten and Lundstrom (1976) point out, somewhat different estimates would have resulted had it been feasible at that time to start revision with corrections to local data by sex and age, allowing total population figures to be flexible, rather than starting with a fixed total population and adjusting within its framework.

Sundbärg's (1907) revised figures for 5-year age groups and 5-year periods up to 1860 have been adopted as the official statistics and have generally been used for research purposes, in conjunction with more recent data. Age-specific fertility rates calculated from these data and shown in Fig. 2.1 begin our overview of fertility change and are used later in this chapter to demonstrate some preliminary steps of exploratory analysis. In Chapters III–VII, however, we return to the unadjusted "Grunddragen" data, in combination with more recent single-year data, for our detailed time-sequence analysis by the methods of EDA.

Marital Fertility   The data needed to calculate age-specific marital fertility rates are available for census years beginning in 1870 and yearly beginning in 1892. Although the total number of confinements for legitimate births is available from the earliest years of data collection, recording of confinements by both the legitimacy of the birth and the age of the mother did not begin until 1868. Recording of the corresponding population data by age, sex, and marital status combined began with the 1870 census. Hofsten and Lundstrom (1976, p. 29) point out that Sundbärg's estimates of marital fertility rates by the 5-year age groups 20–24 to 45–49 for earlier 5-year periods "are based on rough calculations" for both the age distribution of confinements within marriage and the age distribution of married women. In the exploratory analyses of marital fertility in the following chapters, we shall concentrate on the yearly rates beginning in 1892.

Nonmarital conception has been common in Sweden and has traditionally accounted for a high proportion of all first births. The number of conceptions leading to illegitimate births is available yearly by age of mother beginning in 1868, and accounts for 10 to 15 percent of all births in each of the years 1892–1959. Beginning in 1911, when legitimate births were first recorded by duration of marriage and age of mother combined, it is possible to approximate the number of premarital conceptions legitimated by marriage before the birth of the child. From 1911 until the beginning of the 1960s, about 70–80 percent of all births to married women aged 15–19 and about 30–40 percent of all births to married women aged 20–24 are reported to have occurred within 8 months after marriage. Noting that in Sweden it has always been "more common for conception to be the reason for a marriage than vice versa," Hofsten and Lundstrom (1976, pp. 28–29) observe that "what looks like a change in legitimate or illegitimate fertility may, in actual fact, be a change in the habit of marrying among pregnant women." Sweden's experience in recent decades emphasizes the pertinence of this observation. Family formation has preceded or been dissociated from marriage to an increasing degree since the mid-1960s. Births outside of legal marriage accounted for 18 percent of all births in 1970 and 36 percent of all births in 1978. The exploratory analyses in the following chapters develop an approach for examining the interface of nonmarital and marital fertility in time sequence.

Overview of Fertility Change

Change can be viewed from a cross-sectional perspective or a cohort perspective. In which time periods has change occurred? Or which women, proceeding together through various time periods in the process of their childbearing years, effected change from the childbearing behavior of the women who preceded them? Here, we summarize change in Swedish fertility from both of these perspectives. In the following chapters, we shall merge the two views on the basis of exploratory analysis results.

We shall concentrate on two types of rates: one, age-specific fertility rates calculated from births by age of mother and from female population by age, mostly by 5-year age groups from 15–19 to 45–49; and two, total fertility rates—the sum of age-specific rates across all childbearing ages. (See Chapter III, Note 2, on the calculation of total fertility rates and the differences in their interpretation depending on whether the rates are for cohort or cross-sectional fertility and for overall or marital fertility.) These fertility rates, often expressed in terms of births per 100 or 1000 women, will be shown in the figures and tables of this book in terms of births per women.

Cross-sectional Perspective   The major stages of fertility change in Sweden are apparent in the age-specific fertility rates for 5-year periods, which include Sundbärg's aggregated and adjusted rates up to 1860 (Fig. 2.1). The early period of fluctuation for age groups 20–24 to 40–44 is followed by an 1810–1825 increase in rates across this broad age range, then a decline for ages below 30, which is attributed to later marriage. For

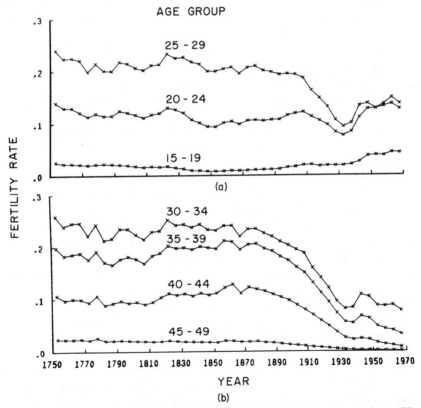

Fig. 2.1   Age-specific overall fertility rates (births per woman) for Sweden from 1751–1755 to 1966–1970: (a) age groups 15–19 to 25–29; (b) age groups 30–34 to 45–49.

ages 30 and above the higher rates were sustained until about 1880. The subsequent decline accelerated about 1910, and at that time ages 20–29 also joined in the reduction of fertility rates, helping to carry the total fertility rate below replacement level in the 1930s. Total fertility rates for the quinquennial periods can be examined in Fig. 2.5a. These expressions of total fertility equal five times the sum of the age-specific rates shown in Fig. 2.1 because the rates are for 5-year age groups (see Chapter III, Note 2).

Except for the brief prominent increase in childbearing at ages 30–39 in the 1940s, the partial and temporary recovery of the total fertility rate from the low levels of the 1930s depended on women below age 30. The first notable increases in childbearing at ages 15–19 occurred during the recovery period and supplemented the prominent increases for women aged 20–29. Temporary departure from a late age pattern of marriage was one factor in the higher rates. The first indications of such a change in marriage age appeared about 1935 (see Fig. 7.9)—following the 1934 publication of a book by Alva and Gunnar Myrdal, "Kris i Belfolkningsfragen" ("Crisis in the Population Question") and slightly preceding the 1937 beginning of government pronatalist efforts to encourage marriage in some segments of the population (Glass, 1967, pp. 316–317, 327–331). Within 15 years the proportion of women married at all childbearing ages above 19 increased dramatically—from .17 to .40 for those aged 20–24 and from .48 to .72 for those aged 25–29. These increases were accompanied by a small change in the proportion of women aged 15–19 who were married—from .02 to .05 by 1959.

Sweden's experience in the 1950s, similar to that of other Northern and Western European countries, involved a much less pronounced "baby boom," however, than occurred in the U.S., Canada, Australia, and New Zealand (Teitelbaum, 1973; Campbell, 1974). The differences between the U.S. and Sweden, measured in the total fertility rates for the 1945–1965 period, can be examined in Fig. 8.1. Since that period, the low fertility rates in Sweden occur in a new context: the proportions of women married at the younger ages have returned to the levels of the 1930s, but the increasing popularity of nonmarital cohabitation has contributed to an unprecedented increase in the proportion of births that occur outside of legal marriage. (See Gendell, 1980, for further discussion of these changes.)

Cohort Perspective   When we return to the beginning of the time sequence in 1775 for the cohort perspective on fertility change over two centuries, the average number of births per woman over the childbearing years becomes a useful indicator of change. (These data can be examined in Fig. 6.10 for all but the most recent cohorts and, for the latter, in Fig.

6.3.) The mean age of childbearing summarizes additional information about change (see Fig. 6.7).

Women who reached the beginning of childbearing ages between about 1805 and 1825 appear to have had the highest rates of total fertility recorded for Sweden—an average of about 4.6 to 4.7 births per woman. That total fertility never reached a higher level has generally been attributed to the adoption of Malthusian control of fertility—postponement of marriage and maintenance of never-married status for a significant fraction of the population. Ideas that anticipated Malthus's early nineteenth-century writings already had wide acceptance in the Swedish upper classes in the last quarter of the eighteenth century, according to Utterstrom (1962), and were entered into legislative debates on a new Servants Act as early as the Estates sessions of 1778/1779.[2] Variations on the pattern of relatively late and nonuniversal marriage persisted well into the twentieth century, continuing to contribute to variation in the level of completed fertility long after neo-Malthusian control, the control of childbearing within marriage, became a prominent factor in Swedish fertility change.

The decline from the highest fertility levels of the early nineteenth-century cohorts has been attributed to an increase in the age at marriage. Following this decline a plateau at an average of about 4.3 to 4.4 births per woman lasts for almost 30 cohorts. The earliest evidence of fertility limitation (or a consistent increase in fertility limitation) within marriage is usually associated with the cohorts of women who reached childbearing ages about 1865 (Hofsten and Lundstrom, 1976). These cohorts initiated the gradual but sustained decline in total rate, which became more pronounced with the cohorts aged 15 about 1890. Over the next 30 cohorts the mean age of childbearing dropped from 31.6 to 29.0 years and then rose again to 29.9 years, while the average number of births per women declined steadily to its lowest level—1.8 for the cohorts aged 15 in the period 1917–1921. Subsequent cohorts provide an example of marked variation in the timing of childbearing with little change in the level of cohort completed fertility. The mean age of childbearing gradually declined from 29.9 to 27.7 years, while the total fertility rate remained about 1.9–2.0 births per woman for cohorts reaching age 50 in the period 1957–1974.

Important regional differences in both of the major determinants of fertility patterns— marriage and control of marital fertility—have probably been obscured in the national aggregates. For the eighteenth and much of the nineteenth centuries, marriage differences might be traced to regionally distinct social structures that were based on the social class of the landholders, the size of the holdings, and the proportion of adult men in

each of the three principal rural population social groups: peasants, croft-
ers and married farm workers, and unmarried farm hands (Utterstrom,
1954). The possibility that neo-Malthusian control of fertility began earlier
in eastern Sweden, and particularly in the city of Stockholm, than in other
parts of the country has been suggested by Hofsten and Lundstrom (1976)
and Utterstrom (1954). Eriksson and Rogers (1978, pp. 134–146) consider
evidence for fertility limitation in relation to socioeconomic status in two
nineteenth-century cohorts selected from parish registers for one rural
district in eastern Sweden.

   Research interests in Swedish fertility with a longitudinal emphasis,
whether cross-sectional or cohort (for example, Hofsten, 1971; Hyrenius,
1951), have most often centered on the rate of natural increase in the
population and the identification of factors underlying the onset and progression of the sustained decline in fertility. Some summary measure of
total fertility—number of births, crude birth rate, net reproduction rate—
has usually been the chosen indicator in these studies. The lack of a well-
fitting, interpretable model of age-specific fertility in time sequence has
hampered more detailed examination of aggregate fertility change and its
relation to social and economic change.

   The two perspectives—cross-sectional and cohort—guide the modeling of the age pattern of fertility reported in Chapters III–VII. In preparation for this detailed analysis of two centuries of fertility change, we shall
consider next the philosophy of the EDA approach and shall demonstrate
some of the tools to be used.

Exploratory Data Analysis—
The Philosophy and the Tools

Exploratory data analysis is described by Tukey (1977) as systematic
"detective work . . . [that] needs both tools and understanding." It starts
from the premise that there can be many valid perspectives on the same
set of data, that is, many angles from which the same body of information
can be examined. The view from some angles will be more informative
than from others. The value to us of a particular view will depend on our
purposes—how we want to use what we have seen. A particular view
can, however, have unexpected value if it suggests the presence of a
pattern that we had not previously suspected. Often, simply removing
from the data some central tendency, such as the median, allows us to
"stand inside" and provides a rewarding new perspective on the data.

Stepwise Dissection and Residuals

The knowledge that we already have about the data can guide choices at the start of exploration and at each later step. To begin, will amounts, rates, or differences be a more appropriate form in which to examine the data? Will patterns be more apparent if the data are first ordered in some manner? Which aggregations of data may obscure valuable information and which are less apt to do so? Will frequency distributions or cumulative distributions suit our purposes better?

The exploration begins without detailed assumptions about the data or the patterns that underlie its variability. The analysis develops an increasingly complete description of the patterns by repeatedly removing regularities from the data (often starting by removing the median) and then looking at what is left over (the residuals). At each step two questions are asked: "How far have we come? Can we go further in developing a useful description of what is going on in the data?" This iterative dissection is continued until the amount of additional regularity removed in a step is negligible. The final fitted description is simply the combination (often the sum) of all the successive fits. Sometimes, of course, insights at a later stage leads us to return and handle an earlier stage differently.

Because data are almost always the result of indirect and imperfect measurement and, therefore, can be expected to fall at best "just *near* a line or curve" (Tukey, 1977), residuals of varying sizes are an expected result of the exploration. A distinctive feature of the EDA approach is that nothing is discarded. The analysis does not stop with a "model" and a statement of the percentage of total variation in the data explained by the description. Instead, the residuals are not only examined for further pattern at each stage of the analysis but are also retained and examined in detail at the end to see where and in what way the data depart from the fitted description; for example, in specific years? at specific ages?

The examination of residuals guides both interpretation and further exploratory analysis. It often leads to the identification of major transitions in the underlying pattern. It may also add to the understanding of the effects of singular events. For example, within the context of a population's trend in the age pattern of fertility, what effects did a war or a period of increased emigration have on childbearing patterns? Examination of residuals can also aid in identifying departures due to errors or misclassifications and then in estimating the appropriate corrections. In a complete EDA, such a process may need repetition, particularly after "fine tuning" the expression of the data.

Among the tools of exploration, four in particular have been used in the analyses of the Swedish fertility time sequences in the following chapters:

1. numeric and graphic summaries of original data, residuals, and fitted descriptions,
2. linearizing re-expressions,
3. robust–resistant interative fitting procedures, and
4. re-presentation of fitted descriptions.

In this chapter we provide an introduction to each of these tools.

Numeric and Graphic Summaries

We can use the Swedish age-specific overall fertility rates shown in Fig. 2.1 to illustrate numeric and graphic summaries in the process of data dissection. The accompanying tabulation of these rates $f_i(a_j)$ for each period i and age group j has 44 rows for the 5-year periods 1751–1755 to 1966–1970 and 7 columns for age groups 15–19 to 45–49.[3] The steps of dissection summarized here provide the background against which more complex analyses of more detailed fertility sequences are carried out in the following chapters.

				Age group			
Period	*15–19*	*20–24*	*25–29*	*30–34*	*35–39*	*40–44*	*45–49*
1751–1755	.0246	.1399	.2396	.2588	.1978	.1066	.0240
⋮	⋮	⋮	⋮	⋮	⋮	⋮	⋮
1966–1970	.0419	.1272	.1373	.0771	.0322	.0076	.0005

Rates and Cumulative Rates   A logical starting point for discussing rates is a summary of the rates for each age group across time (Table 2.1), including the median, minimum, and maximum rates and the interquartile range of rates in each group. The interquartile range is the numerical spread of the central half of the rates for an age group when the rates are ordered from lowest to highest, rather than ordered in time sequence.

Turning a numeric summary into a graphic summary is useful for quick comparisons. Schematic plots are one convenient way of doing this (Tukey, 1972). Such plots for the fertility rates of Table 2.1 are given in Fig. 2.2, which shows as a box the interquartile range of rates for each age group, with the location of the median rate for each age group indicated by a dash in the box. Using the interquartile range of rates as the unit of measure, the relative positions of the highest rate within one interquartile

TABLE 2.1

Numeric Summary of Overall Fertility Rates by Age Group: Sweden, 1751–1755 to 1966–1970

			Rate		
Age group	Minimum	Lower quartile	Median	Upper quartile	Maximum
15–19	.0074	.0112	.0175	.0209	.0428
20–24	.0762	.1054	.1151	.1235	.1399
25–29	.0934	.1561	.2007	.2142	.2396
30–34	.0771	.1492	.2223	.2381	.2588
35–39	.0322	.1207	.1803	.1953	.2105
40–44	.0076	.0640	.0967	.1076	.1270
45–49	.0005	.0077	.0181	.0203	.0260

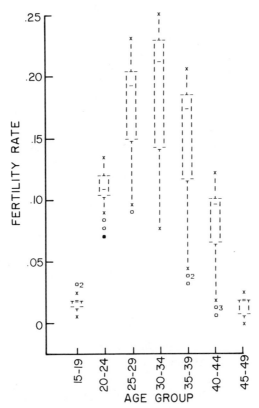

Fig. 2.2 Schematic plots of overall fertility rates by age group for Sweden from 1751–1755 to 1966–1970.

distance of the upper quartile and the lowest rate within one interquartile distance of the lower quartile are shown by an x beyond each end of the box. Outlying rates between these positions and one and a half times the interquartile distance are shown by open circles, whereas rates further out are shown by filled circles. A number to the right of a circle indicates more than one outlier in that position. The plot emphasizes some of the characteristics of the fertility sequence:

1. the very small variation of rate in age group 15–19 over more than two centuries—hardly more than in age group 45–49, where one expects the rates to be consistently quite low;
2. the relatively narrow range of rates for age group 20–24 with a few prominent outliers;
3. the wide range of rates for the other four age groups, with age group 30–34 reaching a higher level than any other and age group 25–29 never falling as low as all of the others do;
4. the very low levels reached at one extreme by age groups 35–39 and 40–44;
5. the location of the median rate well above the middle of the inter-quartile range for all but age group 20–24, reflecting the predominance of higher over lower rates in all but one age group in this time sequence, even in age groups with a wide range of rates.

We shall also want to look at cumulative rates, the sum of the fertility rates for women a given age and younger in each period, as shown in the accompanying tabulation. In this case we speak of "age cuts," for example, "cut at 24/25" to indicate the inclusion of rates for women aged 24 and lower and the exclusion of rates for women aged 25 and above.

				Age cut			
Period	19/20	24/25	29/30	34/35	39/40	44/45	49/50
1751–1755	.0246	.1645	.4041	.6629	.8607	.9673	.9913
⋮	⋮	⋮	⋮	⋮	⋮	⋮	⋮
1966–1970	.0419	.1691	.3064	.3835	.4157	.4233	.4238

The numeric summary of cumulative rates for the sequence can also be viewed conveniently in schematic plots (Fig. 2.3). Because the rate at age cut 49/50 is proportional to the total fertility rate (shown for each of the 44 periods in Fig. 2.5a)[4], the schematic plot summary indicates the moderately wide range in total fertility rate over two centuries—from 4.95 to

2.00. The relative compactness of the range of rates at age cuts 19/20 and 24/25, and also at age cut 29/30 except for a few large outliers, directs attention to the role of age groups 30–34 and 35–39 in determining period differences in total fertility rates in this time sequence.

Normalized Rates   If we are interested not only in fertility rates by age but also in the age pattern of fertility, our first step of dissection should be to normalize the cumulative rates. That is, the cumulative fertility rate at each of the seven age cuts in a period is divided by the rate at age cut 49/50, giving the proportion of total fertility in each period that can be attributed to women a given age and younger, as shown in the accompanying tabulation. Because the division always gives a value of one at the seventh age cut, 49/50, we can reduce the 44 × 7 table of rates to a 44 × 6 table for further dissection. We use the designation f_{ij} for period i and age cut $j = 1, 2, \ldots, 6$ for these cumulated, normalized rates.

	Age cut						
Period	19/20	24/25	29/30	34/35	39/40	44/45	49/50
1751–1755	.0248	.1659	.4076	.6687	.8683	.9758	1.0
:	:	:	:	:	:	:	:
:	:	:	:	:	:	:	:
1966–1970	.0989	.3990	.7230	.9049	.9809	.9988	1.0

The normalizing of rates greatly reduces their variability at each age cut across the 44 periods (Fig. 2.4). An underlying pattern of cumulation of births with age apart from the level of fertility begins to emerge. The number of large positive outliers at all age cuts except 44/45 and the pronounced asymmetry in the spread of the interquartile range of rates around the median rate at age cut 29/30 are clues to variability that remains to be described.

Removal of Age Cut Effects and Year Effects   A second step of dissection might be to remove some central value for each age cut (such as the median rate) from each of the period-specific normalized rates in that age cut:

Age cut	19/20	24/25	29/30	34/35	39/40	44/45
Median rate	.0220	.1584	.4016	.6622	.8666	.9798

This would result in period-independent age-cut effects and produce a set of residual rates with greatly reduced variability (Fig. 2.6). However, the

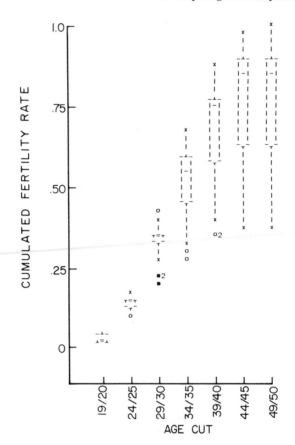

		Rate		
Age cut	Minimum	Lower quartile	Median	Upper quartile	Maximum
---	---	---	---	---	---
19/20	.0074	.0112	.0175	.0209	.0428
24/25	.0940	.1153	.1336	.1419	.1797
29/30	.1874	.3025	.3260	.3473	.4041
34/35	.2682	.4353	.5461	.5766	.6629
39/40	.3243	.5535	.7283	.7682	.8607
44/45	.3500	.6174	.8337	.8811	.9673
49/50	.3530	.6251	.8518	.8997	.9913

Fig. 2.3 Schematic plots of cumulated overall fertility rates by age cut for Sweden from 1751–1755 to 1966–1970.

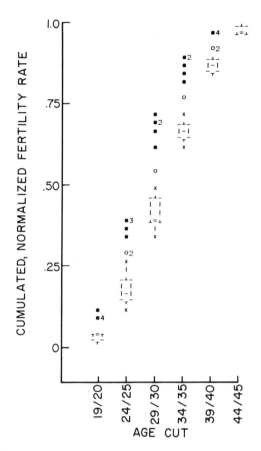

Age cut	Rate				
	Minimum	Lower quartile	Median	Upper quartile	Maximum
19/20	.0086	.0129	.0220	.0291	.0989
24/25	.1184	.1411	.1584	.2044	.3990
29/30	.3473	.3794	.4016	.4541	.7230
34/35	.6120	.6402	.6622	.6928	.9049
39/40	.8400	.8569	.8666	.8855	.9809
44/45	.9716	.9769	.9798	.9877	.9988

Fig. 2.4 Schematic plots of cumulated, normalized overall fertility rates by age cut for Sweden from 1751–1755 to 1966–1970.

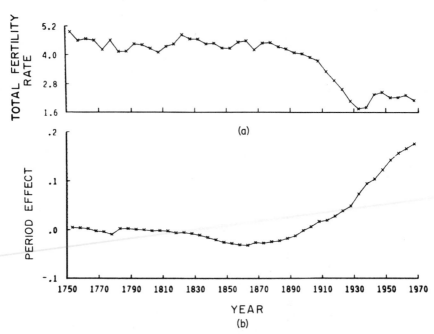

Fig. 2.5 (a) Total fertility rates and (b) age-independent period effects from median polish of cumulated, normalized overall fertility rates for Sweden from 1751–1755 to 1966–1970.

large number of positive outliers and the asymmetry of residual spread are still prominent.

Our third step of dissection might be to remove an age-independent period effect from the residuals by subtracting the median residual for each period from each of the six residual rates in that period. The two-way table of fertility rates would then be described by

$$f_{ij} = \text{(total rate) (age-cut effect + period effect + residuals)}.$$

Such a "sweeping out" of age-cut effects and period effects can be improved upon, "polished," by repeating the last two steps iteratively until both the residual age-cut medians across all periods and the residual period medians across all age cuts are zero. This procedure has been termed "median polish" (Mosteller and Tukey, 1977, pp. 178–181; Tukey, 1977, pp. 363–367). When the median value for the entire table of fertility rates is removed first, before the removal of age-cut effects and period effects, the procedure can be thought of as an iterative analysis of variance based on medians.[5]

Median polish of the 44 × 6 table of cumulated, normalized fertility rates gives a common value of 0.6202 and the following period-independent age-cut effects:

Age cut	19/20	24/25	29/30	34/35	39/40	44/45
Age-cut effect	−.5987	−.4599	−.2184	.0420	.2468	.3582

Adding the overall median to each of these period-independent age-cut effects gives

Common value + age-cut effect	.0216	.1604	.4019	.6622	.8671	.9784

These values are very similar to the age-cut medians that we removed previously:

Median rate	.0220	.1584	.4016	.6622	.8666	.9798

Because the age-independent period effects resulting from median polish of the two-way fertility table have a definite pattern across time (Fig. 2.5b), it is not surprising to find that their removal reduces the size of the residuals and spreads them more evenly across the age cuts (Fig. 2.7). There are, however, still many large outliers with negative values at age cuts 19/20, 39/40, and 44/45, and positive values at the three age cuts in between. Considerable pattern still remains to be described.

The iterative fitting procedures, termed empirical higher rank (EHR) analysis, that are used to search for more complex patterns in the data (for example, age cut by period interactions) are based on the median-polish approach. However, EHR analysis uses a refined measure of the "center" of the entire table, age cut, or period rather than median or trimmed mean rate.[6]

To obtain more information about the patterns not yet removed from the data by median polish, we shall want to display the residuals in several ways. If we plot the residuals for each age cut against time, one plot above the other, some systematic variation may be very evident. Figure 3.4 is an example of such plots, which will be used extensively in the following chapters. We can also summarize in a scatter plot any tendency for the residuals at a pair of age cuts to vary together by year in a systematic way.

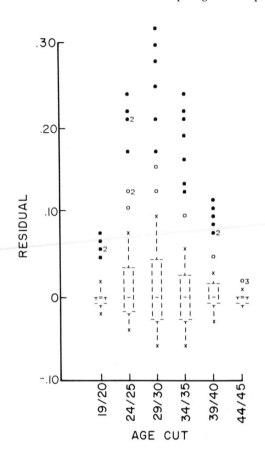

Age cut	Minimum	Lower quartile	Median	Upper quartile	Maximum
19/20	−.0134	−.0091	.0000	.0071	.0769
24/25	−.0399	−.0172	.0000	.0460	.2407
29/30	−.0544	−.0222	.0000	.0525	.3214
34/35	−.0502	−.0221	.0000	.0304	.2427
39/40	−.0265	−.0097	.0000	.0190	.1143
44/45	−.0080	−.0029	.0000	.0079	.0190

Fig. 2.6   Schematic plots of residuals after the removal of age-cut effects from cumulated, normalized overall fertility rates for Sweden from 1751–1755 to 1966–1970.

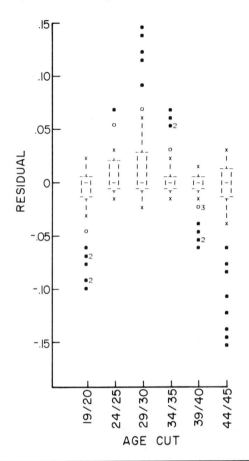

		Residual			
Age cut	Minimum	Lower quartile	Median	Upper quartile	Maximum
19/20	−.0989	−.0181	.0000	.0068	.0200
24/25	−.0173	−.0051	.0000	.0189	.0679
29/30	−.0241	−.0090	.0000	.0273	.1446
34/35	−.0191	−.0089	.0000	.0075	.0667
39/40	−.0618	−.0065	.0000	.0054	.0134
44/45	−.1548	−.0144	.0000	.0174	.0330

Fig. 2.7 Schematic plots of residuals after median polish of cumulated, normalized overall fertility rates for Sweden from 1751–1755 to 1966–1970.

For example, the residuals may be negative at both age cuts in many years and positive at both age cuts in many other years. Figure 4.4 shows evidence of such a tendency for systematic variation in even the very small residuals remaining after EHR analysis of the full fertility time sequence for 185 single years.

What are the appropriate responses to evidence of structure remaining in the residuals? One response is to consider a linearizing re-expression of the data before beginning exploration. A second response is to extend the exploration to more complex descriptions of the data using EHR analysis. We shall talk first about re-expression of the data, taking two examples from the fertility data used in the following chapters.

Shape of the Data and Re-expression
to Increase Linearity

Linear relations are easier to examine than nonlinear ones and departures from linearity are easy to note. Thus, re-expression (or transformation) of data to improve linearity is a practice well established in demographic research (for example, Brass, 1975; Coale and Demeny, 1966). It is usually a preliminary step in exploratory analysis. Re-expression simply alters the scale without altering the order relations of the members of the data set.

Use of $\log y$ is a familiar procedure. A re-expression involving y^2, $\sqrt{y}$, or $1/y$ may be a less familiar but more appropriate choice for a particular data set. Inspection of the general shape of the data can suggest some types of re-expression to try. A ladder of re-expressions will be useful in making choices:

$$y^3 \left| y^2 \right| y \left| \sqrt{y} \right| \sqrt[3]{y} \left| \log y \right| - \frac{1}{\sqrt[3]{y}} \left| - \frac{1}{\sqrt{y}} \right| - \frac{1}{y} \left| - \frac{1}{y^2} \right| - \frac{1}{y^3} .$$

If one expression is straight, those before it are hollowed upward $\smile$ and those after it are hollowed downward $\frown$ (Tukey, 1977, p. 173). Whether a log, reciprocal, power, or more complex re-expression is used to simplify the data's behavior for analysis, de-transformation can readily return the results to the original, raw scale.

Example 1 Age-specific marital fertility schedules $f_i(a_j)$ are examples of a shape commonly found in demographic data—a curve hollowed upward $\smile$. To linearize this curve, we could change the fertility rate scale, the age scale, or both. We would probably first try re-expressing the rates only. The schedule for Sweden in 1959 is shown in Fig. 2.8 with several re-expressions. Substituting $[f_i(a_j)]^2$ for $f_i(a_j)$ obviously increases the curvature. Using $\sqrt{f_i(a_j)}$ moves the expression in the desired direction

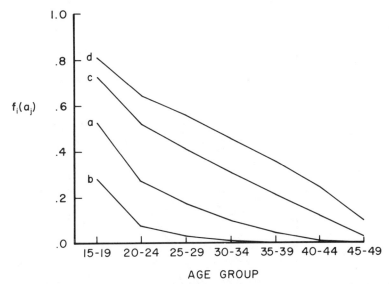

Fig. 2.8 Effect of re-expression on an age-specific marital fertility schedule for Sweden, 1959: curve a, no re-expression; b, square; c, square root; d, cube root.

to decrease the curvature, but using $\sqrt[3]{f_i(a_j)}$ as a linearizing re-expression does better. We might be able to improve on this, but experience shows that perfection is not necessary.[7]

We may also prefer to work with forms of the marital fertility schedules for which other linearizing re-expressions are appropriate. In the following chapters we shall analyze not the age-specific rates illustrated here, but cumulated, normalized rates (see Fig. 3.3 for examples) on the folded square root scale described in the following example.

Example 2 Cumulative age distributions of fertility f_{ij} are examples of another shape commonly found in demographic data—a more or less s-shaped curve ⌒. Such a configuration, hollowed upward in one tail, hollowed downward in the other, calls for a different type of re-expression. The following class of folded re-expressions suggested by McNeil and Tukey (1975):

$$F_{ij} = (f_{ij})^\lambda - (1 - f_{ij})^\lambda, \qquad \text{where} \quad \lambda = 1, \frac{1}{2}, \frac{1}{3}, \ldots, \frac{1}{n}$$

proves to be a frequently satisfactory answer. Other re-expressions may prove to be even better.

The cumulated, normalized overall fertility schedule for Sweden in 1860 is used in Fig. 2.9 to illustrate several folded re-expressions. The simplest,

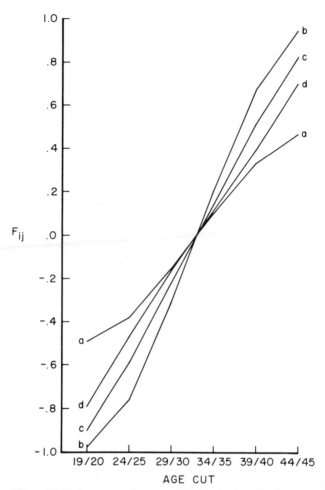

Fig. 2.9 Effect of folded re-expression on a cumulated, normalized age-specific fertility schedule for Sweden, 1860: curve a, centered on median age, no re-expression; b, folded proportion; c, folded square root; d, folded cube root.

the folded proportion

$$F_{ij} = (f_{ij}) - (1 - f_{ij})$$

has the effect of stretching both ends of the distribution. It indicates how far below or above the median is the proportion of the year's fertility achieved by a given age. However, a sigmoid configuration remains apparent in the re-expressed schedule. In contrast, both the folded square root of f_{ij}

$$F_{ij} = (f_{ij})^{1/2} - (1 - f_{ij})^{1/2}$$

and the folded cube root of f_{ij}

$$F_{ij} = (f_{ij})^{1/3} - (1 - f_{ij})^{1/3}$$

perform quite well in straightening out both ends of the distribution. In addition, they stretch the distribution to different degrees in both directions from the median rate at zero. The folded log, or logit, of f_{ij}

$$F_{ij} = \tfrac{1}{2} \ln (f_{ij}) - \tfrac{1}{2} \ln (1 - f_{ij}),$$

which Brass has used productively with other demographic data having a sigmoid configuration (for example, see Brass, 1974, 1975), goes too far with the cumulated fertility distributions (Fig. 2.10). Whether the schedule has a high median age as in 1860 or a median age several years lower as in 1939, the folded square root performs better than the logit as a linearizing re-expression.[8]

Linearizing re-expression of the data before analysis may not, by itself, be sufficient to bring the remaining regularities into a simple additive fitted description. This is true for the Swedish fertility time sequences analyzed in the following chapters. Even though this is the case, re-expression will still be an important tool as we move to EHR analysis.

More Complex Descriptions of Data Using Empirical Higher Rank Analysis

Empirical higher rank analysis is concerned with fitted descriptions that include one or more multiplicative terms, such as an interaction term in a classical analysis of variance $y_{ij} = \mu + A + B + CD$ or the series of multiplicative terms in a principal components analysis $y_{ij} = AB + CD + EF$.

In EHR analysis as initially developed by McNeil and Tukey (1975), the iterative removal of regularities from the data and the examination of residuals at each step are central to the analysis, just as they are in median polish. The analysis incorporates some extensions and refinements of procedure, however, that can be particularly effective in dealing with such demographic data as fertility time sequences. The effectiveness comes from two properties of the estimation procedure:

1. robustness—which means that the validity and efficiency of the estimations are not affected by nonnormality in the distribution of the

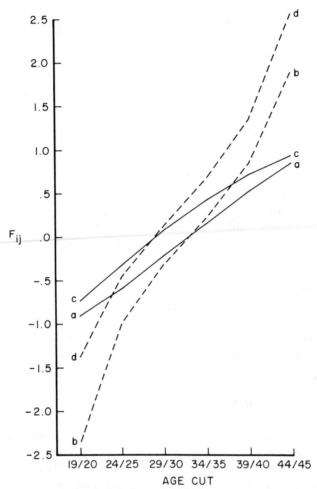

Fig. 2.10 Folded square root and logit re-expressions of cumulated, normalized age-specific fertility schedules for Sweden: curve a, 1860, folded square root; b, 1860, logit; c, 1939, folded square root; d, 1939, logit.

observations making up the data set; thus no detailed assumptions need be made about the distribution of the data or residuals;

2. resistance—which means that even a drastic change in any small part of the data will not substantially alter the summary statistics used to describe the data (Mosteller and Tukey, 1977, pp. 203–205); thus data points that may be far outside the "true" underlying pattern in the set due to singular circumstances or inaccuracies do not hinder the identification of the underlying pattern.

Least squares estimates of fit are taken as the departure point for the EHR procedures. Because ordinary least squares fitting gives equal weight to all residuals, it gives undue influence to extreme outliers that occur in data sets containing unusual observations or sizable errors. It often fails, therefore, to provide the best description of the bulk of the data. To downgrade the effect of outlying observations and provide better estimates, weighted least squares procedures rely on a priori assignment of a set of fixed weights that reflect judgments about the reliability of individual observations. This type of weighting is a method of dealing with known variability in the data.

EHR analysis is a weighted fitting procedure of a different kind, although its purpose is the same—better estimation. The difference lies in technique and interpretation. Fitting in EHR analysis starts without assumptions about the importance of particular observations.

In searching for the patterns underlying a data set, the EHR procedures repeatedly remove an additive or multiplicative factor from the rows or columns of the data or residuals from the preceding step of the analysis. This proceeds until the amount of additional regularity removed in a step is negligible. Cellwise weights are given to the residuals at each iteration (step in the fitting) before searching for further adjustments to the fit. The weights are not fixed, however, but are updated at each iteration on the basis of the incomplete description of the data developed to that point and the size of the deviations from the fit. Thus, an observation that may be given partial weight through the early steps of the fitting may be given zero weight in the final steps if it proves to be an outlier of the developed fit. Also, an observation that may be given only partial weight when an additive factor is being identified may move to full weight once a multiplicative pattern in the data is sought.[9]

The choice of weight function becomes very important if one is simultaneously to ensure resistance to outliers and avoid giving undue weight to small residuals. The iterative fitting procedures of EHR analysis using one weight function of choice are described in detail in Chapter III and Appendix B.

Re-presentation of Fits

So far we have talked about some of the tools of EDA that help us find closely fitted descriptions of data and leave true irregularity in the residuals as

$$data = fit + residuals.$$

Re-presentation of fits is a very different kind of tool. It takes the fitted description and asks: Which of the algebraically equivalent forms of this fitted description will best suit our purposes? For the fertility sequences, which form will best permit us to see change in demographically interpretable terms and compare change in different sequences? Three examples of such equivalent forms will illustrate the idea.

Example 1   In median polish we often first extract a "common value," the median value for the entire data set, and then proceed to extract a row-independent column effect for each column in the data and a column-independent row effect for each row. Every cell of the data is thus described by

$$\text{fit} = \text{common value} + \text{row effect} + \text{column effect}.$$

For a particular time sequence of age-specific fertility rates, we might find that we gain a much better feel for the year-to-year rate changes (the row effects) if we combine the common value (the median fertility rate across all age groups and across all years) with the age (column) effects so that every cell of the data is described by

$$\text{fit} = \text{common value} + \text{column effect} + \text{row effect}$$
$$= \text{column effect*} + \text{row effect},$$

where column effect* = common value + column effect. At another time we might find it more useful to add the common value to each row effect:

$$\text{fit} = \text{column effect} + \text{common value} + \text{row effect}$$
$$= \text{column effect} + \text{row effect*},$$

where row effect* = common value + row effect. Here we have three different presentations of the same fit, all of which are algebraically equivalent.

Example 2   We might find that a better-fitting description of the data would include a positive interaction term:

$$\text{fit} = \text{common value} + \text{row effect} + \text{column effect}$$
$$+ \frac{\text{row effect} \times \text{column effect}}{\text{common value}},$$

which is equivalent to

$$\text{fit} = (\text{common value})\left[1 + \frac{\text{row effect}}{\text{common value}} + \frac{\text{column effect}}{\text{common value}}\right.$$
$$\left. + \frac{\text{row effect} \times \text{column effect}}{(\text{common value})^2}\right].$$

Factoring would give

$$\text{fit} = (\text{common value}) \left[1 + \frac{\text{row effect}}{\text{common value}}\right]\left[1 + \frac{\text{column effect}}{\text{common value}}\right]$$

$$= (\text{common value})\,(\text{row effect*})\,(\text{column effect*}).$$

Here we see that an additive fit has been turned into an algebraically equivalent multiplicative fit. In both of these examples we have neither taken anything away from nor added anything to the fitted description. We have just looked at the same fit in different ways.

Example 3   In commenting on the importance of re-presentation for the more complex descriptions reported in the following chapters, Tukey (Appendix A) gives another simple illustration of algebraically equivalent forms:

Consider a fit $2A_iB_j + 2C_iD_j$, which can also be written as $(A_i + C_i)(B_j + D_j) + (A_i - C_i)(B_j - D_j)$. These two forms are algebraically identical, as can easily be seen by multiplying out the second form. Here there is no question of changing the fit, only of rewriting the fit.

If we are to compare the results of such a fit applied to two or more sets of data, we need to seek out a distinguished re-presentation of each fit so that the results will at least be conveniently comparable. If one fit looks like

$$2A_iB_j + 2C_iD_j$$

when the other looks like

$$(A_i + C_i)(B_j + D_j) + (A_i - C_i)(B_j - D_j),$$

we may miss an instance of a striking resemblance, something we should take only the least possible chance of doing.

In the process of using EHR analysis to generate more complete descriptions of the patterns in a data set, we shall have the choice of a number of algebraically equivalent forms in which to look at each fit. Knowledge of our data and our purposes in fitting the data will help us decide between the different standard forms. For example, for each age-specific fertility time sequence analyzed in the following chapters, we have chosen a standard form that separates into one fitted age parameter and one fitted time parameter as much as possible of the relation to change in total fertility rate. This leaves a second (and sometimes a third) time parameter relatively free of association with total fertility change. The long-term trend of change in the age pattern of fertility as total fertility declines would be more difficult to identify if, instead, both (or all) time parameters varied systematically with the total fertility rate. Some demographically significant choices for re-presentation of EHR fits will be discussed in detail in Chapter V.

Summary

This chapter accomplishes two purposes.

1. It provides an overall view of fertility experience recorded for Sweden across two centuries—information that will help guide the modeling of age-specific fertility change using exploratory data analysis (EDA) methods.
2. It provides an overall view of the flexible, data-guided EDA approach to modeling, which has two valuable outcomes for this fertility analysis: an interpretable description of the patterns underlying each long data time sequence and the identification of the nature and timing of departures from the developed model.

The first section of the chapter reveals a population in which overall fertility ranged from an average of 4.7 births per woman for women who entered childbearing ages in the first quarter of the nineteenth century to a low of 1.8 births per woman, well below replacement level, for women who reached age 15 in the period 1917–1921. Marriage patterns continued to be strongly related to fertility change long after the control of fertility within marriage became prominent. Premarital conception, particularly of first births, has always been common. We thus have an opportunity to model changes in overall and marital fertility patterns that have varied causes and that may or may not be accompanied by a change in the level of fertility. An unusual circumstance, the availability of two centuries of single-year overall fertility schedules by 5-year age groups, permits the construction of closer approximations of cohort experience than have commonly been analyzed and thus allows more detailed comparisons of cohort and cross-sectional change. By bringing under consideration the 85 years of little-analyzed pre-1860 data from "Grunddragen," this long sequence of single-year schedules also directs our attention to one of the strengths of the selected analytic approach—the detection of underlying patterns, even in flawed data. Single-year-of-age cohort overall fertility data, beginning with the birth cohort of 1870, and eight decades of detailed marital fertility data enrich the possibilities for cross-sequence comparisons.

The second section of the chapter presents the philosophy and some of the tools of EDA in enough detail that the reader should be able to visualize their application to other data sets. Partial dissection of a small data set of Swedish fertility rates illustrates the basic stepwise approach to modeling and emphasizes the central role of residuals in the modeling process. At each step of dissection, residuals are used as indicators of further pattern that we may choose to bring into a fitted description. At the end of fitting, residuals become a part of the full description of a data set, identifying the nature and location of departures from the fitted model. For pattern detection, the value of graphic summaries of data, fits, and residuals becomes readily apparent. When the EDA median polish procedure, which is similar to an iterative analysis of variance procedure based on medians, is applied to the small fertility tabulation, the residuals reveal the type of nonlinear relation that is brought into fitted descriptions of fertility in the following chapters.

The greater ease of examining linear relations, as opposed to nonlinear ones, and the frequent need to describe nonlinear relations in demographic data lead to consideration of the shape of data distributions and the choice of an appropriate linearizing re-expression as early steps in exploratory analysis. Uncommon re-expressions, as well as familiar ones, are proposed to simplify pattern detection.

The fact that linearizing re-expression alone may not make data patterns amenable to simple additive fitted description leads to a brief introduction to empirical higher rank (EHR) analysis, the iteratively weighted fitting procedure used in the following chapters to detect the more complex patterns underlying fertility time sequences. For this purpose, the effectiveness of the fitting procedures comes from two properties:

1. robustness, which means that nonnormality in the data does not affect the validity and efficiency of the estimations, and
2. resistance, which means that data points far outside the "true" underlying pattern in the data, because of unusual circumstances or inaccuracies, do not hinder the identification of the underlying pattern.

Discussion of weighting distinguishes from other types the flexible data-guided weighting of EHR analysis, which achieves resistance to outliers by updating the weights at each step of the fitting process. The updating is based on the incomplete description of patterns fitted up to that point and the size of deviations from that fit.

The final section of the chapter introduces the idea that a fitted description of data can be presented in many algebraically equivalent forms, and that the analyst should explore which form will best permit change or difference to be seen in useful terms. When fits for two or more data sets are to be compared, selection of a standard form becomes essential.

Notes to Chapter II

1. For further description of the sources of Swedish population statistics and for a more detailed discussion of the quality of the data and the adjustments made to early data, see Hofsten and Lundstrom (1976, Appendix 1).

2. Indeed, laws affecting marriage might be considered to have been relatively restrictive in Sweden even during the Age of Freedom (1721–1772), although restrictions on the subdivision of land were eased at that time and some new rights were given to the landless.

3. We have two reasons for adopting the designation $f_i(a_j)$ for age-specific fertility rates. We want to clarify the relation of this work to models that use $f(a)$ to designate fertility rates by age. At the same time we want to emphasize that we are dealing here with rates in time sequence or for a series of populations ($i = 1$ to m) and rates for more than one age group ($j = 1$ to n) (see Chapter VII and Appendix A).

4. Total fertility rate is $5 \Sigma_{j=1}^{7} f_i(a_j)$ in this case because we are using rates for 5-year age groups.

5. A related procedure, trimmed mean polish, was used by Page (1977) in her investigation of the effects of marriage duration on marital fertility patterns. Instead of the median, the mean of the central two-thirds of a distribution was used in the successive approximations (see Note 6).

6. The EHR procedures also differ from these "polishing" procedures in another important regard—the weighting of the residuals in the iterative fitting procedure. In median polish no weighting occurs; in trimmed mean polish a fixed and predetermined percentage of residuals from each tail of the distribution is given zero weight at every iteration and all other residuals are given full weight. The more flexible, data-guided weighting incorporated in the EHR procedures updates the weights at each iteration on the basis of the *size* of the deviations from the incomplete description developed up to that point. It also assigns partial weights as well as weights of 0 or 1 in seeking improvements to the fit. See the section titled More Complex Descriptions of Data Using EHR Analysis and Chapter III for further discussion of weighted fitting.

7. The cube root also proves to be an appropriate linearizing re-expression for the cumulative probability of marital dissolution before the use of median polish to identify cohort and duration effects (McCarthy, 1977).

8. Detailed guidance in approaching a variety of shapes can be found in Mosteller and Tukey, 1977, pp. 79–118, and Tukey, 1977, pp. 169–199.

9. The same analysis can make use of both preassigned weights to deal with known variability and iteratively assigned weights to ensure robustness in the fitting procedure. In this case the weight of one kind is multiplied by the weight of the other kind to determine the complete weight to use for an observation (Mosteller and Tukey, 1977, pp. 256–258).

III

Starting an Exploratory Analysis: Choices and Procedures

Introduction

Using the tools of EDA, including EHR analysis, our first goal is to describe our data as closely as we can in a small number of parameters. Several choices must be made to start the exploratory process. These are pro tem choices that can be modified at any step of exploration. Some modifications will be improvements, and these are incorporated into the subsequent steps. Some modifications will be detrimental when judged by the dual criteria of the size of the residuals and the evidence of pattern left in the residuals. When this occurs, we return to a previous step and try again. The important idea is to think of the choosing as an iterative data-guided process.

In Chapter IV we shall look at the results of one combination of choices that seem to work particularly well, for our purposes, with a specific set of age-specific fertility time sequences. Here we shall talk about the kinds of preliminary and intermediate choices that are made to arrive at such a combination:

1. Which fertility sequences will be analyzed?
2. Which form of the data will be used?
3. Which re-expression of the data will be carried through the full set of analyses?
4. Which patterns will be sought in the data? Asked another way, which models will be examined for fit to the sequences?

5. Which procedures will be used for the resistant iterative fitting of these models?
6. How resistant to outliers should the fitting be?
7. What measures and indications of goodness-of-fit will be relied upon?
8. How can procedures be adapted to available computer capabilities?

Selected Time Sequences of Age-specific Fertility

The primary analyses are based on the 12 fertility time sequences listed here. More detailed comments on these sequences and their construction follow the list. The designation for each sequence involves certain conventions, combining one or more letters with a number.

Basic letter:

>   X   Cross-sectional sequence
>   C   Cohort sequence

Letter prefix to X or C:

>   M   Marital fertility sequence of the designated type
>   SYA   Sequence of fertility rates by single year of age; all other rates are by 5-year age groups
> N, X, or C   Sequence modified in a described way

Number suffix to X or C:

> nonitalicized numbers   Youngest age for which fertility rates are included
> *italicized numbers*   Number of years included in a sequence of the designated type (following an *italicized* *X* or *C*)

Comparative analyses of cross-sectional and cohort overall fertility are based on the following sequences:

>   X15   Cross-sectional overall fertility for ages 15–49 by 5-year age groups and by 185 single years, 1775–1959
>   X20   Cross-sectional overall fertility for ages 20–49 only, 1775–1959
> *X202*   Extension of the X15 sequence to 202 years, 1775–1976

C15   Cohort overall fertility for ages 15–49 by 5-year age
       groups, with 155 cohorts designated by year at age 15–19,
       1775–1929

C20   Cohort overall fertility for ages 20–49 only, with cohorts
       designated by year at age 15–19, 1775–1929

SYAC13 Cohort overall fertility by single year of age for ages 13–
       50, with 55 cohorts designated by year at age 15, 1885/
       1886–1939/1940

Coordinate analyses of marital and overall fertility are based on the following sequences:

MX15   Cross-sectional marital fertility for ages 15–49 by 5-year age
       groups and by 68 single years, 1892–1959

MX20   Cross-sectional marital fertility for ages 20–49 only, 1892–
       1959

NX15   Cross-sectional marital fertility for births occurring at mar-
       riage durations of 9 months or more, for ages 15–49 by 5-
       year age groups, 1911–1963 with 1921–1923 missing

XX15   Cross-sectional overall fertility for ages 15–49 by 5-year age
       groups and by 68 single years, 1892–1959

XX20   Cross-sectional overall fertility for ages 20–49 only, 1892–
       1959

MC15   Cohort marital fertility for ages 15–49, with 42 cohorts desig-
       nated by year at age 15–19, 1892–1933

Data used to calculate these rates are taken from publications of the
National Central Bureau of Statistics (Sweden, 1878, 1875–1910, 1911–
1959, 1960–1976, 1976).

*Overall Fertility Sequences—Cross-sectional and
Cohort*

Analyses of the overall fertility sequences beginning in 1775 are central
to our study and allow it to be based on the most general consideration of
changes in the age distribution of fertility over an extended period of time.
Yearly age-specific fertility rates are calculated from confinements by
year and by age of mother in 5-year age groups, 15–19 to 45–49, and from
recorded estimates of mean female population by year in each of these age
groups. (See Chapter II for a discussion of the sources of these data.) Up
to 1955, the yearly number of confinements is recorded by age of mother;
from 1955 onward the number of confinements is calculated from the

recorded number of live, multiple, and still births. Emphasis on the number of confinements, rather than the number of births, is maintained throughout these analyses because our interest lies in the evidence of women's behavior affecting the fertility rate, rather than the fertility rate per se.

This $m \times n$ matrix of age-specific fertility rates for m years and n age groups is analyzed for the full age range 15–49 and for the age range 20–49 only, from two perspectives:

1. in cross section, primarily in the 185-year X15 and X20 sequences, 1775–1959, and in the 202-year *X202* sequence, 1775–1976, but also in five 30–40 year segments at the earliest stages of exploration;
2. by cohort in the C15 and C20 sequences, for 155 cohorts with completed childbearing experience, beginning with the cohort aged 15–19 in 1775, and therefore aged 20–24 in 1780, 25–29 in 1785, . . . and 45–49 in 1805, and ending with the cohort aged 15–19 in 1929, and therefore aged 20–24 in 1934, 25–29 in 1939, . . . and 45–49 in 1959.[1]

A primary interest is to discover how much can be learned, using this exploratory approach, from fertility data in one of its most widely available forms, rates by 5-year age groups. Considerable real irregularity is averaged out in the use of these groups. Substantial change, for example in marriage patterns, can also occur within such age groups. Some irregularity is also created by the age grouping, particularly by the artificial barriers at 19/20 and 24/25. For example, in Figs. 6.7 and 6.17 note that the progression of the mean age of childbearing at a standard level of fertility is smoother for cohorts by single year of age than for cohorts by 5-year age groups. The principal analyses are therefore also carried out for the SYAC13 time sequence of fertility schedules for the birth cohorts of 1870/1871–1924/1925, with fertility histories completed at age 50 in 1920/1921–1974/1975 (Sweden, 1976; see Chapter IV, Note 1, on the dual year designation for these cohorts). The results of the SYAC13 analyses provide a basis for the interpretation of fitted parameters for all other sequences.

To examine the geographic differences underlying the EHR analysis description of cross-sectional overall fertility change for the entire country, time sequences of overall fertility rates covering the period 1860–1970 are analyzed for each of the 25 counties. These rates, computed by Hofsten and Lundstrom (1976) from census data and birth data for the 2 years before and after each census, provide for each county a total of 15 age-specific fertility schedules by 5-year age groups, from 15–19 to 45–49 at 5- to 10-year intervals.

Matched Marital and Overall Fertility Sequences

Age-specific marital fertility rates are calculated from the number of confinements for legitimate births by year and by age of mother in 5-year age groups (15–19 to 45–49) and from recorded estimates of the mean number of married women by year in each age group.

For the comparative analysis of overall and marital fertility, four basic time sequences are selected—the MX15 and MX20 cross-sectional marital fertility sequences and the corresponding XX15 and XX20 overall fertility sequences. These sequences begin with the first year for which recorded data allow the calculation of yearly age-specific marital fertility rates. The marital fertility sequences are terminated in 1959 to include in the EHR analysis only the age patterns of childbearing that preceded the prominent increases in family formation outside of legal marriage from the mid-1960s onward. Further EHR analyses, as proposed in Chapter VII, would include the most recent available data in a three-way time-sequence analysis. Such analyses could relate change in marital fertility patterns and change in nonmarital childbearing patterns to overall fertility patterns across nine decades.

The EHR parameters derived for the 68-year sequences of overall fertility can be expected to differ in some details from those derived for the 185-year sequences and the 202-year sequence. This occurs because the parameters are developed by fitting the fertility experience of the 68 years alone, divorced from the experience of the preceding 117 years or the subsequent 17 years. Fitting the shorter sequence alone contributes to the fine tuning of the fit for that portion of the longer sequence.

The construction of the NX15 sequence, for confinements occurring at marriage durations of 9 months or more, is made possible by the recording of legitimate births by duration of marriage from 1911 onward. Duration categories are in months up to 1 year and thereafter in number of years. For each calendar year in the sequence, the numbers of confinements for the 5-year age groups 15–19, 20–24, and 25–29 are adjusted to omit confinements occurring less than 9 months after marriage. The number of married women in these three age groups is also adjusted to omit women having a confinement in that year less than 9 months after marriage. The NX15 sequence rates for the first three age groups are calculated from these adjusted data. For age groups 30–34, 35–39, 40–44, and 45–49, the marital fertility rates from the MX15 sequence are used without adjustment because births occurring less than 9 months after marriage make only a negligible contribution to rates at the higher ages. The NX15 sequence is used here with the MX15 sequence to illustrate how coordinate

EHR analyses of related fertility sequences can reveal information about the nature of change and lead to estimates of missing data. The NX15 sequence should be viewed as only one of a group of sequences that can be constructed from the available data and profitably analyzed. Another prominent member of such a group would be a sequence for confinements occurring 8 months or more after marriage. This sequence could be presumed to include all but a small fraction of postmaritally conceived childbearing (Leridon, 1977) but to have more contamination by premarital conceptions than the NX15 sequence. To extract different information, other analysts might choose to base the sequence construction on different adjustments than those we have incorporated in the NX15 sequence for the results reported in Chapter VII.

The 42-cohort marital fertility sequence MC15 is the shortest sequence fitted. It is constructed from yearly age-specific marital fertility rates in the same way that the cohort overall fertility sequences were constructed from yearly age-specific overall fertility rates. Beginning with the cohort aged 15–19 in 1892, and therefore aged 20–24 in 1897, 25–29 in 1902, . . . , and 45–49 in 1922, and ending with the cohort aged 15–19 in 1933, and therefore aged 20–24 in 1938, 25–29 in 1943, . . . , and 45–49 in 1963, the MC15 sequence covers the last 38 cohorts in the 155-cohort overall fertility sequence and four additional recent cohorts.

Truncated Sequences

For the various fertility time sequences, analyses restricted to the 20–49 age range are included for two reasons:

1. to enhance comparisons with studies and models that exclude age 15–19 fertility directly or exclude it indirectly through the choice of external standards;
2. to test the relative capability of the EHR approach to describe, empirically and demographically, fertility sequences with full variability and sequences with some of the known causes of irregularity removed.

In an extended EHR analysis, the value of various truncations of the fertility distribution should be explored. For example, truncation of single-year-of-age schedules at age 30 to concentrate on the changing age distribution of childbearing below that age could be informative.

Form of the Data

All fitting procedures are carried out on cumulated, normalized age-specific fertility schedules f_{ij} for cohort i or year i and age cuts $j = 1, 2, \ldots,$ n. This allows us to focus first on the age pattern of fertility and change in this pattern over time. In later steps of analysis we examine the relation of change in pattern to change in fertility level.

To calculate cumulated normalized rates, we start with schedules of age-specific rates $f_i(a_j)$ for age groups $j = 1, 2, \ldots, n$, such as the cohort and cross-sectional overall fertility schedules by 5-year age groups shown in Figs. 3.1a and 3.2a. Each schedule is first cumulated to give the fertility rates for women a given age and younger. Age cuts are at 19/20, 24/25, . . . , 49/50 for schedules by 5-year age groups beginning with ages 15–19 (Figs. 3.1b and 3.2b); age cuts are at 13/14, 14/15, . . . , 49/50 for schedules by single year of age beginning with age 13. Schedules restricted to the age range 20–49 begin the cumulation of rates with age group 20–24 and have their first age cut at 24/25.

Each schedule is then normalized, that is, the rate at each age cut is divided by the sum of the age-specific rates expressed in the rate for women at age cut 49/50 as

$$T_i = \sum_{j=1}^{n} f_i(a_j).$$

For a cohort fertility schedule the cumulated normalized rates at age cuts $j = 1, 2, \ldots, n$ give the proportion of the cohort's total childbearing up to age 50 that has been achieved by the designated age. For example Fig. 3.1b reveals that the cohort aged 15–19 in 1910 completed almost 60 percent of its childbearing below age 30, whereas the cohort aged 15–19 in 1895 completed less than 50 percent below age 30. For cross-sectional fertility the cumulated normalized schedule gives the proportion of the total childbearing in a given year that can be attributed to women a given age or younger in that year (Fig. 3.2b). Note the following details in Figs. 3.1b and 3.2b:

1. the similar sum of rates for the year 1923 and the cohort aged 15–19 in 1910 ($T_i = .51$ and .49, respectively) but their dissimilar age patterns of fertility as revealed in the cumulated normalized rates;
2. the dissimilar sum of rates for the year 1923 and the cohort aged 15–19 in 1895 ($T_i = .51$ and .68, respectively), but their similar age patterns of fertility as revealed in the cumulated normalized rates;

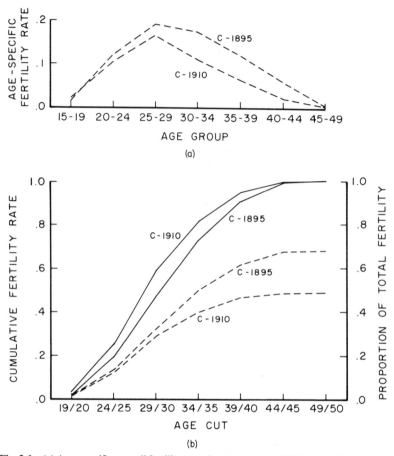

Fig. 3.1 (a) Age-specific overall fertility rates by age group and (b) cumulative rates (——) and proportion of total fertility (——) by age cut for the cohorts aged 15–19 in 1895 and 1910.

3. the centering of the cumulated normalized rates for the year 1895, with the proportion equal to .5 approximately midway between age cut 29/30 and age cut 34/35 and the near symmetry of the cumulative pattern from this center down to age cut 19/20 and up to age cut 44/45.

It is the description of these patterns that we develop with the EHR procedures. Variations in the patterns are subsequently related to variations in the level of fertility as indicated by T_i.[2]

The decision to concentrate on fitting the age pattern of fertility apart from level is consistent with the current body of work on models of

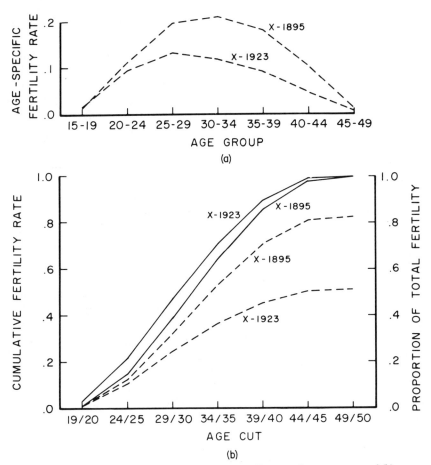

Fig. 3.2   (a) Cross-sectional age-specific overall fertility rates by age group and (b) cumulative rates (———) and proportion of total fertility (——) by age cut for the years 1895 and 1923.

aggregate demographic data for fertility, marriage, and mortality. Examples of such work include Brass's (1974) description of overall fertility, which relates the configuration of observed cumulative normalized distributions to any selected standard fertility distribution; the Coale–Trussell (1974) model schedules for the age pattern of overall fertility; the Coale–McNeil model of the age pattern of entry into marriage (Coale, 1971; Coale and McNeil, 1972); and model life tables based on similarities and differences in the age pattern of mortality (Brass, 1975; Coale and Demeny, 1966; Ewbank, Gomez de Leon, and Stoto, 1983).

The EHR analyses demonstrate that *demographic interpretation of fer-*

tility change across time requires the consideration of both change in pattern and change in total rate (see Chapters VI and VII). This should not be surprising. The biological and social factors that influence fertility can affect its age distribution, its level, or both. For example, the Swedish cohorts aged 15 in the years 1926–1939 differed from each other considerably in their age patterns of childbearing but experienced little difference in their levels of completed fertility (see Fig. 6.3). Similarly, a cross-sectional view of U.S. fertility (Fig. 8.1) reveals that change in pattern occurred with relatively little change in level during the period 1933–1940, whereas change in level occurred with relatively little change in pattern during the period 1956–1964. In addition, the same type of change in pattern can occur with either increasing or declining total rates. For example, a cross-sectional view of twentieth-century Swedish overall fertility data indicates increasing skew toward a younger pattern of childbearing. However, a declining total rate accompanies this change from 1925 to 1933 and 1945 to 1951, whereas an increasing total rate is associated with the change from 1942 to 1945 and 1960 to 1964 (see Fig. 8.1). Parameters fitted to the age pattern of fertility do not distinguish between a younger pattern related to decreased childbearing at higher ages, one related to increased childbearing at younger ages, and one related to both factors. We need to retain the total rate as one dimension in a time-sequence model of fertility change, even as we take advantage of the better detection of underlying age patterns achieved by fitting normalized rates.

Following a standard demographic procedure, cumulative fertility distributions, rather than frequency distributions $f_i(a_j)$, are used throughout the analyses in the following chapters. The reasons for making this choice are that:

1. it is easier to fit the class of distributions that differ in centering and scale;
2. the nature of any systematic bias in the data will be more apparent in the cumulative distribution at the same time that the influence of singular departures will be diminished.

As a result of this second advantage cumulative distributions have come into common usage in the demographic analysis of incomplete or defective data (for examples, see Brass, 1975; United Nations, 1967). In an expanded EHR analysis, fits to frequency distributions would be tested as well.

Re-expression of the Data

The folded square root F_{ij} of the cumulated, normalized fertility distribution f_{ij}:

$$F_{ij} = (f_{ij})^{1/2} - (1 - f_{ij})^{1/2}$$

for year or cohort i and age cuts $j = 1, 2, \ldots, n$ is the linearizing re-expression adopted for all fertility sequences in the analyses reported here. This re-expression centers the distribution on the median age of the schedule and transforms the values for a given schedule from a range of 0 to 1.00 to a range of -1.00 to 1.00 before fitting.[3] (See Figs. 2.9 and 2.10 for examples of re-expressed overall fertility schedules.)

To arrive at the choice of the folded square root, preliminary analyses were carried out both with no linearizing re-expression of the data and with a variety of folded and trigonometric re-expressions. The folded square root consistently performed as well as or better than any of the others when tried in combination with different models and fitting criteria for the various fertility sequences. Although the cumulative marital fertility distributions tend to lack the lower tail of the sigmoid configuration commonly seen in overall fertility distributions, they are sufficiently lin-

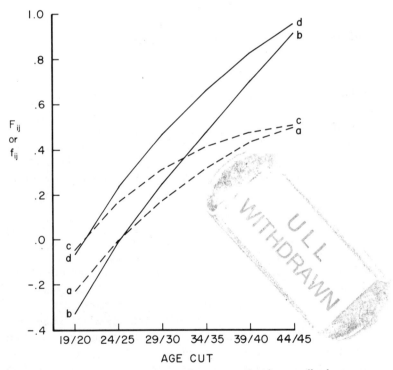

Fig. 3.3 Effect of folded square root re-expression on cumulated, normalized age-specific marital fertility schedules for selected years: curve a, 1895, centered on median age, no re-expression; b, 1895, folded square root; c, 1939, centered on median age, no re-expression; d, 1939, folded square root.

earized by folded square root re-expression (Fig. 3.3) to provide the very close fits reported in Table 4.1 and shown in Fig. 4.10.

If we were interested in marital fertility only, additional types of re-expressions not as well suited to linearizing overall fertility distributions would also be considered. For example, a re-expression that stretches and straightens the upper portion of the cumulative distribution more than the lower portion would be particularly well suited to marital fertility distributions. Such a re-expression should also perform well for those truncated or full-range overall fertility distributions in which a relatively high proportion of total fertility is accounted for by women below age 30. However, at the present stage of exploration of fertility distributions, a single broadly appropriate re-expression is more useful because it allows direct comparison of the fitted parameters for different types of data sequences. An expanded EHR analysis would continue the search for effective re-expressions of each sequence.

Selection of Models for Fitting to Fertility Data

A variety of models will describe with varied success the underlying patterns in an $m \times n$ fertility rate matrix for m years (or m cohorts) and n age cuts. Choices of the patterns to look for in the Swedish data were guided by the preliminary analyses of twentieth-century U.S. data in which the potential of EHR analysis was first indicated (McNeil and Tukey, 1975). These analyses showed that changing overall fertility patterns can be well-described in several forms based on the simple additive model

$$f_{ij} = \mu + \alpha_i + A_j + z_{ij}, \tag{1}$$

where μ refers to any overall measure of center, whether the mean or median fertility rate for the matrix or a refined measure of the center of the matrix identified in an iteratively weighted fitting procedure (Mosteller and Tukey, 1977, pp. 203–207).

With the matrix centered on μ this model, which is analogous to the classical analysis of variance, describes the remaining variability in each cell in terms of a single additive effect α_i of being in year (or cohort) i and a single additive effect A_j of being in age cut j.[4] The part of the fertility rate in a cell that is not described by this sum appears in the residual term z_{ij} for that cell.

We should expect to need a more complex model than (1) to describe the patterns in a time sequence of changing age-specific fertility rates, because these rates are influenced by two major variables—the proportion of women cohabiting at each age and the degree of control exercised by cohabiting women over their fertility.[5] Indeed, when this simple additive model was demonstrated in Chapter II, using the set of aggregated Swedish cross-sectional fertility rates and the iterative fitting procedure median polish, considerable pattern was left in the residuals. Four models that introduce a second year (or cohort) parameter and/or a second age parameter are therefore considered as:

$$f_{ij} = \mu + \alpha_i + A_j + \beta_i B_j + z_{ij}, \tag{2}$$

where $\Sigma \alpha_i = \Sigma A_j = 0$, $\Sigma B_j^2 = 1$;

$$f_{ij} = \mu + \alpha_i + \beta_i B_j + z_{ij}, \tag{3}$$

where $\Sigma \alpha_i = 0$, $\Sigma B_j^2 = 1$;

$$f_{ij} = \mu + A_j + \beta_i B_j + z_{ij}, \tag{4}$$

where $\Sigma A_j = 0$, $\Sigma B_j^2 = 1$;

$$f_{ij} = \alpha_i A_j + \beta_i B_j + z_{ij}, \tag{5}$$

where $\Sigma A_j^2 = \Sigma B_j^2 = 1$.

Model (2) carries model (1) a step further in describing the variance of the fertility rate matrix. Having related every cell to the matrix common value μ, a central value A_j for each age cut $j = 1, 2, \ldots, n$, and a central value α_i for each year (or cohort) $i = 1, 2, \ldots, m$, it seeks additional pattern in the residuals, looking specifically for an age-by-year (or age-by-cohort) interaction term. In geometric terms model (2) examines the residuals z_{ij} that are centered on $\mu + \alpha_i + A_j$ at m points in n-dimensional space (that is, in age space). It asks what rotation of the mean age coordinate system, represented by the A_j vector, will bring it in line with the direction of maximum variance in z_{ij}. The direction cosine of this rotation determines the coordinates of a second vector B_j whose multipliers, the β_i vector, express the variance of the age vector in year (or cohort) space. Models (3) and (4) are special cases of model (2), differing in the way the residuals are centered before additional pattern is sought. All three models may be thought of as similar to selecting a principal component of the fertility rate matrix, a B_j vector (and the component's multipliers β_i), after variously centering (or mean correcting) the matrix.

Model (5) differs from the other four in that it does not identify the matrix common value as the central value for each cell from which age-specific and year-specific (or cohort-specific) deviations occur. Instead, in geometric terms, it identifies the principal axis of matrix variance in age space with no prior mean correction or centering. The coordinates of this axis determine the first age vector A_j whose multipliers, the α_i vector, express the variance of the age vector in year (or cohort) space. The A_j vector is then rotated to the next most prominent axis of matrix variance. The direction cosine of the rotation determines the coordinates of a second age vector B_j. The β_i multipliers express the variance of B_j in year (or cohort) space. Model (5) may be thought of as similar to selecting the first two principal components of the fertility rate matrix, the A_j and B_j age vectors, and the components' multipliers, α_i and β_i.[6] The part of the total variance of the fertility rate matrix that is unexplained by these two age parameters and their year-specific (or cohort-specific) multipliers is left in the residuals z_{ij}. In model (5) all the cells at a given age cut have the same A_j and B_j values but differ from each other in the size of the multipliers α_i and β_i and the size of the residuals z_{ij}. However, all of the cells for a given year (or cohort) in this model have the same multipliers but differ from each other in the age parameters and the size of the residuals. In the accompanying tabulation, a cellwise description of the fitted $m \times n$ matrix of age-specific fertility rates f_{ij} helps to clarify these relations.

Year ($i = 1$ to m)	Age cut ($j = 1$ to n)			
	1	2	$\cdots$	n
1	$\alpha_1 A_1 + \beta_1 B_1 + z_{11}$	$\alpha_1 A_2 + \beta_1 B_2 + z_{12}$	$\cdots$	$\alpha_1 A_n + \beta_1 B_n + z_{1n}$
2	$\alpha_2 A_1 + \beta_2 B_1 + z_{21}$	$\alpha_2 A_2 + \beta_2 B_2 + z_{22}$	$\cdots$	$\alpha_2 A_n + \beta_2 B_n + z_{2n}$
$\vdots$	$\vdots$	$\vdots$		$\vdots$
m	$\alpha_m A_1 + \beta_m B_1 + z_{m1}$	$\alpha_m A_2 + \beta_m B_2 + z_{m2}$	$\cdots$	$\alpha_m A_n + \beta_m B_n + z_{mn}$

Fitting model (5) to the fertility rate matrix can also be viewed as an iterative multivariate regression that chooses from the matrix the independent variables, A_j and B_j and then determines their regression coefficients α_i and β_i. If the A_j and B_j vectors are known or specified in advance, the model is fit through a series of multiple regressions in which the dependent variable, the fertility rate vector f_{ij} for each year (or cohort) i, is regressed on two independent variables, the age effects A_j and B_j. This approach will be used in the Swedish county comparisons in Chapter VI, the natural fertility comparisons in Chapter VII, and the preliminary cross-population comparisons in Chapter VIII. The regressions are carried out under the constraint of a zero intercept because model (5) does not have a constant term.

The double multiplicative description (5) performed the best overall with the various fertility sequences in preliminary tests of various combinations of data re-expression and weighting of residuals (Breckenridge, 1976). Model (5) was used, therefore, to develop the closely fitting two-component descriptions reported for both overall and marital fertility sequences in Chapters IV–VII.

The possibility that more complex models incorporating a third year or cohort effect and/or a third age effect would better describe the underlying pattern in a fertility rate matrix was investigated extensively by Orav (1977) for the X15 sequence. He used the folded square root re-expression and various degrees of resistance to outliers in the iteratively weighted fitting procedures. Of the models tested, the one that gave the most satisfactory overall performance with this sequence was the triple multiplicative model with three age-by-time components

$$f_{ij} = \alpha_i A_j + \beta_i B_j + \gamma_i C_j + z_{ij}, \qquad (6)$$

where $\Sigma A_j^2 = \Sigma B_j^2 = \Sigma C_j^2 = 1$.

This model is carried forward into analysis of the *X202* sequence, representation of fitted parameters in a standard form, and comparisons across time and populations.

Robust–Resistant Iterative Fitting Procedures

Basic to an effective robust–resistant iteratively weighted fitting procedure is a weight function that both ensures resistance to outliers and avoids giving undue weight to small residuals. One weight function of choice appears to be the biweight (or bisquare) function of the residuals:

$$w(z) = \begin{cases} [1 - (z_{ij}/cS)^2]^2 & \text{for} \quad |z_{ij}| \le cS, \\ 0 & \text{otherwise}, \end{cases}$$

where S is the median absolute value of the residuals z_{ij} at each iteration, and c is the tuning constant (a parameter with assigned value). At each iteration the cellwise weights are updated so that residuals greater than c times the median absolute deviation from the previous step of fitting are ignored at the next step, whereas residuals less than about $c/2$ times the median absolute deviation are given about the same weight. Least squares estimates of fit would result if $c \to \infty$ so that $w(z) \to 1$, giving all residuals equal weight regardless of size. Detailed consideration of the desirable properties of the biweight function in robust–resistant fitting procedures is found in the work of Mosteller and Tukey (1977, pp. 351–358) and McNeil (1977, pp. 152–158).

The procedure that incorporates the biweight function in the fitting of two or three multiplicative components to each of the fertility sequences is outlined in Appendix B. The order of fitting emphasizes the patterns in the age dimension of the fertility matrix. The procedure for two components can be summarized as follows:

1. Iterative selection is made of a central value for the distribution of fertility within each age cut across time. An age vector A_j is formed from these biweight centers and its variability in the time dimension is determined.
2. From the residuals, iterative selection is made of a second central value for each age cut. A second age vector B_j is formed from these biweight centers, and its variability in the time dimension is determined.
3. From successive sets of residuals, iterative improvement is made in the two age vectors and their time vectors of multipliers until convergence in A_j and B_j.

If the fitting had started with the time dimension of the matrix instead of the age dimension a similar but probably not precisely equivalent fitted description would have been generated.

The choice of c for the fitting process is of considerable importance, to ensure that neither too many nor too few residuals are removed from consideration during efforts to extract the regularities underlying a given data set. Values between 6 and 9 are usually effective choices at the beginning of exploration. However, the optimal choice of the value of c depends on the data and also on the analyst's purpose—to find a general description for the whole data set or to identify logical subgroups of the data with variations on a general underlying pattern. For all of the fertility time sequences, increasing c to a value of 12 proved appropriate to draw most of the systematic variability in the full sequence into a single fitted description and to leave irregular deviations in the residuals. Setting $c = 6$ helped identify the logical division points in a time sequence and effectively provided evidence of major transitions in the type of pattern underlying the age distribution of fertility (see Fig. 3.4 as an example). A general rule is to try a series of values of c, beginning perhaps with $c = 6$ and examine the residuals for any remaining pattern using the procedures outlined in the following section.

The iteratively weighted fitting of models (1)–(5) to the Swedish fertility time sequences was based on the algorithms implemented by McNeil in

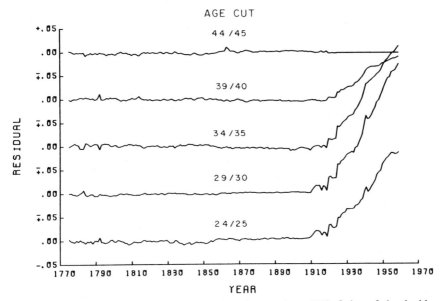

Fig. 3.4 Time-sequence plot of residuals by age cut from EHR fitting of the double multiplicative model to the X20 sequence, 1775–1959, with data expressed on the raw fraction scale and $c = 6$ in the biweight.

APL for use with an interactive computer (McNeil and Tukey, 1975). Satisfactory performance was obtained for all of the sequences analyzed. Orav (1977) used extensions of these algorithms to test more complex models for fit to the X15 sequence. His experience indicates that modification of the convergence criterion could improve performance. In practice, a guided start to the fit as well as modification of the convergence criterion may be necessary with certain data sets.

Measures of Goodness-of-Fit

Two criteria for judging fit are the size of the residuals and the amount of structure or pattern left in the residuals. There are several ways of looking at each.

Size of Residuals

We are concerned with the size of residuals on two levels: the amount of variability in a whole time sequence that is explained by the fitted description and the closeness of fit to individual schedules in the sequence. For summary measures of fit there are several choices. The familiar measure based on the sum of the squared deviations,

$$\text{proportion of variation explained} = 1 - \frac{\sum(z_{ij})^2}{\sum(F_{ij} - \text{mean } F_{ij})^2},$$

proved to be a less useful measure than others for comparing various combinations of data re-expression and fitting conditions. This measure gives undue weight to a small number of large residuals and does not distinguish effectively between fits when the residuals are all relatively small. For example, fits of 99.96 to 99.99 percent were common in the stages of exploration leading to the choice of the one combination of conditions (model, re-expression, and weighting) to be carried forward into the full set of analyses (Breckenridge, 1976).

The measure of fit based on the sum of the absolute deviations,

$$\text{proportion of variation explained} = 1 - \frac{\sum|z_{ij}|}{\sum|F_{ij} - \text{median } F_{ij}|},$$

is a measure that is less sensitive to large residuals. This measure proved to be more useful in exploration. However, a misleading impression of poor fit due to a very good overall fit with a few outliers is still possible. This measure is best used, therefore, in conjunction with a detailed examination of residuals to determine the nature of departures from fit.[7]

In some contexts, a measure of quality of fit that is highly resistant to outliers may be desirable. A recently developed robust measure of variance based on biweighted residuals provides such a criterion. This measure, denoted by s_{bi}^2, is described by Mosteller and Tukey (1977, pp. 207–208) and was used in slightly modified form by Orav (1977) to simplify the choice between complex fits to the X15 sequence (see Appendix B for a detailed description).

Such summary measures of fit, whether based on squared deviations, absolute deviations, or robust variance, tell only part of what we want to know about the size of residuals when fitting is completed. We also want to know about the closeness of fit to individual schedules. Some schedules may be considerably less well fit than others, and we may have achieved extremely close fits to a small portion of the schedules. But for the majority of the schedules, those between the worst and the best fits, how closely do the fitted parameters describe the data? Before comparisons are made, we need to de-transform the fitted distributions from the folded square root scale used in the fitting to the original raw fraction scale of the reported distributions (see Chapter VIII for an outline of the simple de-transformation procedure).

Structure in Residuals

In practice, examination of the residuals for structure is the first step in deciding between various combinations of re-expression and fitting conditions. For data in time sequence, large residuals with a truly irregular distribution suggest either the presence of errors in the data, the inclusion of some observations in the wrong category, or the impact of singular events. At another extreme, large and highly patterned residuals, perhaps for the end of a time sequence after an extended period of very close fit, indicate a major transition in the underlying patterns. This outcome suggests the need for alteration in the specified combination of re-expression and fitting conditions to accommodate the new pattern and/or division of the sequence at the transition to analyze the periods separately. Also frequently encountered are residuals of intermediate size and irregular enough distribution that existing pattern is not readily seen. For this case a detailed examination of the residuals is necessary to both bring out any hidden regularities and indicate what change in data re-expression or fitting conditions can accommodate the additional pattern detected.

In these three examples of irregular and patterned residuals, the sum of the absolute deviations from fit may actually be the same. However, it is the location of the deviations that determines the analyst's response and leads to a better understanding of the data. Identified structure in even very small residuals can suggest directions to move in seeking still sharper and more informative descriptions of the data. Useful procedures for detecting structure include schematic, diagnostic, scatter, and time-sequence plots of residuals.

Schematic plots were described and illustrated in Chapter II. With the residuals ordered by size for each column across all rows, the plots summarize the distribution of the residuals within each column. When schematic plots are used with the fertility data to decide between various combinations of data re-expression and weighting of residuals in the fitting procedures, the age cuts are considered as columns. Such plots give a convenient picture of the degree of symmetry in the spreading of residuals around the median residual for each age cut, the degree of agreement between age cuts concerning the extent of spread of the residuals, and the number, location, and relative size of the outliers.

Diagnostic plots of the residuals allow a more detailed examination of the type of structure remaining and, in particular, can demonstrate the presence of tilts in the distribution of the residuals. In the simplest type of diagnostic plot, the residuals from fitting any of models (1)–(6) to the fertility rate matrix are plotted against the corresponding values of (year effect) (age effect)/(common value) obtained from fitting the simple addi-

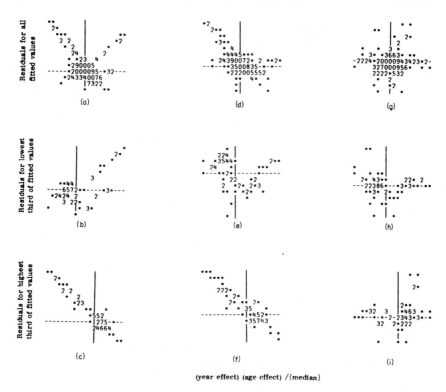

Figure section	Range of X		Range of Y		Figure section	Range of X		Range of Y	
	From	To	From	To		From	To	From	To
(a)	−.0252	.0263	−.0117	.0315	(f)	−21.25	15.11	−.0280	.0458
(b)	−.0168	.0263	−.0115	.0243	(g)	−21.25	22.30	−.0138	.0193
(c)	−.0252	.0161	−.0117	.0315	(h)	−15.85	22.30	−.0138	.0163
(d)	−21.25	22.30	−.0292	.0458	(i)	−21.25	15.11	−.0122	.0193
(e)	−15.85	22.30	−.0292	.0145					

Fig. 3.5 Diagnostic plots of residuals from EHR fitting of selected models to selected expressions of the 1811–1850 cross-sectional overall fertility sequence. (a)–(c): no re-expression of data, $f_{ij} = \mu + \alpha_i + A_j + z_{ij}$. (d)–(f): folded square root re-expression, $f_{ij} = \mu + \alpha_i + A_j + z_{ij}$. (g)–(i): folded square root re-expression, $f_{ij} = \alpha_i A_j + \beta_i B_j + z_{ij}$. Single entries at a location are indicated by dots, 2–9 entries by the appropriate number, and 10 entries by 0.

tive model (1) to the matrix. Evidence that the residuals follow the distribution of these interaction terms indicates the presence of a power function in the residuals. Such a power function could be removed by an appropriate re-expression of the data (Tukey, 1949) or the fitting of an additional multiplicative term to the data.

For our data, a modification of the diagnostic plots identifies more clearly the presence of a pattern that McNeil and Tukey (1975) call "astig-matic"—a tendency for residuals to concentrate near two straight lines of opposite slope. To detect this pattern the residuals are divided into three groups on the basis of the size of the fitted values. By doing separate diagnostic plots for the residuals corresponding to the lowest third and to the highest third of the fitted values, any tendency for the plots for the lowest third to tilt in one direction and the plots for the highest third to tilt in the opposite direction is clearly shown. Such a pattern of crossed tilts is often associated with a sigmoid configuration in the data and signals the need to try either further power re-expression of the data or other models.

Figure 3.5, taken from early stages of exploratory analysis of the fertil-ity time sequences (Breckenridge, 1976), illustrates the diagnostic plot evidence of structure remaining in the residuals after fit of the simple additive model (1) without data re-expression. It also shows the succes-sive steps of improvement in fit obtained through data re-expression and fitting a model with multiplicative terms.

Scatter plots summarize any systematic variations across time in both size and sign of residuals for pairs of age cuts. The residuals ordered in time sequence for each age cut are plotted against the residuals ordered in time sequence for every other age cut. Tilts in these scatter plots (see Fig. 4.4) again signal the need to consider other data re-expressions and fitting conditions.

Time-sequence plots of residuals by age cut provide more detail about the remaining structure by placing in the time dimension the systematic variations detected by other means. They help to answer several ques-tions: Does systematic variation occur as short-period fluctuations or as a pattern over extended periods? Does the variation come after a period of very close fit, indicating a major transition in fertility pattern (as in Fig. 3.4)? Do systematic variations in overall fertility residuals coincide in time with those for marital fertility residuals? Time-sequence plots of residuals may also contribute significantly to the interpretation of fitted time parameters. They are an essential tool in the consideration of singu-lar departures from fit.

Adapting to Computer Capabilities

When an interactive computer system provides a sufficiently large active workspace for the iterative fitting of long fertility time sequences such as the *X202* sequence and large sequences such as the SYAC13 sequence, models are first fit directly to the entire fertility rate matrix, and any indications for division of the sequence into dissimilar segments are then sought in the fitted parameters and the residuals. Most of the work reported in the following chapters was carried out in this way.

However, workspace of sufficient size is not always available. In fact, the early stages of this exploratory analysis of changing age patterns of fertility were carried out with a much smaller interactive workspace than became available in the later stages. To demonstrate the accommodation of exploratory analysis methods to practical limitations, alternative procedures used with large matrices are described here.

Fitting Segments of a Long Sequence

To begin the exploration, a 177-year sequence of cumulated, normalized overall fertility distributions for the years 1775–1951 was divided into convenient segments of about 35–40 years. Preliminary resistant fitting of these segments with several of the described models located times of apparent transition in the age pattern of fertility. For example, grouping the years 1811–1814 with 1815–1850 in fitting model (5) only slightly altered the age parameter B_j for the period 1815–1850, whereas grouping the years 1811–1814 with 1775–1810 considerably altered the B_j parameter for the period 1775–1810.

With the transitions used as more logical points of division, the sequence was divided into five segments: 1775–1810, 1811–1850, 1851–1890, 1891–1920, 1921–1951. These segments were then subjected to extensive comparative fitting with models (1)–(5), various re-expressions of the data, and resistant fitting procedures with $c = 6$. On a squared scale, fits explaining 99.97–99.99 percent of the variation were usual; on a linear scale, fits explaining greater than 98 percent of the variation were common.

When both the amount of variability explained and the amount of structure remaining in the residuals were the criteria of fit, the double multiplicative model (5) combined with the folded square root re-expression appeared to have small but clear advantages over other model and re-expression combinations, even for the short segments. The resulting fitted age vectors A_j and B_j are shown in Fig. 3.6. Values for corresponding age cuts of the A_j vectors are joined by dashed lines to emphasize the small but progressive changes in the last two periods in contrast to the constancy in the first three periods. The variety in the B_j vectors is more prominent. Such variation in both the A_j and B_j vectors makes apparent the difficulty in comparing fertility patterns for the different periods without taking some further steps. The following two steps are proposed:

1. finding a single fit for the full sequence, using the procedures outlined in the next section to counteract limitations on workspace size;

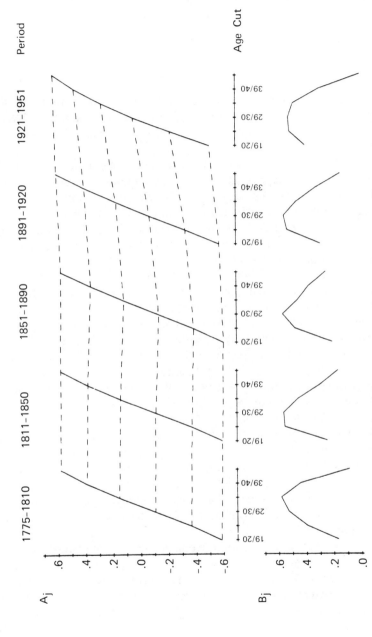

Fig. 3.6 Age parameters A_j and B_j from EHR fitting of the double multiplicative model to successive segments of a 177-year cross-sectional overall fertility sequence from 1775–1810 to 1921–1951 (from Breckenridge, 1976). Age cuts on the X axis range from 19/20 to 44/45.

2. re-presentation of fitted descriptions in a demographically guided standard form, as outlined in Chapter V, before attempting comparisons.

Two-stage Fitting of a Long Sequence

To find a single combination of age-cut and year effects that will describe the changes in the age pattern of fertility over the entire 177-year span, an alternative procedure to direct fitting, involving five steps, is proposed.

Step 1   The first 175 years of the time sequence of cumulated, normalized fertility rates (re-expressed on the folded square root scale) are divided into five quinquennial matrices of single-year fertility rates. The first matrix includes every fifth year beginning in 1775 and ending in 1945, the second matrix includes every fifth year beginning in 1776 and ending in 1946, . . . , and the last matrix includes every fifth year beginning in 1779 and ending in 1949.

Step 2   The double multiplicative model (5) is fitted to each of these five matrices, giving for each matrix a six-member vector for the first age effect A_j and a six-member vector for the second age effect B_j (where j refers to age cuts 19/20–44/45). We want each of the five matrices to pick up as well as possible the underlying pattern of changes in the whole time sequence. Therefore, by varying the value assigned to the tuning constant c, we explore different weightings of the intermediate residuals generated at each iteration of the fitting procedure. We then choose the weighting that comes closest to minimizing the differences among the five A_j vectors and among the five B_j vectors.

Step 3   An additive model (1) is then fitted to the matrix formed by the five A_j vectors and to the matrix formed by the five B_j vectors (Tukey, 1962). This model represents each A_j (or B_j) vector as common value + row effect + column effect + residual. It determines, in effect, the correction (the corresponding residual) that must be applied to each value of A_j (or B_j) for the five A_j vectors (or the five B_j vectors) to be expressions of the same model.

Step 4   Each schedule in a quinquennial matrix from Step 1 is then regressed on that matrix's two fitted age effects (A_j vector and B_j vector) from Step 3, with the constraint that the regression lines have a zero intercept. The two resulting regression coefficients for each year are then expressions of the two year effects α_i and β_i in the double multiplicative model

$$F_{ij} = \alpha_i A_j + \beta_i B_j + z_{ij}.$$

TABLE 3.1

Age Parameters A_j and B_j from Two-stage Fitting of the Double Multiplicative Model to Quinquennial Matrices of Cross-sectional Overall Fertility Schedules, 1775–1949

Parameter	Matrix	Age cut					
		19/20	24/25	29/30	34/35	39/40	44/45
A_j							
Before	1	−.5864	−.3577	−.0975	.1545	.3893	.5859
second	2	−.5880	−.3588	−.0982	.1534	.3882	.5845
fitting	3	−.5873	−.3581	−.0980	.1532	.3885	.5855
	4	−.5856	−.3550	−.0938	.1574	.3916	.5866
	5	−.5855	−.3556	−.0957	.1562	.3905	.5871
After	1	−.5868	−.3574	−.0971	.1546	.3892	.5857
second	2	−.5880	−.3585	−.0983	.1534	.3881	.5846
fitting	3	−.5876	−.3581	−.0978	.1539	.3885	.5850
	4	−.5845	−.3550	−.0947	.1570	.3916	.5881
	5	−.5854	−.3559	−.0957	.1560	.3907	.5871
B_j							
Before	1	.2597	.4981	.5435	.4787	.3531	.1877
second	2	.2786	.5049	.5454	.4745	.3412	.1689
fitting	3	.2625	.4963	.5455	.4794	.3514	.1843
	4	.2626	.4956	.5443	.4806	.3525	.1842
	5	.2724	.4944	.5448	.4803	.3514	.1745
After	1	.2630	.4967	.5451	.4799	.3518	.1843
second	2	.2604	.4942	.5425	.4774	.3493	.1817
fitting	3	.2625	.4963	.5446	.4794	.3514	.1838
	4	.2629	.4967	.5450	.4798	.3518	.1842
	5	.2627	.4964	.5448	.4796	.3515	.1840

TABLE 3.2

Percentage of Variation Explained by Fitting the Double Multiplicative Model, with Selected Weightings, to Quinquennial Matrices of the Cross-sectional Overall Fertility Sequence, 1775–1949

	Percentage of variation explained			
	with $c = 6$ in biweight		with $c = 12$ in biweight	
Matrix	Linear scale	Squared scale	Linear scale	Squared scale
1	93.96	98.19	99.05	99.99
2	93.57	98.01	99.05	99.99
3	93.13	97.85	99.03	99.99
4	94.34	98.28	99.04	99.99
5	85.98	82.08	98.97	99.99

Step 5   The five resulting matrices of residuals z_{ij} are then collated, as are the five sections of paired regression coefficients, so that both residuals and year effects can be examined in single-year sequence for the entire 175 years.

The fitting of model (5) to the quinquennial matrices in Step 2 was carried out first with the parameter $c = 6$ in the resistant fitting procedure used to fit models to the shorter segments of the time sequence. Although the resulting five A_j vectors showed only a small amount of variability (for example, the values of A_j for age cut 39/40 ranged from 0.3771 to 0.3848), the five B_j vectors varied considerably (with B_j for age cut 39/40, for example, ranging from -0.0253 to 0.4569). This indicates that the degree of resistance with $c = 6$ in the fitting eliminates too many residuals from consideration in the intermediate steps for the underlying pattern of the whole sequence to be identified. Because each matrix spans in the same way a 170-year period from the same 175 years, the underlying pattern should be common to all matrices.

The fitting was therefore repeated with other weights. Setting the parameter $c = 12$ results in a set of A_j vectors and a set of B_j vectors with only slight variability, even before the further fitting in Step 3. This second fitting brings the five A_j vectors (and the five B_j vectors) still closer together (Table 3.1). For example, the range of B_j for age cut 39/40 has been narrowed from .3412–.3531 to .3493–.3518. Least squares fitting of the quinquennial fertility rate matrices results in a similar set of A_j vectors but a set of B_j vectors with somewhat greater variability than those for resistant fitting with $c = 12$.

The much higher proportion of the variation in each of the quinquennial fertility rate matrices explained by resistant fitting with $c = 12$ than by fitting with $c = 6$ is shown in Table 3.2. A time-sequence plot of the residuals from $c = 6$ fitting is particularly revealing. Such a plot, similar to Fig. 3.4, shows that, if the sequence had run only from 1775 to about 1914, then setting $c = 6$ would have been adequate to pull most of the systematic variation in the data into the fitted description. This finding, among others, points to the period 1910–1920 as one of major transition in cross-sectional fertility age patterns as well as rates (see Chapters VI–VII).

Summary

This chapter serves two purposes.

1. It outlines the choices to be made in an exploratory analysis of any data set and describes generally useful analytic procedures.

2. It discusses the choices made in carrying out the analyses that lead to very close fits of all the fertility time sequences.

Decision making is presented as an iterative, data-guided process to be modified at any step of exploration.

The purpose of the exploration—modeling the age pattern of fertility change—determines the selection of Swedish single-year data sequences ranging from 52 to 202 years and 55 to 155 cohorts in length. These sequences emphasize fertility by 5-year age groups to demonstrate how much can be learned from an exploratory analysis of fertility data in one of its most widely available forms. A single-year-of-age cohort sequence is an important addition for confirming the interpretation of five-year-age-group parameters. The selection of related groups of sequences—giving both cross-sectional and cohort perspectives on overall and marital fertility—permits a more detailed consideration of trends and transitions in fertility patterns than would otherwise be possible. Overall fertility sequences for the 25 counties of Sweden are included for two purposes: to test the suitability of standard patterns derived for the entire country for use in the description of subpopulation experience and to seek information about subpopulation contributions to national change.

The choice of fitting cumulative fertility distributions that are normalized to concentrate on pattern apart from level is related to standard demographic procedures and the current body of work on models of aggregate demographic data. The retention of total fertility rate as a separate dimension of the data for use in further dissection of the model parameters is a departure from usual modeling practice. Selection of the folded square root as a single, broadly appropriate, linearizing re-expression for all of the fertility schedules permits the direct comparison of fitted parameters for one type of fertility sequence with the parameters for any other type. Refinements of re-expression for specific sequences are to be expected in later stages of exploration.

The evidence from Chapter II that models with more than one age parameter and/or more than one time parameter will be needed to describe the full range of fertility patterns leads to the discussion of two types of models: one, models that center or mean-correct the data in some way before seeking row-by-column (time-by-age) interaction terms are considered in the context of the analysis of variance; two, models that do not center the data before seeking row-by-column interactions are considered in the contexts of principal components analysis and multivariate regression.

Discussion of robust–resistant iteratively weighted fitting procedures focuses on the models that have two or three multiplicative components fitted directly, with no preliminary centering of the data matrix. These models, in which each component is made up of an age parameter and its year- or cohort-specific multiplier, are the basis of the descriptions reported in Chapters V–VIII for all the fertility time sequences. Two choices in the fitting procedures receive particular attention:

1. choice of a weight function—the biweight of the residuals, in our case—that both ensures resistance to outliers and avoids giving undue weight to small residuals;
2. choice of the degree of resistance to incorporate in the fitting procedure to meet the analyst's purposes, whether it is desired to develop a general description of the whole data set or identify subgroups having related variations in pattern.

Discussion of goodness-of-fit in exploratory analysis emphasizes the greater value of identification of pattern in the residuals and the lesser value of summary measures of residual size. Four procedures are described for the detection of hidden structure in residuals and the indication of what change in data re-expression or fitting conditions would bring detected pattern into a fitted description. On the basis of sensitivity to large residuals and insensitivity to differences in small residuals, summary measures of residual size are ranked as follows.

1. A measure of squared deviations is least useful by both criteria.
2. A measure of absolute deviations is more useful, particularly when used in conjunction with a detailed examination of residuals to determine the nature of departures from fit.
3. A robust measure of variance of the residuals is more useful than either of the other measures when high resistance to outliers is desirable.

The final section of the chapter considers ways of adapting fitting methods to computer capabilities in the exploratory analysis of large data sets.

Notes for Chapter III

1. Note, however, that the fertility rates are constructed from data that relate childbearing to a woman's age at the time of confinement but not to her year of birth and that aggregate confinements by 5-year age groups on a cross-sectional basis. Therefore, we do not have true cohort fertility rates—the data needed to calculate these rates for birth cohorts of Swedish women are available only from 1955 onward. Instead, we are working with approximations of cohort experience. We recognize that the designation of cohorts by "year at age 15–19" is a simplified description that does not apply precisely.

2. The significance of the total fertility measures

$$5T_i = 5 \sum_{j=1}^{n} f_i(a_j)$$

for schedules by 5-year age groups and

$$T_i = \sum_{j=1}^{n} f_i(a_j)$$

for schedules by single year of age varies with the type of sequence. For *cohort overall fertility* schedules, these expressions of total rate represent the average number of births per woman by the time the cohort reaches the end of the childbearing years. For *cross-sectional overall fertility* schedules, these are the conventional expressions of total fertility rate (TFR), or the average number of births per woman over the childbearing years of a synthetic cohort. In other words, they represent the sum of the average fertility experience of women in a number of different age cohorts at a given time as if it were the childbearing experience of a single cohort over time. For *cohort marital fertility* schedules, these expressions of total rate as the mean number of births per married woman are synthetic in another sense—they sum the average fertility experience by age of those women who were then married as if all of the women had been in the same marriage cohort and had borne children at each age at the same rate as those who were actually married at that age. For *cross-sectional marital fertility* schedules, the expressions of total rate are synthetic in both senses—they sum the average fertility experience of women in a number of different age cohorts and a number of different marriage cohorts at a given time as if it were the experience of a single cohort of women passing through time after entering marriage at the same age. These differences in meaning influence the interpretation of relations between EHR-measured change in the age pattern of fertility and change in the level of fertility for the different types of sequence.

3. If we had been interested in fitting the changes in rates rather than the changes in age pattern of fertility, we could have re-expressed the cumulative rates $T_i f_{ij}$ as

$$F'_{ij} = (T_i f_{ij})^{1/2} - (T_i - T_i f_{ij})^{1/2},$$

where $T_i = \sum_{j=1}^{n} f_i(a_j)$ for year or cohort i and age groups $j = 1, 2, \ldots, n$. This also centers the distribution on the median age of the schedule but transforms the values for a given schedule from a range of 0 to T_i to a range of $-T_i$ to T_i. Factoring this re-expression gives

$$F'_{ij} = T_i^{1/2}[(f_{ij})^{1/2} - (1 - f_{ij})^{1/2}].$$

It is now apparent that $F'_{ij} = T_i^{1/2} F_{ij}$ expresses the relation between the normalized and nonnormalized schedules on the folded square root scale.

4. Roman letters will be used throughout for age parameters, with corresponding Greek letters representing the associated year or cohort parameters.

5. Such a two-factor decomposition is the basis of the Coale–Trussell (1974) model fertility schedules, which express the age pattern of overall fertility in two age parameters and three cohort parameters.

6. The constraint that $\Sigma A_j^2 = \Sigma B_j^2 = 1$ obtains uniqueness for each component vector, except for sign. Analysis for two principal components is ordinarily carried out under the further constraint that $\Sigma A_j B_j = 0$, which imposes orthogonality on the two components.

7. With either the squared variation or absolute variation criterion of fit, the percentage of variation explained should be viewed in relation to the percentage of variation that would

have been explained if identical fitted descriptions had been given to every vector member of the data set. For example, for the X15 time sequence of cumulative fertility distributions, about 97 percent of the squared variation and about 86 percent of the absolute variation are explained when every year is assigned the same time-independent fit defined by the (common value + age effect) vector from median polish of the sequence. (See Chapter II for an illustration of median polish).

IV

Residuals: The Evidence of Goodness-of-Fit

Introduction

The choice of discussing residuals before presenting the parameters of the fitted descriptions may seem to be a reversal of the usual priorities. However, this is the appropriate order in which to consider the results of an exploratory analysis. At every step, successful exploration relies heavily on the examination of residuals not only in terms of their size and distribution but more importantly their pattern.

The simplest description of a data set,

$$\text{data} = \text{median} + \text{residuals},$$

leaves all of the existing pattern in the residuals. A data set can also be expressed in terms of *any* selected model, even a highly inappropriate one, plus the residuals:

$$\text{data} = \text{fit} + \text{residuals}.$$

The value that a particular set of fitted parameters has for data interpretation depends heavily on how well we have considered what is left in the residuals.

We shall test in detail the goodness-of-fit of the descriptions, developed using two multiplicative components and the folded square root re-expression, of the 185-year cross-sectional overall fertility sequences (X15 and X20), the 155-cohort overall fertility sequences (C15 and C20), and the 68-year marital fertility sequences (MX15 and MX20). Two-component fits to the 55-cohort single-year-of-age overall fertility sequence

(SYAC13), the 42-cohort marital fertility sequence (MC15), and the 50-year sequence for births occurring 9 months or more after marriage (NX15) are also examined.

The success of the fitting, by several criteria of the size of residuals, becomes apparent upon examination of Table 4.1. The more important matter of detecting pattern in residuals from two-component fits receives the greater emphasis, both as background for considering improvements made by fitting a third multiplicative component and as an aid in interpretation of the fitted parameters (Chapters VI–VII). Size of the residuals is mentioned first only because it is important for the reader to have in mind just how small are the residuals then being examined for structure. Those readers who want only to verify the closeness of the fitted descriptions should examine Tables 4.1 and 4.2 and Figs. 4.5–4.7 for an impression of the differences between cross-sectional and cohort residuals. They may then proceed to Chapters V–VII to consider the demographic implications of the fitted parameters presented in a standard form.

Size of Residuals

At all but two of the 1110 cross-sectional age cuts and 63 of the 930 cohort age cuts, the difference between the reported and fitted values for two-component descriptions of overall fertility by 5-year age groups does not exceed the third decimal place on the original scale of the cumulative fertility distributions. The original scale is in terms of the proportion of a year's or cohort's total fertility that can be attributed to women below a given age. Even using the complete marital fertility distribution, including age 15–19 births, results in very close fits that depart from reported values by no more than .007 on the original scale at any age cut. We shall refer to the original scale as the "raw fraction scale" to distinguish it from the folded square root scale of the re-expressed data used in the fitting procedures.

The difficulties that many models have in fitting the tails of fertility distributions have often been dismissed as relatively unimportant. However, good fit in the tails may be particularly important to useful description when the total fertility rate is low, the age pattern of entry into childbearing is changing, or the focus is on the nature of brief departures from trend. Using EHR procedures, close fits are obtained for the age 15–19 tail of very disparate fertility distributions in which age group 15–19 accounts for less than 1 percent to more than 10 percent of overall fertility and 26–48 percent of marital fertility. As we shall see later, the fits to the

TABLE 4.1

Features of Residuals from EHR Fitting of Double and Triple Multiplicative Models to Cumulated, Normalized Age-Specific Fertility Rates Expressed on the Folded Square Root Scale for Selected Time Sequences: 1775–1976

| Sequence[a] | Percentage of variation explained | | ns^2_{bi} (10^{-5}) | Residuals (folded square root scale) | |
	Linear scale	Squared scale		Median absolute	Upper 90%
X15	99.0	99.98	4.14	.0046	.0101
X20	98.9	—	—	—	—
X202	99.5	—	0.93	.0017	.0065
C15	98.5	99.79	8.07	.0057	.0160
C20	98.3	—	—	—	—
SYAC13	98.2	99.95	19.23	.0077	.0266
MX15	98.9	99.98	1.76	.0026	.0072
MX20	99.1	—	—	—	—
NX15	98.6	—	4.01	.0039	.0107
MC15	97.1	99.88	13.63	.0071	.0193

[a] Two-component fits are used for all sequences except *X202*, for which a three-component fit is used.

lower tail are sufficiently close that years are identified in which child-bearing behavior at ages 15–19 appears to make an aberrant contribution to total fertility. Examples include the period 1964–1968 for cross-sectional overall fertility (Fig. 4.6) and 1937, 1949, and 1960–1962 for confinements occurring 9 months or more after marriage (Fig. 4.11). It is apparent that we need to look at the size of residuals on two levels: the amount of variability in a whole time sequence explained by its fitted description and the difference between individual reported and fitted schedules.

Summary Measures of Fit

We shall consider first the evidence of close fit summarized in a measure based on the sum of the absolute deviations:

$$\text{Proportion of variation explained} = 1 - \frac{\sum |z_{ij}|}{\sum |F_{ij} - \text{median } F_{ij}|}.$$

All of the basic cross-sectional and cohort sequences of overall and marital fertility are shown in Table 4.1 to have a very high proportion of their total variability explained by the fitted parameters. The nature of the less close fits for the cohort sequences is most profitably examined in the time-sequence plots of residuals (Figs. 4.7–4.8) discussed later in this chapter.

For a measure of fit that is highly resistant to outliers, we turn to the robust estimate of the variance of the residuals—s_{bi}^2 (see Appendix B). This measure provides information about the relative compactness of the main body of the residuals for the various sequences and aids the comparison of two-component and three-component fits. A few values of the percentage of squared variation explained are also included in Table 4.1 to reiterate the point made in Chapter III that this measure of fit is not a very useful one for our present purposes.

Fits to Individual Schedules

Table 4.2 illustrates the close fits to individual schedules in four different sequences. Reported and fitted distributions for representative years with very different age distributions of fertility and some years of "worst fit" are given on both the folded square root and the raw fraction scales. The reported and fitted cumulative rates for each of these schedules can be calculated by multiplying the raw fraction at each age cut by $T_i = \Sigma_{j=1}^7 f_i(a_j)$. Fits to selected individual schedules in the single-year-of-age cohort sequence are shown on the raw fraction scale in Fig. 4.1a for representative cohorts and Fig. 4.1b for a cohort of "worst fit." No effort has been made to choose "best fits" for any of these sequences. By referring to the original data and the procedure outlined in Chapter VIII, the reader can check the fits for other years or cohorts of interest. Close fits in two components tend to be improved by the introduction of a third component (compare the X15 and *X202* residuals for 1957 and also for 1890 in Table 4.2). The singular nature of such distributions as that for 1792 is evident in a two-component fit and is further emphasized by the continued presence of a prominent residual at age cut 39/40 in a three-component fit.

Two points should be kept in mind when examining this table. The first point concerns residuals on the folded square root scale. With a folded linearizing re-expression that centers the distribution on its median, the rates near the median are changed less during re-expression than are higher or lower rates. Therefore a residual of given size for a rate much higher or lower than the median rate will have relatively less significance for the fitted distribution on the raw fraction scale than will a residual of the same size for a rate near the median. For example, with the folded square root re-expression, a residual of .01 will have its highest de-transformed value .007 at the center of the cumulated, normalized fertility

TABLE 4.2

Reported and EHR-Fitted Fertility Distributions on Folded Square Root and Raw Fraction Scales; Selected Sequences and Selected Years: 1775–1976

Distribution	Age cut						T_i
	19/20	24/25	29/30	34/35	39/40	44/45	
X15 (1890)							
Folded square root							
Reported	−.8774	−.5528	−.1774	.1869	.5424	.8536	
Fitted	−.8781	−.5579	−.1801	.1933	.5467	.8467	
Residual	.0007	.0051	.0027	−.0064	−.0043	.0069	
Raw fraction							
Reported	.0134	.1402	.3755	.6310	.8542	.9813	.8295
Fitted	.0133	.1375	.3737	.6354	.8565	.9795	
Residual	.0001	.0027	.0018	−.0044	−.0023	.0018	
X202 (1890)							
Raw fraction							
Reported	.0134	.1402	.3755	.6310	.8542	.9813	.8295
Fitted	.0137	.1406	.3727	.6319	.8555	.9811	
Residual	−.0003	−.0004	.0028	−.0009	−.0013	.0002	
X15 (1957)							
Folded square root							
Reported	−.6669	−.1751	.2548	.5696	.8018	.9509	
Fitted	−.6587	−.1650	.2498	.5649	.8060	.9630	
Residual	−.0082	−.0101	.0050	.0047	−.0044	−.0121	
Raw fraction							
Reported	.0841	.3771	.6773	.8687	.9670	.9977	.4620
Fitted	.0878	.3841	.6739	.8662	.9683	.9987	
Residual	−.0037	−.0070	.0034	.0025	−.0013	−.0010	
X202 (1957)							
Raw fraction							
Reported	.0841	.3771	.6773	.8687	.9670	.9977	.4620
Fitted	.0845	.3765	.6773	.8689	.9669	.9978	
Residual	−.0004	.0006	.0000	−.0002	.0001	−.0001	
X15 (1792)[b]							
Folded square root							
Reported	−.8410	−.5345	−.1789	.1829	.5610	.8267	
Fitted	−.8516	−.5378	−.1697	.1928	.5352	.8253	
Residual	.0106	.0033	−.0092	−.0099	.0258	.0014	
Raw fraction							
Reported	.0219	.1501	.3745	.6283	.8641	.9743	.9571
Fitted	.0193	.1483	.3809	.6351	.8503	.9739	
Residual	.0026	.0018	−.0064	−.0068	.0138	.0004	
X202 (1792)[b]							
Raw fraction							
Reported	.0219	.1501	.3745	.6283	.8641	.9743	.9571
Fitted	.0207	.1513	.3765	.6265	.8450	.9738	
Residual	.0012	−.0012	−.0020	.0018	.0191	.0005	

(table continues)

TABLE 4.2 (*continued*)

Distribution	Age cut						T_i
	19/20	*24/25*	*29/30*	*34/35*	*39/40*	*44/45*	
C15 (1890)							
Folded square root							
Reported	−.8685	−.5007	.−0854	.2947	.6352	.8947	
Fitted	−.8655	−.4925	−.0875	.2890	.6308	.9047	
Residual	−.0030	−.0082	.0021	.0057	.0044	−.0100	
Raw fraction							
Reported	.0153	.1689	.4397	.7038	.9013	.9899	.7274
Fitted	.0160	.1735	.4383	.7001	.8992	.9917	
Residual	−.0007	−.0046	.0014	.0037	.0021	−.0018	
C15 (1920)							
Folded square root							
Reported	−.7256	−.2852	.1075	.4238	.6934	.9342	
Fitted	−.7264	−.2926	.1067	.4327	.7033	.8837	
Residual	.0008	.0074	.0008	−.0089	−.0099	.0505	
Raw fraction							
Reported	.0596	.3025	.5758	.7859	.9273	.9959	.3705
Fitted	.0593	.2976	.5752	.7913	.9314	.9878	
Residual	.0003	.0049	.0006	−.0054	−.0041	.0081	
C15 (1929)[b]							
Folded square root							
Reported	−.7625	−.3925	.0023	.4608	.7777	.9480	
Fitted	−.7681	−.2969	.1314	.4772	.7616	.9472	
Residual	.0056	−.0956	−.1291	−.0164	.0161	.0008	
Raw fraction							
Reported	.0459	.2334	.5016	.8081	.9593	.9974	.3916
Fitted	.0440	.2947	.5925	.8176	.9538	.9974	
Residual	.0019	−.0613	−.0909	−.0095	.0055	.0000	
MX15 (1905)							
Folded square root							
Reported	−.2868	.0298	.2789	.5023	.7130	.9081	
Fitted	−.2888	.0325	.2789	.4983	.7129	.9094	
Residual	.0020	−.0027	.0000	.0040	.0001	−.0013	
Raw fraction							
Reported	.3014	.5211	.6933	.8320	.9354	.9923	2.041
Fitted	.3001	.5230	.6934	.8298	.9354	.9925	
Residual	.0013	−.0019	−.0001	.0022	.0000	−.0002	
MX15 (1930)							
Folded square root							
Reported	−.1107	.2162	.4395	.6215	.7903	.9349	
Fitted	−.1089	.2091	.4386	.6280	.7941	.9288	
Residual	−.0018	.0071	.0009	−.0065	−.0038	.0061	

TABLE 4.2 (*continued*)

	Age cut						
Distribution	*19/20*	*24/25*	*29/30*	*34/35*	*39/40*	*44/45*	T_i
Raw fraction							
Reported	.4219	.6511	.7954	.8947	.9634	.9960	1.314
Fitted	.4232	.6462	.7948	.8979	.9646	.9953	
Residual	−.0013	.0049	.0006	−.0032	−.0012	.0007	
MX15 (1955)[b]							
Folded square root							
Reported	−.0345	.2999	.5397	.7211	.8652	.9620	
Fitted	−.0254	.3029	.5328	.7147	.8635	.9731	
Residual	−.0091	−.0030	.0069	.0064	.0017	−.0111	
Raw fraction							
Reported	.4756	.7072	.8528	.9386	.9839	.9986	1.182
Fitted	.4820	.7092	.8490	.9361	.9835	.9993	
Residual	−.0064	−.0020	.0038	.0025	.0004	−.0007	

[a] Two-component fits are used for all sequences except *X202*, for which a three-component fit is used.
[b] This is a year of "worst fit".

distribution and progressively lower de-transformed value toward either tail of the distribution.

The second point concerns residuals on the raw fraction scale. With the reported and fitted distributions expressed on the raw fraction scale, a residual of a given size indicates less of a difference between fitted and reported rates at an age cut when the total rate of fertility is low than when it is high. For example, when the sum of age-specific rates $T_i = 1.5$ is multiplied by a raw fraction residual of .01, the result is a difference of .015 between the reported and fitted rates at that age cut. When $T_i = .5$, one-third as much, a residual of .01 means a difference of only .005 between reported and fitted rates.

Structure in Residuals

Of the many informative ways of looking at residuals for structure or pattern, three will be illustrated from analyses of the X15, *X202*, C15, SYAC13, MX15, and NX15 sequences:

1. schematic plots that order by size the residuals for each age cut and summarize their distribution within an age cut;

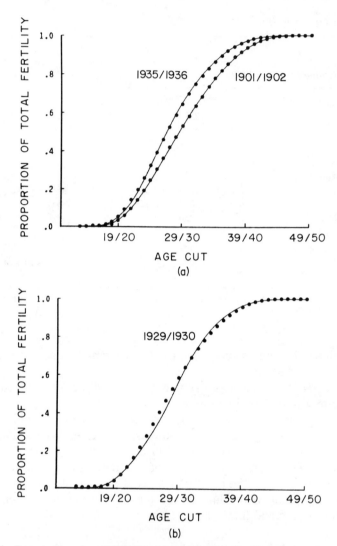

Fig. 4.1   Reported (——) and EHR-fitted (● ● ●) fertility distributions (raw fraction scale) from double multiplicative fits to the SYAC13 sequence, selected cohorts by year at age 15: (a) 1935/1936 and 1901/1902; (b) 1929/1930 (a "worst fit").

2. scatter plots that summarize the size and sign relations of residuals ordered in time sequence for pairs of age cuts;
3. time-sequence plots for all age cuts that allow the examination of changes in residual patterns by age cut from one time period to another.

These plots demonstrate, in different ways, the extent to which the developed descriptions have captured the underlying structure of the fertility sequences.

Schematic Plots

Schematic plots are described and illustrated in Chapter II for some preliminary steps of dissection of a simplified time sequence of age-specific fertility rates (see Chapter II for a definition of schematic plot symbols). For the two-component fits to the single-year sequences beginning in 1775, we concentrate on two properties of the fit: the degree of symmetry in the spreading of residuals around the median residual for each age cut and the degree of agreement between age cuts in the amount of spreading of the residuals. Both of these properties indicate the extent to which pattern remains in the residuals. For the C15 sequence (Fig. 4.2), 90 percent of the residuals (and all residuals within the range from one interquartile distance of the upper quartile to one interquartile distance of the lower quartile) are similarly and evenly distributed for all age cuts. However, the outliers are predominantly positive for the first two and last two age cuts, predominantly negative for the two central age cuts. In contrast, the X15 residuals (Fig. 4.3) are more compact. Although symmetrically distributed around the median for the first four age cuts, they show dissimilarity between age cuts in the amount of spread, particularly in the interquartile range. At even this early stage of examination, we can conclude that some structure remains in both cohort and cross-sectional residuals from two-component fits; and the most visible structure lies in the outliers for the cohorts but appears in the main body of the residuals for the cross-sectional sequence.

Scatter Plots

Scatter plots reveal a tendency for the residuals at some pairs of age cuts in the cross-sectional fertility sequences to vary together by year in some systematic way. For example, for two-component fits the X15 residuals for age cut 24/25

1. show no systematic variation over time with the residuals for age cut 29/30 (Fig. 4.4a);
2. tend to be of opposite sign by year from the residuals for age cut 39/40 (Fig. 4.4b);
3. tend to be of the same sign by year as the residuals for age cut 44/45 (Fig. 4.4c).

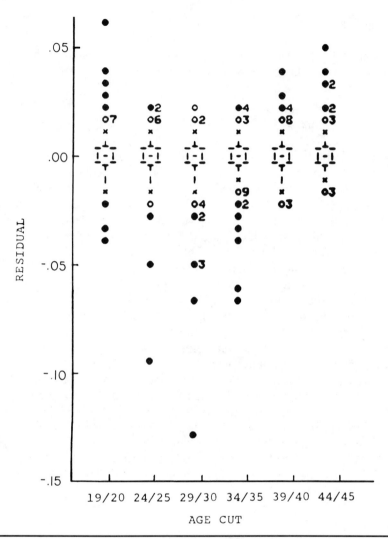

Fig. 4.2 Schematic plots of residuals by age cut (folded square root scale) from EHR fitting of the double multiplicative model to the C15 sequence: cohorts aged 15–19 from 1775 to 1929.

		Residual		
Age cut	Minimum	Lower quartile	Median	Upper quartile	Maximum
19/20	−.0366	−.0060	−.0012	.0042	.0637
24/25	−.0956	−.0062	−.0015	.0054	.0240
29/30	−.1292	−.0068	.0004	.0058	.0236
34/35	−.0670	−.0048	.0000	.0062	.0265
39/40	−.0223	−.0057	.0002	.0057	.0390
44/45	−.0180	−.0054	.0011	.0044	.0515

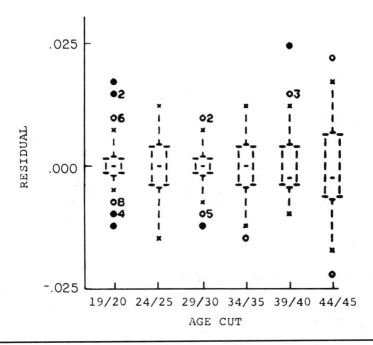

Fig. 4.3 Schematic plots of residuals by age cut (folded square root scale) from EHR fitting of the double multiplicative model to the X15 sequence: 1775–1959.

Age cut	Minimum	Lower quartile	Median	Upper quartile	Maximum
			Residual		
19/20	−.0138	−.0022	.0004	.0029	.0170
24/25	−.0157	−.0052	.0000	.0056	.0119
29/30	−.0136	−.0032	.0006	.0029	.0109
34/35	−.0152	−.0052	−.0008	.0051	.0128
39/40	−.0109	−.0051	−.0015	.0040	.0258
44/45	−.0234	−.0069	−.0017	.0068	.0241

When an appropriate compound nonlinear smoothing procedure (Tukey, 1977, pp. 205–264 and 523–542) is applied to the residual vectors by age cut to de-emphasize irregular fluctuations and provide more sensitive detection of patterns of covariation, the tilts in the scatter plots of Figs. 4.4b and 4.4c persist. This result further supports the presence of some remaining underlying structure in the small residuals.

Scatter plots of the cohort residuals from two-component fits do not reveal a relation between age cuts across cohorts until the residuals for an age cut are shifted forward 5 years before comparison with the residuals

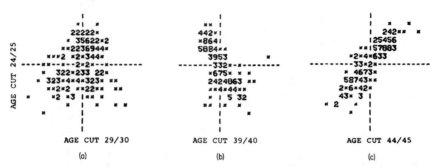

Fig. 4.4   Scatter plots of residuals (folded square root scale) for pairs of age cuts from EHR fitting of the double multiplicative model to the X15 sequence: 1775–1959. Age cut 24/25 residuals are plotted against (a) age cut 29/30 residuals, where the range of X is $-.015$ to $.015$; (b) age cut 39/40 residuals, where the range of X is $-.02$ to $.03$; and (c) age cut 44/45 residuals, where the range of X is $-.04$ to $.04$. The range of Y is $-.02$ to $.015$ for all three plots.

for the preceding age cut. This lagged relation between residuals for cohort age cuts is seen vividly in time-sequence plots of residuals (Figs. 4.7 and 4.8 and Fig. 7.13). Its significance as an indicator of period effects on cohort fertility is discussed in the following section.

Time-sequence Plots

Time-sequence plots of residuals by age cut provide more detail about the remaining structure. Such plots are presented with the final set of residuals expressed on the raw fraction scale so the relative importance of any residual can be judged directly. To emphasize the nature of the small deviations, the residuals have also been coded:

○ $<(M - \frac{1}{4}I)$
− $(M - \frac{1}{4}I)$ to $(M + \frac{1}{4}I)$
+ $>(M + \frac{1}{4}I)$
M Median residual across all years and age cuts
I Absolute range between the values of the residuals at the lower and upper 25 percentage points when the residuals are ordered by value

For example, when the $n = 1110$ residuals for X15 fits are ordered by value alone, from the largest negative residual to the largest positive residual across all years and age cuts, the median residual value is $M = -.000058$. To determine the value of I, the residuals at the $n/4$ and $3n/4$ points in the order are identified. Then I is the absolute range between the value $-.0021$ of residual number 278 and the value $.0019$ of residual

TABLE 4.3

Basis of Coding Raw Fraction Scale Residuals in Time-Sequence Plots (Fig. 4.5–4.8, 4.10, 4.11)

	Residual					
Sequence	M	$n/4$	$3n/4$	I	$M - \frac{1}{4}I$	$M + \frac{1}{4}I$
X15	−.000058	−.00214	.00191	.00404	−.00107	.00095
X202	.000002	−.00072	.00088	.00159	−.00040	.00040
C15	−.000057	−.00215	.00256	.00471	−.00124	.00112
SYAC13	−.000032	−.00199	.00226	.00425	−.00110	.00103
MX15	.000047	−.00099	.00121	.00220	−.00050	.00060
NX15	−.000243	−.00155	.00163	.00318	−.00104	.00055

number 832. Coding values are shown in Table 4.3 for all sets of residuals to be examined in time-sequence plots.

Cross-sectional Overall Fertility For the X15 residuals, a time-sequence plot (Fig. 4.5) confirms the schematic plot impression of few singular departures from fit at any age cut. The years 1783 and 1792 stand out as deviant. The plot also locates in the time dimension a pattern of departures from random distribution that was detected in the scatter plots of the pairs of X15 residual vectors. Age cuts 34/35 and 39/40 tend to have residuals $>(M + \frac{1}{4}I)$ before 1855, then $<(M - \frac{1}{4}I)$ until about 1937. Age cuts 24/25 and 44/45 show the reverse tendency, with residuals $<(M - \frac{1}{4}I)$ before 1855, then $>(M + \frac{1}{4}I)$ until about 1937. This means, for example, that before 1855 a slightly lower proportion of births is reported to have occurred at ages 20–24 in most years than the fit would have predicted. The X20 residuals by age cut have the same systematic variations as the X15 residuals, indicating that departure from fit is not greatly influenced by age 15–19 fertility in this time sequence.

The capacity of a third component to draw much of the remaining cross-sectional pattern into a fitted description is illustrated with the X202 sequence, which includes the most recent changes in fertility patterns. Fitting a triple multiplicative model to the folded square root re-expression of this 202-year sequence, using $c = 12$ in the weight function, leaves the residuals shown in Fig. 4.6. Note that the scale is expanded in comparison to Fig. 4.5 to emphasize the nature of the departures from fit that remain in the further diminished residuals. The 1964–1968 period stands out with higher than predicted proportions of total fertility at ages 15–19. The 1930–1950 period contains much of the remaining systematic departure from fit, whereas the pre-1815 period contains the most prominent

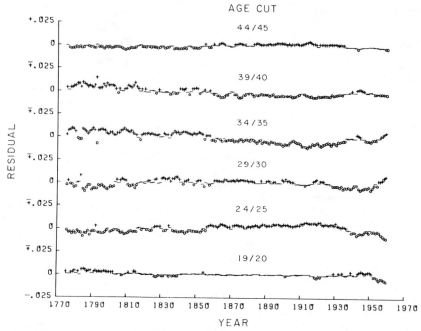

Fig. 4.5 Time-sequence plot of coded residuals by age cut (raw fraction scale) from EHR fitting of the double multiplicative model to the X15 sequence: 1775–1959.

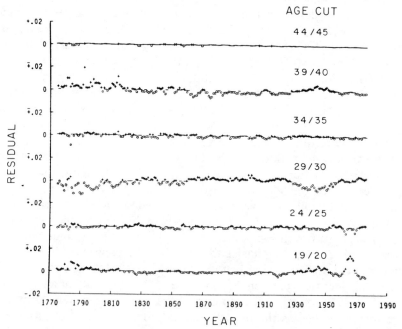

Fig. 4.6 Time-sequence plot of coded residuals by age cut (raw fraction scale) from EHR fitting of the triple multiplicative model to the *X202* sequence: 1775–1976.

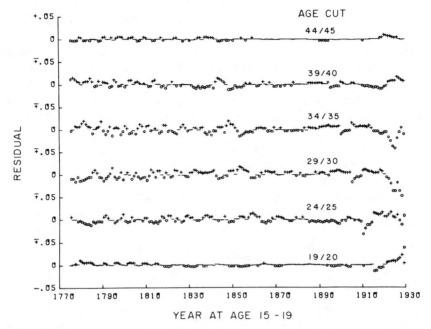

Fig. 4.7 Time-sequence plot of coded residuals by age cut (raw fraction scale) from EHR fitting of the double multiplicative model to the C15 sequence: cohorts aged 15–19 from 1775 to 1929.

irregularities. Note that many of the irregular departures are more clearly identifiable in Fig. 4.6 than in Fig. 4.5 because additional pattern has been removed by the third component.

Thus, fitting a third component can be a useful step of exploration even when we later use only the first two fitted time parameters to describe trends and major transitions. In general, we first want to see what can be learned from a relatively simple EHR description of each fertility time sequence. The decision to go to a more complex model seeks an appropriate balance between parsimony and completeness of description. A model sufficiently complex to give an excellent mathematical description of almost all variation in a data set can usually be found. However, such a model would be more likely to have lost the demographic significance of its parameters (Anscombe, 1967).

Cohort Overall Fertility Time-sequence plots of cohort residuals for the C15 sequence, shown in Fig. 4.7 in coded form on the raw fraction scale, present a very different picture from plots of the X15 residuals (Fig. 4.5). When the vector of residuals for any age cut (such as 29/30) is compared with the vector of residuals for the next age cut (34/35) shifted to the right by five cohorts, the fluctuations appear to be highly correlated. This visual impression is reinforced by both scatter plots of shifted residual vectors for pairs of age cuts and calculated correlation coefficients (.63–.83) for pairs of lagged residual vectors on the folded square root scale used in the fitting. However, fluctuations, peaks of positive residuals and valleys of negative residuals, are less pronounced for about a 40-year span (for example, 1870–1910 for cohorts at age cut 24/25).

Residuals by age cut for the C20 sequence have the same pattern as those for the C15 sequence indicating that fertility at ages 15–19 is not a major determinant of this pattern of departures from fit. Residuals from EHR analysis of the cohort marital fertility sequence MC15, using the same combination of re-expression and fitting as for the C15 sequence, exhibit the same lagged pattern (see Fig. 7.13). The relation of the corresponding C15 and MC15 residuals will be considered in Chapter VII in conjunction with the corresponding sets of fitted time parameters.

At least two questions about the systematic lagged variations in cohort residuals need to be explored. First, has the construction of cohort sequences from cross-sectional data in 5-year age groups contributed to the variation? Second, does the lagged pattern represent period effects on cohort fertility patterns? Does it represent either the influence of real events that have affected the childbearing of all age groups to some extent in particular years or the dissemination of cross-sectional data errors to a number of cohorts?

EHR analysis of the single-year-of-age cohort sequence SYAC13 provides a partial answer to the first question—lagged pattern in cohort residuals is not an artifact of age grouping or the method of sequence construction, at least for the cohorts aged 15 after 1884. Residuals from a two-component fit to this sequence reveal peaks of positive residuals on a 1-year diagonal and valleys of negative residuals on a 1-year diagonal (Fig. 4.8). For a matrix with 37 age cuts, the residuals can not be conveniently graphed. Instead, they are shown in coded form according to the table accompanying Fig. 4.8. The similarity of the SYAC13 pattern to that for the C15 residuals on a 5-year diagonal (Fig. 4.7) is readily apparent.

The backward lag of the pattern and its relation to period effects on cohort fertility patterns can be more easily understood from a diagram, viewed first in cross-sectional perspective (Fig. 4.9a) and then in cohort perspective (Fig. 4.9b)[1]. In Fig. 4.9a, age-specific fertility in 1920 is emphasized as a composite of a portion of the childbearing experience of many cohorts of women who entered their childbearing ages in various calendar years in the past. When we rotate this diagram 45° counterclockwise

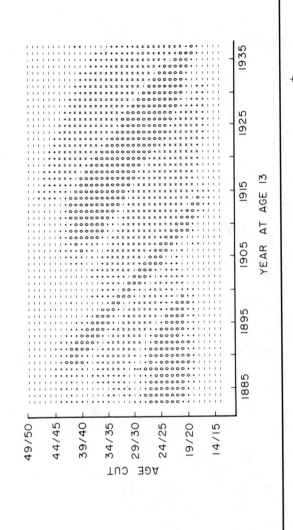

Fig. 4.8 Coded residuals by age cut (raw fraction scale) from EHR fitting of the double multiplicative model to the SYAC13 sequence: cohorts aged 15 from 1885/1886 to 1939/1940.

0				•			−				+			x	
$<(M - \frac{3}{4}I)$			$(M - \frac{3}{4}I)$	to	$(M - \frac{1}{4}I)$		$(M - \frac{1}{4}I)$	to	$(M + \frac{1}{4}I)$		$(M + \frac{1}{4}I)$	to	$(M + \frac{3}{4}I)$		$>(M + \frac{3}{4}I)$
$<(-.00322)$			$(-.00322)$	to	$(-.00110)$		$(-.00110)$	to	$(.00103)$		$(.00103)$	to	$(.00316)$		$>(.00316)$

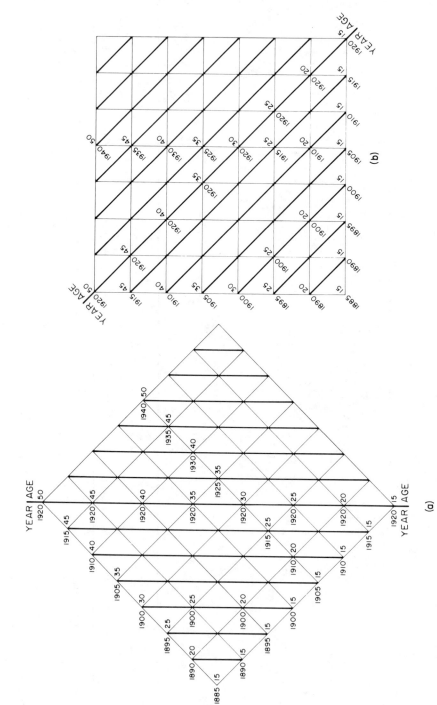

Fig. 4.9 Relations of cohort and cross-sectional age-specific fertility rates: (a) cross-sectional perspective, (b) cohort perspective.

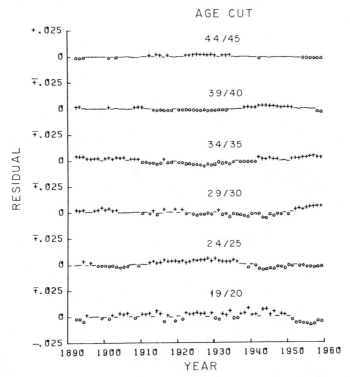

Fig. 4.10 Time-sequence plot of coded residuals by age cut (raw fraction scale) from EHR fitting of the double multiplicative model to the MX15 sequence: 1892–1959.

(Fig. 4.9b), the calendar years of entry into childbearing ages form a horizontal axis, emphasizing the cohort perspective. We see that any period influence of the year 1920 on the childbearing of all cohorts passing through it at various ages would appear on a backward-rising diagonal.

Returning to Figs. 4.7–4.8, we find in the cohort residuals the same positive or negative effect of a given period whether cohort fertility has been analyzed by single-year-of-age or 5-year age groups:

1. the negative influence below age 27 in the 1892–1907 period, the positive influence above age 25 in the 1907–1914 period, the negative influence of World War I on fertility;
2. the positive effect of the 1919–1932 postwar period, followed by the negative effects of 1933–1944;
3. the positive influences of 1945 to 1959, if we extrapolate the diagonals to an extended baseline.

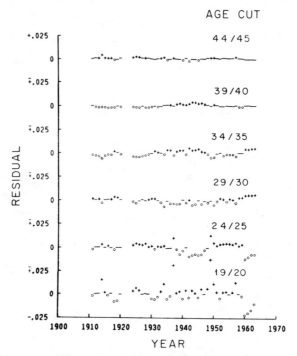

Fig. 4.11 Time-sequence plot of coded residuals by age cut (raw fraction scale) from EHR fitting of the double multiplicative model to the NX15 sequence: 1911–1963, with 1921–1923 missing.

The cohort residuals, representing only a small portion of the variability in the data, nevertheless reveal an interesting additional aspect of the data's systematic variation.

Cross-sectional Marital Fertility The very small MX15 residuals (shown in Fig. 4.10) and the corresponding set of MX20 residuals include no prominent isolated departures from fit. However, some tendency is apparent at all age cuts for stretches of residuals to lie either above or below the central interval, and these stretches are similar in sign to those for the two-component fits to the overall fertility sequence for the same years (Fig. 4.5).

For the NX15 sequence of confinements occurring 9 months or more after marriage, the residuals shown in Fig. 4.11 are similar to those for the MX15 sequence at the higher age cuts, but they exhibit some differences from the MX15 sequence at age cuts 19/20 and 24/25. The differences include prominent departures from fit in specific years, which will be discussed in conjunction with the fitted time parameters in Chapter VII.

Summary

This chapter tests how well we have met our first goal in the description of fertility change—"to make our fit to the diversity of the real world as good as possible, subject to holding the number of parameters to a minimum" (Tukey, Appendix A). We have examined residuals for size and, more importantly, for structure in testing the goodness of EHR fits to 10 time sequences of age-specific fertility schedules, including both cross-sectional and cohort perspectives on overall and marital fertility. The schedules had been cumulated, normalized, and re-expressed on a folded square root scale before fitting. The sum of the absolute deviations from fit and a robust measure of the variance of residuals have been the preferred bases of comparison for the amount of variability in a whole sequence explained by the fitted description. The differences between individual reported and fitted schedules have also been considered for both typical fits and "worst fits." The testing of residuals for remaining structure has been illustrated with schematic plots, scatter plots, and time-sequence plots.

The thorough examination of residuals supports the following conclusions. By all criteria of residual size and structure, the descriptions developed in two components for all the overall and marital fertility sequences meet the first goal of the analyses: to bring into a small number of parameters most of the systematic variability in each sequence and to identify in the residuals the nature and timing of departures from these patterns. The fits in the two age parameters and two time parameters are sufficiently close to be carried forward to Chapter V for re-presentation of the fits in a demographically guided standard form. Two-component fits leave some structure in the small residuals of each of the fertility time sequences, both overall and marital. The diagonal pattern in residuals for cohort sequences, different from the structure remaining in residuals for cross-sectional sequences, provides an indicator of positive or negative period effects on cohort fertility patterns.

Extensions of EHR analysis naturally ask, Are more complex descriptions of fertility distributions appreciably better? Do other re-expressions of the data result in still better fits? Fitting three components to the folded square root re-expression of the 202-year cross-sectional sequence brings into the fitted description most of the structure not captured in two components. There are certain advantages to fitting the additional component. One, bringing more of the systematic variation into the fits makes the nature of isolated deviations more evident in the residuals. This helps to identify a response to unusual circumstances or the existence of data errors. Two, having three components to submit to the re-presentation procedures (Chapter V) permits standardization of the form of two age parameters. This can enhance cross-sequence comparisons even if the analyst decides to retain only the first two of the three re-presented components. Three, having one more component than might be preferred for the final fit gives the analyst more information for use in simplifying the description or seeking an appropriate balance between parsimony and completeness of description. Exploration of other data re-expressions will be more profitable after examination of the folded square root results for Sweden (Chapters VI–VII) and the preliminary cross-population comparisons that use the age standards derived on the folded square root scale from the Swedish data (Chapter VIII).

Notes for Chapter IV

1. Figure 4.9 is a simplified diagram that places emphasis on the nature of the residual pattern. However, the fertility schedules that we are analyzing relate childbearing to a woman's age at the time of confinement rather than the age that she reaches in a specific calendar year. "Year at age 15" is assigned approximately from the fertility schedules and for single-year-of-age schedules should be understood to refer to two years (aged 15 in 1920/1921, for example). See Note 1 in Chapter III for the designation of year and age relations for cohorts by 5-year age groups.

V

Re-presentation of Fits: Demographically Guided Standard Forms

Introduction

We have concentrated first on obtaining optimal descriptions of the regularities in long and diverse time sequences while holding the number of parameters to a minimum. The residuals have been reserved for detailed examination to see what they suggest about unusual circumstances affecting specific data points and about errors in the data for which we may want to consider revisions. Now we focus on the fitted descriptions of all the fertility sequences, including both cross-sectional and cohort perspectives on overall and marital fertility for age ranges 15–49 and 20–49. We want to examine the descriptions individually and then compare them with each other for interpretation. Therefore, we need to re-present all of the fitted descriptions in a demographically guided standard form.

Major considerations in our choice of a standard form include:

1. simplifying the description to come as close as possible to describing the variability in the data with one less parameter, for either a whole time sequence or parts of it;
2. making the standard form relate to the patterns in demographic processes that are expected to underlie the cumulative age distribution of fertility—among others, age patterns of entry into childbearing, age patterns of change in fecundity, and age patterns of limitation of fertility;
3. incorporating in a single time parameter, as far as possible, the long-term trend of change in the age pattern of fertility that is associated with decline in the level of fertility.

A guided re-presentation of fit is possible because a final fitted data description is just one of many algebraically equivalent combinations of the parameters (see Chapter III and Appendix A). This circumstance is not peculiar to EHR analysis, although other procedures may place more or different constraints on the fitting. For example, fitting by least squares in a traditional principal components analysis would require the age vectors A_j and B_j to be orthogonal. Once the fitting is complete, however, the fitted description would remain only one of many algebraically equivalent combinations of the parameters. To re-present a least squares fit the constraint of orthogonality might have to be abandoned to impose other selected combinations of constraints, but this would be a valid procedure for efforts to enhance the interpretation or comparability of fitted descriptions.

Depending on the constraints selected for the standard form, we should expect some sets of fitted parameters to be relatively unchanged by re-presentation and other sets to be changed substantially. Re-presentation begins with the set of EHR-fitted age vectors shown in Table 5.1 for each fertility sequence and the corresponding sets of fitted time parameters (whose ranges are also shown in Table 5.1). Because EHR analysis places few constraints on the fitting procedure, we know it is possible for age vectors within a set to vary together in some way and for the year or cohort effects (the multipliers of the age vectors) to be more or less linearly related. This linear relation occurs most noticeably when the distributions have appreciable variation over time at the first age cut (for example, the X20, MX15, and MX20 sequences), in contrast to variation largely confined to the central age cuts (for example, the X15 sequence in which age 15–19 fertility is always low and the SYAC13 sequence in which fertility at age 13 is always close to zero).[1] The MX20 fitted time parameters before re-presentation (Fig. 5.1) and after re-presentation (Fig. 7.4) illustrate a linear relation and its removal in the standard form selected for the parameters. This standardization permits the useful comparisons made in Chapter VII between the marital fertility patterns and the corresponding overall fertility patterns.[2]

We shall first discuss the form of re-presentation chosen for the EHR double multiplicative fits of all the fertility sequences and the related form selected for the triple multiplicative fits. We shall then consider in more detail the demographic logic of the choices involved, turning finally to the results of re-presentation—the characteristics of the standard-form parameters carried into Chapters VI–VIII. Some readers may want to scan the last section of this chapter on the characteristics of the parameters before considering the details of their derivation.

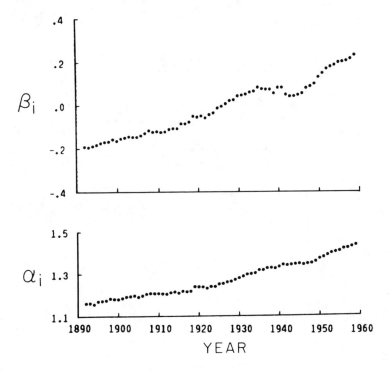

Fig. 5.1   EHR-fitted time parameters α_i and β_i before re-presentation of fits in a standard form: MX20 sequence, 1892–1959.

Form of Re-presentation of Double Multiplicative Fits

We can refer to the double multiplicative fit

$$\hat{F}_{ij} = \alpha_i A_j + \beta_i B_j$$

as a rank-two fit, where rank-two refers to the sum of two rank-one terms. A rank-one term is the product of a constant by a function of row alone by a function of column alone. Constraints on the standard forms of rank-two fits are of three types:

1. "fixing" a vector—for example, requiring it to be a constant, exactly linear, or as close as possible to a given form;
2. making two vectors orthogonal;
3. avoiding introduction of a mixed row-by-column term $\alpha_i B_j$ or $\beta_i A_j$.

TABLE 5.1

Fitted Age Parameters and Range of Fitted Time Parameters (Folded Square Root Scale) Derived by EHR Analysis of the Age Distribution of Overall and Marital Fertility in Selected Time Sequences, 1775–1976

Sequence	Time parameter	Range From	Range To	Age parameter	Age cut 19/20	24/25	29/30	34/35	39/40	44/45
C15	α_i	1.400	1.546	A_j	−.5810	−.3478	−.0845	.1669	.3986	.5895
X15		1.401	1.496		−.5835	−.3504	−.0889	.1620	.3949	.5888
XX15		1.409	1.535		−.5331	−.2570	.0108	.2453	.4530	.6199
X202		1.398	1.509		−.5721	−.3262	−.0620	.1847	.4112	.5993
MX15		1.245	1.636		−.1093	.1154	.2802	.4190	.5449	.6510
NX15		1.300	1.541		−.2934	−.0263	.1936	.3825	.5405	.6613
MC15		1.356	1.592		−.0982	.1325	.2967	.4319	.5470	.6317
C20		1.151	1.350		—	−.4467	−.1149	.1969	.4829	.7178
X20		1.132	1.420		—	−.4620	−.1323	.1816	.4729	.7159
XX20		1.149	1.354		—	−.3393	−.0055	.2793	.5284	.7264
MX20		1.156	1.433		—	−.1429	.1431	.3661	.5595	.7156
C15	β_i	−.194	.505	B_j	.2177	.4860	.5623	.4976	.3627	.1455
X15		−.172	.707		.2820	.5047	.5522	.4772	.3329	.1493
XX15		−.337	.436		.3579	.5229	.5502	.4639	.2818	.0349
X202		−.236	.799		.2454	.4513	.5709	.5243	.3508	.1109
MX15		−.332	.224		.6627	.5339	.3907	.2171	−.0120	−.2754
NX15		−.170	.202		.4826	.5010	.5283	.3994	.1282	−.2471
MC15		−.279	.174		.7241	.5465	.3255	.1412	.0345	−.2237
C20		−.173	.472		—	.5584	.6029	.4885	.2926	.0217
X20		−.133	.673		—	.6255	.6079	.4404	.1954	−.0834
XX20		−.291	.393		—	.5862	.6048	.4780	.2344	−.0850
MX20		−.194	.231		—	.6314	.5783	.4143	.1175	−.2855
X202	γ_i	−.051	.037	C_j	−.2624	−.6195	−.0079	.3294	.0453	−.6609

TABLE 5.2

Standard-Form Age Parameters and Characteristics of Standard-Form Time Parameters (Folded Square Root Scale) after Re-presentation of EHR Fits to the Age Distribution of Overall and Marital Fertility in Selected Time Sequences, 1775–1976

Sequence	Time parameter	Value μ	Value σ	Age parameter	Age cut 19/20	24/25	29/30	34/35	39/40	44/45
C15	α_i^*	1.479	.030	A_j^*	-.5965	-.3886	-.1337	.1217	.3639	.5728
X15		1.476	.019		-.6016	-.3915	-.1375	.1170	.3600	.5680
XX15		1.468	.013		-.5989	-.3776	-.1292	.1158	.3603	.5821
X202		1.440	.021		-.5822	-.3432	-.1070	.1328	.3807	.6077
MX15		1.226	.018		-.4816	-.2238	-.0058	.2093	.4468	.6888
NX15		1.260	.021		-.3940	-.1374	.0712	.2844	.4990	.7007
MC15		1.363	.016		-.4531	-.1642	.0894	.2996	.4880	.6572
C20		1.203	.023		—	-.5774	-.2775	.0482	.3725	.6697
X20		1.205	.013		—	-.5838	-.2839	.0425	.3699	.6633
XX20		1.187	.011		—	-.5250	-.2206	.0898	.4087	.7075
MX20		1.106	.013		—	-.3428	-.0547	.2102	.4908	.7711

Sequence	Time parameter	Range From	Range To		Age cut 19/20	24/25	29/30	34/35	39/40	44/45
C15	β_i^*	-.062	.633	B_j^*	.2025	.4771	.5603	.5022	.3733	.1610
X15		-.039	.843		.2870	.5074	.5525	.4754	.3291	.1438
XX15		.037	.815		.2801	.4846	.5502	.4983	.3468	.1245
X202		-.124	.931		.2788	.4913	.5648	.4905	.3264	.1217
MX15		.473	1.144		.5056	.5140	.5479	.4042	.2757	.1075
NX15		.133	.565		.2479	.4068	.5479	.5410	.3980	.1476
MC15		.451	.950		.6080	.5495	.4229	.3165	.2090	.0761
C20		.168	.802		—	.4527	.5709	.5273	.3975	.1819
X20		.191	.971		—	.4826	.5802	.5178	.3674	.1654
XX20		.140	.849		—	.4575	.5758	.5408	.3834	.1402
MX20		.204	.711		—	.4521	.5622	.5451	.4008	.1474

Sequence	Time parameter	μ	σ		19/20	24/25	29/30	34/35	39/40	44/45
X202	γ_i^*	.021	.129	C_j^*	-.4560	-.6849	-.0239	.3781	.2036	-.3716

[a] Time parameter α_i^* is shown in terms of μ and σ to indicate how near it is to a constant. Ranges of α_i^* values are shown in Table 5.4 for the C15 and X15 sequences, Table 5.7 for the X202 sequence, and Table 5.9 for the MX15, NX15, MC15, MC15, and MX20 sequences.

A total of four constraints should be selected to ensure uniqueness of the standard-form description. Then each double multiplicative fit

$$\hat{F}_{ij} = \alpha_i A_j + \beta_i B_j$$

is re-presented as an identically equivalent

$$\hat{F}_{ij} = k_1 \alpha_i^{**} A_j^{**} + k_2 \beta_i^{**} B_j^{**} = \alpha_i^* A_j^* + \beta_i^* B_j^*,$$

where $\alpha_i^{**} = p\alpha_i + q\beta_i$, $A_j^{**} = sA_j + tB_j$, p, q, s, and t are constants, k_1 and k_2 can be expressed in terms of p, q, s, and t, and $\Sigma A_j^{*2} = \Sigma B_j^{*2} = 1$ for standardization. For comparisons between time sequences, we incorporate the constants k_1 and k_2 in the time parameters so that, after the normalization of A_j^{**} and B_j^{**}, each element of the ith fitted fertility distribution is expressed as

$$\hat{F}_{ij} = \alpha_i^* A_j^* + \beta_i^* B_j^*.$$

For example, the MX15 fitted rate (expressed on the folded square root scale) at age cut 29/30 in 1910 is

$$\hat{F}_{19,3} = \alpha_{19} A_3 + \beta_{19} B_3$$
$$= (1.3310)(.2802) + (-.1752)(.3907) = .3045.$$

This is re-presented under the selected four constraints in the algebraically equivalent form

$$\hat{F}_{19,3} = \alpha_{19}^* A_3^* + \beta_{19}^* B_3^*$$
$$= (1.2261)(-.0058) + (.6507)(.4788) = .3045.$$

Note that β_i, A_j, and B_j undergo considerable change in the re-presentation.

The constraints chosen (Breckenridge, 1978) for the standard-form representation of all the fitted fertility distributions are:

1. to ensure the absence of the $\alpha_i^* B_j^*$ term in the expression;
2. to ensure the absence of the $\beta_i^* A_j^*$ term in the expression;
3. to make the equation $\alpha_i^{**} = p\alpha_i + q\beta_i$ as constant as possible, using least squares regression (with zero intercept) of a vector of identical constants on α_i and β_i to give the two regression coefficients p and q;
4. to make the equation $A_j^{**} = sA_j + tB_j$ as linear as possible, using one of the alternative procedures described in Appendix C for determining the required values of s and t: a canonical correlation analysis to establish a relation between linearly independent straight lines and the age vectors A_j and B_j or a simple pencil-and-paper procedure to identify what proportion of B_j, when added to A_j, would bring A_j^{**} as close as possible to linearity.[3]

The values of p, q, s, and t for the calculation of A_j^{**} and α_i^{**} and the subsequent calculation of B_j^{**} and β_i^{**} from A_j^{**}, α_i^{**}, B_j, β_i, p, q, s, and t are given in Appendix C, where the following relations are shown to hold:

$$B_j^{**} = B_j - \frac{q}{ps + qt} A_j^{**}, \qquad \beta_i^{**} = \beta_i - \frac{t}{ps + qt} \alpha_i^{**},$$

$$k_1 = \frac{1}{ps + qt}, \qquad k_2 = \frac{ps + qt}{ps}.$$

For each fertility time sequence, the regression to fix α_i^{**} leads to a time vector α_i^* that exhibits only a small amount of variation from a constant value (see Figs. 6.3, 6.10, 6.11, 7.4–7.6, and 7.12). The principal departures are associated with specific periods or groups of cohorts in the time sequences, such as the 1942–1945 period, the post-1960 period, and the cohorts aged 15–19 from 1915 to 1930. For most of the sequences, the narrow range of departure summarized in the standard deviation of α_i^* (Table 5.2) contrasts with the range of α_i before re-presentation of the fitted parameters (Table 5.1).

The age vectors before re-presentation, A_j and B_j, and those after representation, A_j^* and B_j^*, can be examined in Tables 5.1 and 5.2 for all 5-year-age-group sequences and in Table 5.3b for the single-year-of-age cohort sequence. The re-presented age standards for the SYAC13 sequence will also be shown graphically in Fig. 6.1.[4]

With few exceptions—for example, the α_i and B_j parameters for the C15 and X15 sequences—re-presentation results in noticeable change in the age and time parameters. This makes evident the importance of re-presentation of fits in a standard form before the comparison of time parameters for different sequences.

TABLE 5.3a

Time Parameters (Folded Square Root Scale) Before and After Re-presentation of EHR Fits to the SYAC13 Sequence, Cohorts Aged 15 from 1885/1886 to 1939/1940

		Time parameter		
Rank	α_i	β_i	α_i^*	β_i^*
Lowest	4.225	−.658	4.162	.039
Median	4.298	—	4.267	—
Highest	4.431	.683	4.332	1.394

TABLE 5.3b

Age Parameters (Folded Square Root Scale) Before and After
Re-presentation of EHR Fits to the SYAC13 Sequence, Cohorts
Aged 15 from 1885/1886 to 1939/1940

Age cut	Age parameter			
	A_j	B_j	A_j^*	B_j^*
13/14	−.2318	.0332	−.2343	−.0011
14/15	−.2305	.0381	−.2338	.0040
15/16	−.2277	.0432	−.2318	.0094
16/17	−.2219	.0582	−.2286	.0251
17/18	−.2123	.0785	−.2224	.0467
18/19	−.1991	.1035	−.2134	.0733
19/20	−.1828	.1283	−.2014	.1001
20/21	−.1645	.1513	−.1871	.1256
21/22	−.1449	.1730	−.1713	.1499
22/23	−.1243	.1922	−.1541	.1718
23/24	−.1033	.2092	−.1361	.1917
24/25	−.0822	.2245	−.1178	.2099
25/26	−.0615	.2361	−.0992	.2245
26/27	−.0411	.2450	−.0805	.2362
27/28	−.0214	.2508	−.0620	.2448
28/29	−.0021	.2539	−.0435	.2507
29/30	.0164	.2551	−.0254	.2546
30/31	.0344	.2534	−.0074	.2555
31/32	.0517	.2497	.0103	.2543
32/33	.0684	.2427	.0280	.2499
33/34	.0845	.2334	.0454	.2430
34/35	.1000	.2213	.0627	.2334
35/36	.1149	.2075	.0796	.2219
36/37	.1292	.1911	.0965	.2078
37/38	.1429	.1724	.1130	.1913
38/39	.1560	.1524	.1292	.1734
39/40	.1685	.1315	.1449	.1546
40/41	.1802	.1102	.1600	.1353
41/42	.1910	.0874	.1744	.1143
42/43	.2007	.0647	.1877	.0933
43/44	.2091	.0418	.1997	.0718
44/45	.2160	.0229	.2096	.0541
45/46	.2215	.0051	.2179	.0374
46/47	.2255	−.0086	.2240	.0244
47/48	.2283	−.0186	.2284	.0149
48/49	.2301	−.0236	.2311	.0103
49/50	.2313	−.0281	.2330	.0060

Form of Re-presentation of Triple Multiplicative Fits

We shall choose a two-stage re-presentation of a triple multiplicative fit

$$\hat{F}_{ij} = \alpha_i A_j + \beta_i B_j + \gamma_i C_j$$

as an identically equivalent

$$\hat{F}_{ij} = k_1 \alpha_i^{**} A_j^{**} + k_2 \beta_i^{**} B_j^{**} + k_3 \gamma_i^{**} C_j^{**} = \alpha_i^* A_j^* + \beta_i^* B_j^* + \gamma_i^* C_j^*,$$

where $\alpha_i^{**} = p\alpha_i + q\beta_i + r\gamma_i$, $A_j^{**} = sA_j + tB_j + uC_j$, $p, q, r, s, t, u, k_1, k_2$, and k_3 are constants, k_1 can be expressed in terms of p, q, r, s, t, and u, and $\Sigma A_j^{*^2} = \Sigma B_j^{*^2} = \Sigma C_j^{*^2} = 1$ for standardization. For the first stage of re-presentation, the same constraints are selected as for the double multiplicative re-presentation:

1. to avoid the introduction of the mixed terms $\alpha_i^* B_j^*$ and $\alpha_i^* C_j^*$;
2. to avoid the introduction of the mixed terms $\beta_i^* A_j^*$ and $\gamma_i^* A_j^*$;
3. to make the equation $\alpha_i^{**} = p\alpha_i + q\beta_i + r\gamma_i$ as constant as possible;
4. to make the equation $A_j^{**} = sA_j + tB_j + uC_j$ as linear as possible.

The procedures for constraints 3. and 4., analogous to those used with a rank-two fit, are shown in Appendix C.

The calculation of $k_1 = 1/(ps + qt + ru)$ and the determination of any conveniently identified set of β_i'', γ_i'', B_j'', and C_j'' from α_i^{**}, A_j^{**}, β_i, B_j, γ_i, C_j, p, q, r, s, t, and u (see Appendix C) leads to the second-stage re-presentation of the unconstrained portion of the fit

$$\hat{F}_{ij} - k_1 \alpha_i^{**} A_j^{**} = \beta_i'' B_j'' + \gamma_i'' C_j''$$

as an identically equivalent

$$k_2 \beta_i^{**} B_j^{**} + k_3 \gamma_i^{**} C_j^{**} = \beta_i^* B_j^* + \gamma_i^* C_j^*,$$

where $\beta_i^{**} = \beta_i'' - f\gamma_i''$, $B_j^{**} = B_j'' + gC_j''$, f and g are constants, k_2 and k_3 can be expressed in terms of f and g, and $\Sigma B_j^{*^2} = \Sigma C_j^{*^2} = 1$ for standardization. Note that carrying out the re-presentation in two stages allows us to deal with a rank-two portion of the fit in the second stage. The constraints selected for the second stage are:

1. to avoid the introduction of the mixed term $\beta_i^* C_j^*$;
2. to avoid the introduction of the mixed term $\gamma_i^* B_j^*$;
3. to make the equation $B_j^{**} = B_j'' + gC_j''$ as quadratic as possible;
4. to make the equation $\beta_i^{**} = \beta_i'' - f\gamma_i''$ express the major long-term trend of systematic change in the age distribution of fertility by maximizing slow change in β_i^{**} and leaving the remaining systematic variations to the third component $\gamma_i^{**} C_j^{**}$.

The procedures for determining the values of g and f needed to meet these requirements and the calculation of C_j^{**} and γ_i^{**} from B_j^{**}, β_i^{**}, C_j'', γ_i'', g, and f are given in Appendix C, where the following relations are shown to hold:

$$C_j^{**} = C_j'' + \frac{f}{(1 - fg)} B_j^{**}, \qquad \gamma_i^{**} = \gamma_i'' \frac{g}{(1 - fg)} \beta_i^{**},$$

$$k_2 = 1/(1 - fg), \qquad k_3 = 1 - fg.$$

For comparisons between time sequences, the constants k_1, k_2, and k_3 are again incorporated in the time parameters so that, after normalization of A_j^{**}, B_j^{**}, and C_j^{**}, each of the elements in the ith fitted fertility distribution is expressed as

$$\hat{F}_{ij} = \alpha_i^* A_j^* + \beta_i^* B_j^* + \gamma_i^* C_j^*.$$

The *X202* sequence will be used to illustrate three-component fits in the following chapters. The re-presented time parameters α_i^*, β_i^*, and γ_i^* for this sequence will be shown in Fig. 6.12. The age vectors before representation, A_j, B_j, and C_j, and those after re-presentation, A_j^*, B_j^*, and C_j^*, can be examined in Tables 5.1 and 5.2.

Demographic Logic in the Choice of a Standard Form

Recall the considerations in our choice of a standard form outlined at the beginning of this chapter:

1. to simplify the fitted description;
2. to select patterns related to underlying demographic processes;
3. to concentrate in a single time parameter the long-term trend of change in the age pattern of fertility that is associated with decline in the level of fertility.

For all sequences, constraining the first time parameter α_i^* to be as constant as possible provides a direct test of the potential for simplifying the description. Avoiding the introduction of mixed terms such as $\alpha_i^* B_j^*$, $\beta_i^* A_j^*$, $\gamma_i^* B_j^*$, and $\alpha_i^* C_j^*$ in the process of re-presentation helps maintain any simplification achieved. To understand how the selected constraints meet the second and third considerations, however, we need to give separate attention to overall fertility and marital fertility.

*Overall Fertility Patterns and the Choice
of Constraints*

We shall first consider how making one age vector as linear as possible relates the fitted overall fertility descriptions to underlying demographic processes. If both menarche and menopause occurred at fixed ages and if, on the average, women were equally likely to give birth at every age from menarche to menopause, then the cumulative fertility distribution would be linear. Whether the probability of a birth was low or high, and thus whether the number of total births was low or high, the proportion of total births included at a given age cut would always be the same. Also, the proportions would progress from age cut to age cut at a uniform rate.

In actuality, the proportion of women both biologically capable and exposed to the possibility of pregnancy increases over the lowest childbearing ages and declines over the highest ages. Thus, a first natural variation from a linear distribution is a concentration of births in the central ages of the childbearing age range, commonly taken as ages 15–50 but more complete if taken as ages 12–50. This concentration would be reflected in a slower rate of cumulation through the lower ages, a faster rate of cumulation across the central ages and through the mean age of childbearing, and then a slower rate as the cumulative fertility distribution approaches 100 percent. The resulting s-shaped distribution would be similar to those described at the beginning of our analysis. If the birth probabilities declined at the higher ages at the same rate they increased at the lower ages, the s-shaped curve would be symmetric around a mean age of childbearing of 32.5 for births occurring to women between ages 15–50. The extent to which births would be concentrated around this mean age would depend on how rapidly or slowly the birth probabilities changed with age.

When we recall that the folded square root re-expression was used in Chapter II to linearize s-shaped curves, we see that constraining the first standard age pattern (on the folded square root scale) to be as linear as possible is consistent with the first basic pattern that would naturally underlie a cumulative overall fertility distribution. De-transformation of the $\alpha_i^* A_j^*$ component, with the nearly linear A_j^* multiplied by the nearly constant α_i^*, should provide an underlying s-shaped standard pattern of the cumulation of births with age on which are imposed the major variations in the age distribution of fertility and variations in the mean age of childbearing.

The most common variation from the derived standard pattern of cumulation of births with age is asymmetry or skewness, which occurs when the probability of a birth does not increase across the lower ages at the same rate that it declines across the higher ages. At the lower ages, the probabilities depend on the age pattern of entry into childbearing—whether determined by the age pattern of development of fecundity, the age distribution of marriages, or the age pattern of contraceptive practices. At the higher ages, the probabilities depend on the age pattern of decline in childbearing—whether the result of physiological decline of fecundity, conscious use of contraceptive measures, or some other decrease in exposure to the possibility of pregnancy both within marriage and through widowhood or divorce. A high incidence of delay in the onset of childbearing and/or an extension of childbearing to higher ages would contribute negatively to the skewness of the overall fertility distribution. High incidence of early onset of childbearing and/or curtailment of childbearing at higher ages would contribute positively to the skewness of the distribution. The net effect of these opposed influences on the symmetry of the overall fertility distribution is captured in the second component of the fitted description $\beta_i^* B_j^*$, where B_j^* is roughly quadratic in form.[5]

The additional constraints chosen for re-presentation of a triple multiplicative fit establish more systematically our previous accomplishments in double multiplicative fitting. They also allow us to draw into the third component an additional type of demographically interpretable variation in fertility distributions. Whereas the B_j^* vector is roughly quadratic in a two-component fit, B_j^* is fixed to be as quadratic as possible in a three-component fit. This enhances the comparability of fitted descriptions for different sequences. In some instances, the nearly linear A_j^* vector and the nearly quadratic B_j^* vector provide such close fits that the third component $\gamma_i^* C_j^*$ can be dropped for most purposes. One example of such close fits is the description of a 52-year U.S. fertility sequence in terms of the A_j^*, B_j^*, and C_j^* age vectors derived from the Swedish $X202$ sequence (see Chapter VIII). This description supports the demographic appropriateness of the choice of constraints for the first two age vectors.

Once the time parameter α_i^* is constrained to be as constant as possible, the time parameter β_i^* in a two-component fit encompasses the major systematic change over time in the overall fertility distribition. In a three-component fit, the constrained time parameter β_i^* maximally expresses slow change in the sequence and acts in conjunction with the constrained, nearly quadratic B_j^* vector to provide a refined expression of the extent to which the age distribution of childbearing is skewed toward higher or lower ages. The $\beta_i^* B_j^*$ component of two- and three-component fits will be shown in Chapter VI to capture almost all of the association between the long-term trend for fertility decline and the change in the age pattern of childbearing. This component also includes variations in the symmetry of the distribution that are related to change in the timing of births apart from change in the level of fertility. The level-standardization procedures described in Chapter VI permit a separate examination of the timing effects.

The comparatively small amount of systematic variation left for expression in the third component $\gamma_i^* C_j^*$ is shown later in this chapter to have a demographically distinct pattern for the *X202* sequence. The pattern is either an asymmetrical contraction or asymmetrical spreading of the overall fertility distribution across the prime ages of childbearing. Such a pattern appears in Chapters VI–VIII to be associated with variations in the age pattern of entry into childbearing.

The constraints chosen for the re-presentation of EHR fits to overall fertility appear to meet all of the outlined considerations in terms of simplifying the description by fixing one of the time parameters to be as constant as possible and providing a demographically logical standard form in which to examine age and time parameters.

Marital Fertility Patterns and the Choice of Constraints

The set of constraints selected for overall fertility should also be generally appropriate for marital fertility. If marriage and menopause occurred at fixed ages and if, on the average, married women were equally likely to give birth at every age from marriage to menopause, the cumulative marital fertility distribution would be linear. Whether the probability of a birth was low or high, and thus whether the number of total births was low or high, the proportion of total legitimate births included at a given age cut would always be the same and the proportions would progress from age cut to age cut at a uniform rate.

The physiological decline of fecundity of couples with age assures the departure of the cumulative distribution from linearity at the highest ages. High incidence of any behavior that reduces exposure to the possibility of pregnancy even in the absence of conscious efforts to limit fertility—for example, decreased coital frequency with age—supplements the effects of physiological decline. Conscious use of contraceptive measures may further supplement these effects.

At the lowest ages, major influences on the degree of departure from a linear cumulative distribution include the relations between the age distribution of marriages, the age distribution of first births within marriage, and the length of interbirth intervals. When all exposure to the possibility of pregnancy occurs within marriage, the relation of first births to marriages depends on the level of fecundity of those who marry and on any behavior that delays or prevents a first birth. When exposure to the possibility of pregnancy precedes marriage for a significant proportion of women and when "pregnancy tends to drive marriage rather than the other way around," as has traditionally occurred in Sweden (Hofsten and Lundstrom, 1976), the age distribution of first births within marriage is distorted by the selection for marriage of women of proven fecundity.[6] Whatever age distribution of marriage underlies a marital fertility pattern, its effect on the pattern may be transmitted from lower to higher ages by a tendency for fertility to decline by duration of marriage as well as by age. This may occur not only when fertility is controlled at higher ages (Page, 1977) but also in the absence of deliberate limitation of births (Henry, 1979). The factors that influence the spacing of births—length of the postpartum anovulatory period, customs on breast feeding and postpartum resumption of sexual relations, contraceptive delay of a next pregnancy—provide further variation in the aggregate fertility pattern.

The departure of the cumulative marital fertility distribution from linearity is thus influenced by physiological and behavioral factors and dominated by society's customs concerning marriage and sexual intercourse. Two of the EHR-analyzed marital fertility time sequences, the MX15 and MC15 sequences for age 15–49 confinements, express the aggregate effects of all these factors. Two additional time sequences, the MX20 sequence for age 20–49 confinements and the NX15 sequence for confinements occurring 9 months or more after marriage, are only partial expressions of the consequences of these factors.

First Component $\alpha_i^* A_j^*$ For each sequence the first standard-form EHR component $\alpha_i^* A_j^*$, composed of a nearly linear A_j^* age vector multiplied by a nearly constant time parameter α_i^*, provides the underlying pattern of cumulation of births with age on which the major variations in pattern across the sequence are imposed. When de-transformed from the folded square root scale to the raw fraction scale, the $\alpha_i^* A_j^*$ component should describe any tendency for the cumulation of births to accelerate toward the median age of A_j^* and then decelerate over higher ages.

For the MX20 and NX15 sequences, the pattern expressed in the $\alpha_i^* A_j^*$ component proves (see Chapter VII) to be very close to actual marital fertility distributions considered to have a "natural" fertility pattern—the type of aggregate age distribution of births that occurs in the absence of deliberate limitation of births (Henry, 1961). Therefore, $\alpha_i^* A_j^*$ values for the MX20 and NX15 sequences are already established as demographically appropriate bases for comparisons of the major variations in marital fertility pattern across the two sequences.

The patterns expressed in the $\alpha_i^* A_j^*$ components for the MX15 and MC15 sequences are comparable standards that underlie the remaining two sequences. However, the high levels of fertility in age group 15–19, due to the high proportion of premaritally conceived births, act as high levels of fecundity. The selected constraint of making A_j^* as linear as possible then provides in the $\alpha_i^* A_j^*$ component the age pattern of fertility that would have resulted if correspondingly high levels of fecundity were sustained across the entire distribution. Therefore, $\alpha_i^* A_j^*$ values for the MX15 and MC15 sequences, unlike those for the MX20 and NX15 sequences, describe age patterns of fertility that would be expected in actual schedules only if fecundity reached maximum physiological levels at every age. For example, on the basis of actual total fertility rates, the $\bar{\alpha}_i^* A_j^*$ component for the MX15 sequence predicts (see Chapter VII) a total rate of 17.1 births per woman for women married at age 15–19, almost double the rate of 8.8 births per woman that the $\bar{\alpha}_i^* A_j^*$ component for the NX15 sequence would predict. However, the NX15 sequence includes few premarital pregnancies and probably reflects some degree of postpartum subfecundity at the lowest ages.

Second Component $\beta_i^* B_j^*$ An expression of asymmetry should be the most prominent pattern in the departure of marital fertility distributions from the pattern described by the $\alpha_i^* A_j^*$ component. The net effect of two sets of factors determines the degree of this asymmetry. The first set includes those factors that contribute positively to the proportion of births at higher ages—for example, delay between marriage and the onset of legitimate childbearing, high incidence of late marriage, and high fecundity at older ages coupled with high exposure to the possibility of pregnancy at these ages. The second set includes those factors that contribute negatively to the proportion of births at higher ages—for example, frequent selection for marriage by proven fecundity rather than sexual maturity alone, high incidence of early marriage, and limitation of births at older ages. For a population in which the total rate of marital fertility declines over time, the asymmetry expressed in the $\beta_i^* B_j^*$ component should describe a long-term trend of decrease in the proportion of total births that occurs at older ages. The $\beta_i^* B_j^*$ component should also describe variations in symmetry that are *not* expressions of an association between a decline in the level of marital fertility and a decline of fertility rates at higher ages. The amount of variation of each type can be examined separately by the level-standardization procedures described in Chapter VII.

Based on the A_j^* and B_j^* age standards for Swedish data, preliminary cross-population comparisons of marital fertility reveal a third type of systematic variation in recent schedules for some countries (see Chapter VIII). The variation is similar to that captured in the standard-form third component $\gamma_i^* C_j^*$ described for overall fertility—an asymmetrical contraction of the distribution within the 15–30 age range, suggesting the delay and spacing of births at lower ages within marriage. Three-component fits should therefore receive high priority in further EHR analysis of marital fertility.

Functions of the Standard-form Components

With A_j^*, B_j^*, and C_j^* as age standards in the re-presented descriptions

$$\hat{F}_{ij} = \alpha_i^* A_j^* + \beta_i^* B_j^* \qquad \text{or} \qquad \hat{F}_{ij} = \alpha_i^* A_j^* + \beta_i^* B_j^* + \gamma_i^* C_j^*$$

for each fertility time sequence, and α_i^*, β_i^*, and γ_i^* varying from cohort to cohort or year to year we ask, How does a change in α_i^*, β_i^*, or γ_i^* affect the age distribution of fertility in each sequence? The answers establish that the function of each component in describing actual fertility time sequences is that intended when we chose our particular standard-form re-presentation.

Functions of Two Components for Overall Fertility

Five-year-age-group Sequences   For the 155-cohort C15 sequence and the 185-year, cross-sectional X15 sequence, the extreme values of each component are shown in Table 5.4. The $\alpha_i^* A_j^*$ component represents (on the folded square root scale) an underlying pattern of cumulation of births by age. It is centered on zero at the median age of childbearing (32.7 years for both sequences) that would occur if no $\beta_i^* B_j^*$ component were added. The more negative the value of $\alpha_i^* A_j^*$ for an age cut below the median age, the smaller the proportion of total births that is included at that age cut. The more positive the value of $\alpha_i^* A_j^*$ for an age cut above the median age, the higher the proportion of total births that is included at that age cut. For both sequences $\alpha_i^* A_j^*$ has a narrow range, as intended, but the range for the C15 sequence is slightly the wider.

The addition of the $\beta_i^* B_j^*$ component makes a nonlinear alteration in the cumulative fertility distribution as expressed by $\alpha_i^* A_j^*$. The result is a change in the shape and median age of the distribution. A positive value of β_i^* lowers the median age and a negative value raises it. This effect can be tested by taking the median value of $\alpha_i^* A_j^*$ at each age cut for the X15 sequence and adding to it the lowest or highest value of $\beta_i^* B_j^*$ at the age cut. The median age would then vary from 33 years when β_i^* is most negative to 27 years when β_i^* has its highest positive value. The slightly higher and wider range of $\beta_i^* B_j^*$ for the X15 sequence than for the C15 sequence is not unexpected because the X15 sequence includes the partial childbearing experience of 30 additional cohorts that contribute to a progressively younger cross-sectional age pattern of childbearing.

The effect of a small change in α_i^* or β_i^* can be seen by:

1. constructing a series of fertility distributions based on corresponding pairs of A_j^* and B_j^* vectors and uniform increments in the time parameters α_i^* and β_i^*;
2. de-transforming the distributions from the folded square root scale to the raw fraction scale;
3. expressing the distributions in noncumulated form (Table 5.5).

As shown in Table 5.5, a positive change in α_i^* increases the proportion of total fertility in the central age groups at the expense of the two lowest and two highest age groups. In particular, such a change emphasizes age group 30–34. However, any shift in fertility toward or away from the central ages is limited by the narrow range of α_i^*. In fact, the full range of α_i^* for the X15 sequence is shown in Table 5.5. In contrast, a positive change in β_i^* (Table 5.5) decreases the proportion of total fertility in the four highest age groups, particularly in groups 35–39 and 40–44, and increases the proportion in the three lowest age groups, with the most emphasis on age group 20–24. This is precisely the demographically interpretable function that was expected for this second component of the fitted descriptions.[7]

Pronounced similarity for the C15 and X15 sequences is illustrated in the raw scale fertility distributions defined by given levels of α_i^* and β_i^* (compare the $f_i(a_j)$ values in Table 5.5 for the two sequences). The similarity is also shown by the magnitude and direction of change in the distributions when each component is varied in even increments while the other is held constant. This means that change in these two sequences over time can reasonably be compared in Chapter VI using the EHR time parameters. The comparability of the C20 and X20 time parameters can be established in the same way from appropriate pairs of A_j^* and B_j^* age vectors (Table 5.2) and even increments in the values of α_i^* and β_i^*.

Single-year-of-age Sequence The differences among a series of fertility distributions based on the A_j^* and B_j^* vectors and uniform increments in the time parameters α_i^* and β_i^* for the SYAC13 sequence add valuable detail to the 5-year-age-group information, including which ages are positively or negatively affected by a change in α_i^* or β_i^*. A positive change in α_i^* is shown (Table 5.6) to increase the proportion of total fertility occurring at ages 23–39 at the expense of the higher and lower ages. However, any shift in fertility toward or away from the central ages is again limited by the narrow range of α_i^*, 4.16–4.33 (Table 5.3a).[8] A positive change in β_i^*

TABLE 5.4

Range of Values by Age Cut for Components $\alpha_i^* A_j^*$ and $\beta_i^* B_j^*$ of the Fitted Descriptions of the C15 and X15 Sequences, Folded Square Root Scale

| | Time parameter | | | Age cut | | | | | |
Rank	α_i^*	β_i^*	Component	19/20	24/25	29/30	34/35	39/40	44/45
C15 Sequence									
Lowest	1.396	—	$\alpha_i^* A_j^*$	-.8325	-.5424	-.1866	.1699	.5079	.7994
Median	1.480	—		-.8830	-.5753	-.1979	.1802	.5387	.8479
Highest	1.544	—		-.9209	-.6000	-.2064	.1879	.5618	.8843
Lowest	—	-.0624	$\beta_i^* B_j^*$	-.0126	-.0298	-.0350	-.0313	-.0233	-.0100
Highest	—	.6327		.1282	.3019	.3545	.3177	.2362	.1018
X15 Sequence									
Lowest	1.420	—	$\alpha_i^* A_j^*$	-.8543	-.5559	-.1953	.1661	.5112	.8066
Median	1.477	—		-.8886	-.5782	-.2031	.1728	.5317	.8389
Highest	1.518	—		-.9132	-.5943	-.2087	.1776	.5465	.8622
Lowest	—	-.0386	$\beta_i^* B_j^*$	-.0111	-.0196	-.0213	-.0184	-.0127	-.0056
Highest	—	.8427		.2419	.4276	.4656	.4006	.2773	.1212

TABLE 5.5

Noncumulated Fertility Distributions $f_i(a_j)$ (Raw Fraction Scale) Constructed from the Age Parameters A_j^* and B_j^* for Double Multiplicative Fits to the C15 and X15 Sequences: Effect of Increments in the Time Parameters α_i^* and β_i^*

Age group	Change in $f_i(a_j)$ $\alpha_i^* = 1.47$ $\Delta\beta_i^* = +.10$	$f_i(a_j)$					Change in $f_i(a_j)$ $\Delta\alpha_i^* = +.10$ $\beta_i^* = .05$
		$\alpha_i^* = 1.47$ $\beta_i^* = .00$	$\alpha_i^* = 1.47$ $\beta_i^* = .10$	$\alpha_i^* = 1.47$ $\beta_i^* = .05$	$\alpha_i^* = 1.42$ $\beta_i^* = .05$	$\alpha_i^* = 1.52$ $\beta_i^* = .05$	
C15 Sequence							
15–19	.0046	.0135	.0181	.0157	.0230	.0097	−.0133
20–24	.0211	.1169	.1380	.1274	.1307	.1231	−.0076
25–29	.0131	.2319	.2450	.2386	.2327	.2443	.0116
30–34	−.0043	.2631	.2588	.2611	.2523	.2699	.0176
35–39	−.0145	.2247	.2102	.2175	.2118	.2229	.0111
40–44	−.0159	.1282	.1123	.1202	.1224	.1170	−.0054
45–49	−.0039	.0216	.0177	.0196	.0272	.0132	−.0140
X15 Sequence							
15–19	.0063	.0120	.0183	.0150	.0222	.0091	−.0131
20–24	.0209	.1163	.1372	.1267	.1301	.1222	−.0079
25–29	.0110	.2303	.2413	.2359	.2301	.2415	.0114
30–34	−.0055	.2622	.2567	.2596	.2508	.2683	.0175
35–39	−.0150	.2263	.2113	.2188	.2131	.2244	.0113
40–44	−.0140	.1295	.1155	.1224	.1244	.1196	−.0048
45–49	−.0037	.0235	.0198	.0216	.0294	.0149	−.0145

TABLE 5.6

Noncumulated Fertility Distributions $f_i(a_j)$ (Raw Fraction Scale) Constructed from the Age Parameters A_j^* and B_j^* for Double Multiplicative Fits to the SYAC13 Sequence: Effect of Increments in the Time Parameters α_i^* and β_i^*

Age	Change in $f_i(a_j)$ $\alpha_i^* = 4.25$ $\Delta\beta_i^* = +.10$	$f_i(a_j)$ $\alpha_i^* = 4.25$ $\beta_i^* = .00$	$\alpha_i^* = 4.25$ $\beta_i^* = .10$	$\alpha_i^* = 4.25$ $\beta_i^* = .05$	$\alpha_i^* = 4.20$ $\beta_i^* = .05$	$\alpha_i^* = 4.30$ $\beta_i^* = .05$	Change in $f_i(a_j)$ $\Delta\alpha_i^* = +.10$ $\beta_i^* = .05$
13	.00000	.00002	.00002	.00002	.00024	.00006	−.00018
14	.00001	.00002	.00003	.00003	.00008	−.00003	−.00011
15	.00002	.00017	.00020	.00019	.00037	−.00001	−.00039
16	.00012	.00058	.00069	.00063	.00093	.00032	−.00061
17	.00035	.00204	.00239	.00221	.00271	.00168	−.00103
18	.00075	.00508	.00582	.00544	.00606	.00479	−.00127
19	.00121	.01025	.01146	.01085	.01148	.01017	−.00131
20	.00159	.01683	.01842	.01762	.01816	.01705	−.00110
21	.00189	.02375	.02564	.02469	.02505	.02430	−.00075
22	.00203	.03088	.03291	.03189	.03206	.03170	−.00036
23	.00206	.03717	.03923	.03820	.03818	.03820	.00002
24	.00200	.04213	.04414	.04314	.04295	.04331	.00036
25	.00177	.04651	.04828	.04740	.04707	.04772	.00065
26	.00151	.04973	.05124	.05049	.05005	.05093	.00088

27	.00118	.05184	.05301	.05243	.05190	.05295	.00104
28	.00085	.05339	.05424	.05382	.05324	.05440	.00117
29	.00055	.05356	.05411	.05384	.05323	.05445	.00122
30	.00018	.05386	.05404	.05396	.05333	.05459	.00126
31	−.00012	.05318	.05306	.05313	.05250	.05375	.00125
32	−.00050	.05279	.05230	.05255	.05194	.05316	.00122
33	−.00081	.05139	.05059	.05099	.05042	.05157	.00116
34	−.00111	.04987	.04876	.04932	.04878	.04985	.00106
35	−.00132	.04732	.04600	.04666	.04620	.04713	.00093
36	−.00154	.04504	.04350	.04427	.04388	.04466	.00078
37	−.00171	.04207	.04036	.04122	.04092	.04151	.00059
38	−.00176	.03831	.03655	.03743	.03724	.03761	.00037
39	−.00175	.03431	.03256	.03344	.03337	.03349	.00013
40	−.00166	.02948	.02783	.02865	.02871	.02857	−.00014
41	−.00158	.02477	.02320	.02398	.02418	.02376	−.00042
42	−.00135	.01937	.01802	.01869	.01902	.01834	−.00068
43	−.00111	.01431	.01319	.01375	.01418	.01328	−.00090
44	−.00074	.00915	.00841	.00878	.00925	.00827	−.00098
45	−.00051	.00570	.00519	.00544	.00594	.00492	−.00102
46	−.00027	.00292	.00265	.00279	.00322	.00233	−.00089
47	−.00013	.00136	.00123	.00130	.00164	.00093	−.00071
48	−.00005	.00051	.00046	.00048	.00071	.00025	−.00046
49	−.00002	.00022	.00020	.00021	.00039	.00003	−.00036
50	−.00001	.00009	.00008	.00009	.00043	.00001	−.00043

decreases the proportion of total fertility occurring at ages 31–50 and increases the proportion occurring at ages 16–30. In particular, ages 20–26 are favored at the expense of ages 35–42. These effects of incremental change in α_i^* and β_i^* will also be shown graphically in Fig. 6.2. The wide range of β_i^*, .04–1.39 (Table 5.3a), coupled with the results from the even increments of change in β_i^*, confirms again that major differences between fertility distributions are encompassed in the $\beta_i^* B_j^*$ component. Thus the single-year-of-age effects of time-parameter change, although crossing the conventional 5-year-age-group bounds to some extent, demonstrate that the standard form of the parameters based on 5-year age groups (Table 5.5) well represents the nature of the major changes in cohort fertility patterns.

Functions of Three Components for Overall Fertility

As we examine the selected standard form for the three-component fits to the cross-sectional fertility sequence X202, we ask two questions. First, how much have the functions of the first two components $\alpha_i^* A_j^*$ and $\beta_i^* B_j^*$ been changed by fitting a third component and including it in the re-presentation process? Second, what is the function of the third component $\gamma_i^* C_j^*$ in describing change in fertility distributions?

The $\alpha_i^* A_j^*$ component for the X202 sequence (Table 5.7) is centered on a median age of 32.2 years, which is .5 years lower than that for the X15 sequence. This reflects the inclusion in the X202 fitting process of 17 additional recent years with younger childbearing patterns. The extreme values that $\alpha_i^* A_j^*$ assumes for the X202 sequence are slightly lower than those for the X15 sequence (Table 5.4). The extreme values of the $\beta_i^* B_j^*$ component for the X202 sequence cover a wider range than do those for the X15 sequence. However, the effects of uniform increments in α_i^* and β_i^* on change in the fertility distribution for the X202 and X15 sequences are identical in direction and very similar in magnitude (compare Tables 5.8a and 5.5).

Whereas a positive increment in α_i^* concentrates the distribution toward the central age group 30–34 and a positive increment in β_i^* shifts the distribution away from age groups 40–44 and 35–39 and toward age group 20–24, an increment in γ_i^* modifies the fitted description in another demographically important way that should be considered for both $+\Delta\gamma_i^*$ and $-\Delta\gamma_i^*$. A positive increment in γ_i^* shifts the distribution toward age group 25–29 at the greater expense of age group 20–24 and the lesser expense of age groups 35–39 and 40–44 (Table 5.8b). The positive increment thus has

TABLE 5.7

Range of Values by Age Cut for Components $\alpha_i^* A_j^*$, $\beta_i^* B_j^*$, and $\gamma_i^* C_j^*$ of the Fitted Description of the $X202$ Sequence, Folded Square Root Scale

Time parameter		Component	Age cut					
			19/20	24/25	29/30	34/35	39/40	44/45
α_i^*		$\alpha_i^* A_j^*$						
Lowest	1.374		−.7998	−.4714	−.1471	.1825	.5229	.8348
Median	1.443		−.8401	−.4952	−.1545	.1917	.5493	.8769
Highest	1.501		−.8736	−.5149	−.1606	.1993	.5712	.9118
β_i^*		$\beta_i^* B_j^*$						
Lowest	−.1240		−.0346	−.0609	−.0700	−.0608	−.0405	−.0151
Highest	.9311		.2596	.4575	.5259	.4567	.3039	.1133
γ_i^*		$\gamma_i^* C_j^*$						
Lowest	.0213		−.0097	−.0146	−.0005	.0081	.0043	−.0079
Highest	.1294		−.0590	−.0886	−.0031	.0489	.0264	−.0481

a distinctive contracting influence. If we reverse the signs of the change in $f_i(a_j)$ for $\Delta\gamma_i^*$ in Table 5.8b, we see that a negative change in γ_i^* results in an asymmetrical spreading of the fertility distribution. The shift is most strong from age group 25–29 into age group 20–24, but it also positively affects age groups 35–39 and 40–44. Although the arithmetic effect of a given decrement in γ_i^* would be similar at any level of β_i^* (see Note 5), the demographic significance of such a change would strongly depend on the level of β_i^*. When β_i^* is low enough that the median age of childbearing remains within or higher than age group 25–29, a decrement in γ_i^* has an evening effect on the distribution. When β_i^* is sufficiently high that the median age of childbearing falls within age group 20–24, a decrement in γ_i^* further emphasizes age group 20–24, diminishes the importance of age group 25–29, and further decreases the importance of age group 30–34.

Although γ_i^* for the $X202$ sequence passes through small decrements and increments, it always remains positive in value. The possibility of a negative value for γ_i^* occurs when some of the Coale–Trussell (1974) model fertility schedules by 5-year age groups are expressed as weighted sums of the $X202$ age standards (see Table 8.1). A negative value of γ_i^* is associated with model schedules that incorporate a rapid pace of entry into marriage at an early age. The highest positive values of γ_i^* are associated with model schedules that incorporate a slow pace of entry into marriage.

The addition of the third component $\gamma_i^* C_j^*$ does not change the interpretation of the components in a two-component EHR model. Also, this

TABLE 5.8a

Noncumulated Fertility Distributions $f_i(a_j)$ (Raw Fraction Scale) Constructed from the Age Parameters A_j^*, B_j^*, and C_j^* for Triple Multiplicative Fits to the X202 Sequence: Effect of Increments in the Time Parameters α_i^* and β_i^*

Age group	Change in $f_i(a_j)$ $\alpha_i^*=1.44$ $\Delta\beta_i^*=+.10$ $\gamma_i^*=.05$	$f_i(a_j)$ $\alpha_i^*=1.44$ $\beta_i^*=.00$ $\gamma_i^*=.05$	$\alpha_i^*=1.44$ $\beta_i^*=.10$ $\gamma_i^*=.05$	$\alpha_i^*=1.44$ $\beta_i^*=.05$ $\gamma_i^*=.05$	$\alpha_i^*=1.39$ $\beta_i^*=.05$ $\gamma_i^*=.05$	$\alpha_i^*=1.49$ $\beta_i^*=.05$ $\gamma_i^*=.05$	Change in $f_i(a_j)$ $\Delta\alpha_i^*=+.10$ $\beta_i^*=.05$ $\gamma_i^*=.05$
15–19	.0069	.0170	.0239	.0203	.0281	.0136	−.0145
20–24	.0208	.1364	.1572	.1468	.1488	.1439	−.0049
25–29	.0117	.2374	.2491	.2434	.2374	.2493	.0119
30–34	−.0062	.2561	.2499	.2532	.2449	.2614	.0165
35–39	−.0163	.2158	.1995	.2076	.2021	.2129	.0108
40–44	−.0141	.1192	.1051	.1121	.1145	.1086	−.0059
45–49	−.0028	.0181	.0153	.0167	.0242	.0104	−.0138

TABLE 5.8b

Noncumulated Fertility Distributions $f_i(a_j)$ (Raw Fraction Scale) Constructed from the Age Parameters A_j^*, B_j^*, and C_j^* for Triple Multiplicative Fits to the *X202* Sequence: Effect of Increments in the Time Parameter γ_i^*

Age group	$f_i(a_j)$			Change in $f_i(a_j)$
	$\alpha_i^* = 1.44$ $\beta_i^* = .05$ $\gamma_i^* = .05$	$\alpha_i^* = 1.44$ $\beta_i^* = .05$ $\gamma_i^* = .00$	$\alpha_i^* = 1.44$ $\beta_i^* = .05$ $\gamma_i^* = .10$	$\alpha_i^* = 1.44$ $\beta_i^* = .05$ $\Delta\gamma_i^* = +.10$
15–19	.0203	.0263	.0150	−.0113
20–24	.1468	.1605	.1332	−.0273
25–29	.2434	.2245	.2615	.0370
30–34	.2532	.2395	.2668	.0273
35–39	.2076	.2152	.2001	−.0151
40–44	.1121	.1214	.1023	−.0191
45–49	.0167	.0127	.0212	.0085

addition has only slight impact on the effect of increments in the $\alpha_i^* A_j^*$ and $\beta_i^* B_j^*$ components. However, the third component does reflect additional aspects of fertility behavior not considered in the two-component model. Thus the insight gained from the two-component model can be retained in the assessment of the three-component model, increasing the sophistication of the understanding of fertility change. Preliminary cross-population fits (see Chapter VIII) suggest that the type of asymmetrical change or difference captured by the $\gamma_i^* C_j^*$ component is particularly important to the complete description of fertility patterns for several countries, for example, Japan, Korea, Taiwan, and the Netherlands, and, to a lesser extent, also enters into the recent fertility patterns for a number of other countries.

Functions of Two Components for Marital Fertility

For the special cases of the related marital fertility sequences MX15, MX20, NX15, and MC15, we expect similarities in the function of each standard-form component $\alpha_i^* A_j^*$ or $\beta_i^* B_j^*$. We also expect differences determined by the particular section of marital childbearing experience included in each sequence. For example, both the MX15 and MX20 sequences are influenced by premarital pregnancy but to different degrees.[9] Most major aspects of the change in fertility over time are similarly detected in the α_i^* and β_i^* time parameters for the full age 15–49 marital fertility experience or the age 20–49 experience alone. However, some

TABLE 5.9

Range of Values by Age Cut for Components $\alpha_i^* A_j^*$ and $\beta_i^* B_j^*$ of the Fitted Descriptions of the MX15, MX20, MC15, and NX15 Sequences, Folded Square Root Scale

	Time parameter			*Age cut*					
Rank	α_i^*	β_i^*	*Component*	19/20	24/25	29/30	34/35	39/40	44/45
MX15 Sequence									
Lowest	1.193	—	$\alpha_i^* A_j^*$	−.5745	−.2670	−.0069	.2497	.5330	.8217
Median	1.226	—		−.5904	−.2774	−.0071	.2566	.5478	.8445
Highest	1.284	—		−.6184	−.2874	−.0074	.2687	.5737	.8844
Lowest	—	.473	$\beta_i^* B_j^*$	.2391	.2431	.2265	.1912	.1304	.0508
Highest	—	1.144		.5784	.5880	.5477	.4624	.3154	.1230
MX20 Sequence									
Lowest	1.080	—	$\alpha_i^* A_j^*$	—	−.3702	−.0591	.2270	.5301	.8328
Median	1.106	—		—	−.3791	−.0605	.2325	.5428	.8528
Highest	1.138	—		—	−.3901	−.0622	.2392	.5585	.8775
Lowest	—	.204	$\beta_i^* B_j^*$	—	.0922	.1147	.1112	.0818	.0301
Highest	—	.711		—	.3214	.3997	.3876	.2850	.1048
MC15 Sequence									
Lowest	1.333	—	$\alpha_i^* A_j^*$	−.6038	−.2189	.1192	.3992	.6503	.8757
Median	1.363	—		−.6174	−.2238	.1219	.4082	.6649	.8954
Highest	1.398	—		−.6336	−.2296	.1251	.4189	.6823	.9188
Lowest	—	.4510	$\beta_i^* B_j^*$	.2742	.2478	.1907	.1427	.0943	.0343
Highest	—	.9499		.5775	.5220	.4017	.3006	.1985	.0723
NX15 Sequence									
Lowest	1.220	—	$\alpha_i^* A_j^*$	−.4809	−.1677	.0869	.3471	.6090	.8551
Median	1.257	—		−.4952	−.1727	.0895	.3574	.6272	.8806
Highest	1.316	—		−.5187	−.1809	.0937	.3744	.6569	.9224
Lowest	—	.133	$\beta_i^* B_j^*$	.0331	.0543	.0731	.0722	.0531	.0197
Highest	—	.565		.1400	.2298	.3094	.3056	.2248	.0834

aspects of change are missed when age group 15–19 is omitted from the analysis (see Chapter VII).

The extreme values of $\alpha_i^* A_j^*$ and $\beta_i^* B_j^*$ for the marital fertility sequences can be examined in Table 5.9. In each case the $\alpha_i^* A_j^*$ vector has a very narrow range, as intended. Representing the underlying pattern of the cumulation of births with age expressed on the folded square root scale, $\alpha_i^* A_j^*$ is centered on zero at the median age that the fertility distribution would have if no $\beta_i^* B_j^*$ component were added. For the four marital sequences, the differences in median age of the distributions, expressed by (median α_i^*)A_j^* alone and with (lowest β_i^*)B_j^* or (highest

TABLE 5.10

Median Age of the Cumulated Marital Fertility Schedule Implied by (Median α_i^*)A_j^* Alone and with (Lowest β_i^*)B_j^* or (Highest β_i^*)B_j^* Added (Based on Component Values in Table 5.9)

| | | Median age | |
| | | (median α_i^*)A_j^* + (lowest β_i^*)B_j^* | (median α_i^*)A_j^* + (highest β_i^*)B_j^* |
Sequence	(median α_i^*)A_j^*		
MX15	30.2	25.4 $(-4.8)^a$	20.2 $(-5.2)^b$
MC15	28.3	24.7 (-3.6)	20.5 (-4.2)
NX15	28.3	27.0 (-1.3)	24.4 (-2.6)
MX20	31.0	29.4 (-1.6)	25.8 (-3.6)

[a] Values in parentheses are the change in median age caused by adding (lowest β_i^*)B_j^* to (median α_i^*)A_j^*.
[b] Values in parentheses are the change in median age caused by increasing β_i^* from its lowest to its highest value.

β_i^*)β_j^* added (Table 5.10), provide evidence of the prominent role of the $\beta_i^*B_j^*$ component in the description of the two sequences most influenced by premarital pregnancy—MX15 and MC15. The $\beta_i^*B_j^*$ component is much less prominent in the description of the MX20 sequence, which is less influenced by premarital pregnancy, and the NX15 sequence, in which any influence is registered as postpartum subfecundity.

By constructing for each sequence a series of fertility distributions based on uniform increments in the time parameters α_i^* and β_i^*, we can see how each age group is affected by a small change in α_i^* or β_i^* (see Table 5.11). In all four cases a positive change in α_i^* increases the proportion of fertility in the second and later age groups through 35–39 at the expense of the first age group in particular (which is either 15–19 or 20–24 for a given sequence) and also of age groups 40–44 and 45–49. The second and third age groups are emphasized almost equally by a positive change in α_i^* (Table 5.11)—in contrast to the overall fertility descriptions in which age group 30–34 is the focus of positive change in α_i^* for both age 15–49 sequences (Table 5.5) and age 20–49 sequences (Table 5.12). Any contraction of a marital fertility distribution toward the second and third age groups or any spreading away from these age groups is still limited, however, by the narrow range of α_i^*—approximately the range shown in Table 5.11 for the MX15 and NX15 sequences and still less for the MC15 and MX20 sequences (see Table 5.9).

A positive change in β_i^* (see Table 5.11) decreases the proportion of total fertility in the higher age groups and increases the proportion in the lower age groups—the demographically interpretable function expected for the second component. For the NX15 sequence, which includes few

TABLE 5.11

Noncumulated Fertility Distributions $f_i(a_j)$ (Raw Fraction Scale) Constructed from the Age Parameters A_j^* and B_j^* for Double Multiplicative Fits to the MX15, MX20, MC15, and NX15 Sequences: Effect of Increments in the Time Parameters α_i^* and β_i^*

Age group	Change in $f_i(a_j)$	$f_i(a_j)$					Change in $f_i(a_j)$
	$\alpha_i^* = 1.23$ $\Delta\beta_i^* = +.10$	$\alpha_i^* = 1.23$ $\beta_i^* = .50$	$\alpha_i^* = 1.23$ $\beta_i^* = .60$	$\alpha_i^* = 1.23$ $\beta_i^* = .55$	$\alpha_i^* = 1.18$ $\beta_i^* = .55$	$\alpha_i^* = 1.28$ $\beta_i^* = .55$	$\Delta\alpha_i^* = +.10$ $\beta_i^* = .55$
MX15 Sequence							
15–19	.0331	.2669	.3000	.2833	.2992	.2677	−.0315
20–24	.0033	.2202	.2235	.2219	.2140	.2297	.0157
25–29	−.0041	.1749	.1708	.1729	.1652	.1806	.0154
30–34	−.0088	.1453	.1365	.1410	.1347	.1472	.0125
35–39	−.0120	.1175	.1055	.1115	.1081	.1145	.0064
40–44	−.0097	.0663	.0566	.0614	.0643	.0571	−.0072
45–49	−.0017	.0089	.0072	.0080	.0146	.0033	−.0113
	$\alpha_i^* = 1.10$ $\Delta\beta_i^* = +.10$	$\alpha_i^* = 1.10$ $\beta_i^* = .20$	$\alpha_i^* = 1.10$ $\beta_i^* = .30$	$\alpha_i^* = 1.10$ $\beta_i^* = .25$	$\alpha_i^* = 1.05$ $\beta_i^* = .25$	$\alpha_i^* = 1.15$ $\beta_i^* = .25$	$\Delta\alpha_i^* = +.10$ $\beta_i^* = .25$
MX20 Sequence							
20–24	.0303	.3015	.3318	.3166	.3281	.3051	−.0230
25–29	.0093	.2354	.2447	.2402	.2306	.2497	.0191
30–34	−.0050	.1966	.1916	.1942	.1856	.2027	.0171
35–39	−.0157	.1605	.1448	.1527	.1476	.1573	.0097
40–44	−.0159	.0926	.0767	.0845	.0876	.0797	−.0079
45–49	−.0029	.0134	.0105	.0119	.0205	.0054	−.0151

MC15 Sequence

	$\alpha_i^* = 1.35$ $\Delta\beta_i^* = +.10$	$\alpha_i^* = 1.35$ $\beta_i^* = .50$	$\alpha_i^* = 1.35$ $\beta_i^* = .60$	$\alpha_i^* = 1.35$ $\beta_i^* = .55$	$\alpha_i^* = 1.30$ $\beta_i^* = .55$	$\alpha_i^* = 1.40$ $\beta_i^* = .55$	$\Delta\alpha_i^* = +.10$ $\beta_i^* = .55$
15–19	.0405	.2876	.3281	.3077	.3229	.2927	–.0302
20–24	–.0018	.2499	.2481	.2491	.2398	.2584	.0186
25–29	–.0116	.1908	.1792	.1851	.1764	.1937	.0173
30–34	–.0107	.1367	.1260	.1313	.1264	.1361	.0097
35–39	–.0092	.0893	.0801	.0847	.0839	.0850	.0011
40–44	–.0061	.0404	.0343	.0373	.0409	.0327	–.0082
45–49	–.0010	.0052	.0042	.0047	.0098	.0014	–.0084

NX15 Sequence

	$\alpha_i^* = 1.26$ $\Delta\beta_i^* = +.10$	$\alpha_i^* = 1.26$ $\beta_i^* = .15$	$\alpha_i^* = 1.26$ $\beta_i^* = .25$	$\alpha_i^* = 1.26$ $\beta_i^* = .20$	$\alpha_i^* = 1.21$ $\beta_i^* = .20$	$\alpha_i^* = 1.31$ $\beta_i^* = .20$	$\Delta\alpha_i^* = +.10$ $\beta_i^* = .20$
15–19	.0148	.1928	.2076	.2002	.2120	.1885	–.0235
20–24	.0138	.2282	.2420	.2351	.2281	.2419	.0138
25–29	.0090	.1997	.2087	.2043	.1970	.2115	.0145
30–34	–.0059	.1747	.1688	.1719	.1660	.1777	.0117
35–39	–.0155	.1299	.1144	.1221	.1200	.1237	.0037
40–44	–.0139	.0665	.0526	.0594	.0635	.0540	–.0095
45–49	–.0023	.0083	.0060	.0071	.0134	.0026	–.0108

TABLE 5.12

Noncumulated Fertility Distributions $f_i(a_j)$ (Raw Fraction Scale) Constructed from the Age Parameters A_j^* and B_j^* for Double Multiplicative Fits to the XX20 Sequence: Effect of Increments in the Time Parameters α_i^* and β_i^*

Age group	Change in $f_i(a_j)$ $\alpha_i^* = 1.20$ $\Delta\beta_i^* = +.10$	$f_i(a_j)$ $\alpha_i^* = 1.20$ $\beta_i^* = .15$	$\alpha_i^* = 1.20$ $\beta_i^* = .25$	$\alpha_i^* = 1.20$ $\beta_i^* = .20$	$\alpha_i^* = 1.15$ $\beta_i^* = .20$	$\alpha_i^* = 1.25$ $\beta_i^* = .20$	Change in $f_i(a_j)$ $\Delta\alpha_i^* = +.10$ $\beta_i^* = .20$
20–24	.0248	.1357	.1605	.1479	.1624	.1339	-.0285
25–29	.0152	.2392	.2544	.2469	.2401	.2533	.0132
30–34	-.0032	.2575	.2543	.2561	.2453	.2668	.0215
35–39	-.0168	.2248	.2080	.2165	.2087	.2240	.0153
40–44	-.0171	.1278	.1107	.1191	.1218	.1150	-.0068
45–49	-.0029	.0150	.0121	.0135	.0217	.0071	-.0146

premarital pregnancies, a positive change in β_i^* emphasizes age groups 15–19 and 20–24 almost equally, mainly at the expense of age groups 35–39 and 40–44. For the MX15, MC15, and MX20 sequences, there is a particularly strong positive effect on the lowest age group (which is either 15–19 or 20–24 for a given sequence), but the two or three higher age groups affected most negatively differ by sequence. The $\beta_i^* B_j^*$ components for the relatively short cohort marital fertility sequence MC15 and the cross-sectional sequence MX15 (of which the MC15 sequence is a diagonal cut) are less similar than are the $\beta_i^* B_j^*$ components for the much longer cohort (C15) and cross-sectional (X15) overall fertility sequences examined previously. This is not surprising because the completed cohort experience from which the MC15 age standards are derived includes mainly the cohorts that carried out the major fertility transition of the twentieth century (see Chapter VI), whereas the MX15 parameters are influenced by the partial childbearing experience of earlier and later cohorts.

Similarities in the effect of a change in β_i^* should be particularly noted for two pairs of sequences: the NX15 and MX20 sequences for age groups 25–29 and higher (Table 5.11) and the MX20 and XX20 sequences (Tables 5.11 and 5.12) for age groups 30–34 and higher. In Chapter VII we shall take advantage of both the similarities and differences in the EHR descriptions of these related marital fertility sequences to interpret change in marital fertility patterns across time and examine this change in relation to change in overall fertility patterns.

Summary

This chapter applies a very useful concept for modeling: the empirically best-fitting model need not be, and often should not be, the form in which the fitted parameters are examined and interpreted. The opportunity for re-presentation of fits in other forms is inherent in the fact that a fitted description is just one of many algebraically equivalent combinations of the parameters. The need to select carefully a standard form for the parameters comes from our desire to compare the parameters for one sequence with those for other sequences, to simplify the descriptions if possible, and to interpret the parameters for all sequences in demographically understandable terms. In the search for useful standard forms of the EHR fits that express a fertility time sequence in two or three age parameters and their year- or cohort-specific multipliers (the time parameters), this chapter makes several contributions.

1. It illustrates how knowledge of demographic processes that underlie variations in the age pattern of fertility can be used to guide the re-presentation of fit for both overall and marital fertility.
2. It outlines simple procedures for obtaining some commonly useful forms of the fitted description.
3. It identifies sets of overall and marital fertility age standards that become the bases not only of the time-sequence comparisons for the entire population (see Chapters VI and VII) but also of subpopulation comparisons with the entire population (see Chapter VI) and preliminary cross-population comparisons (see Chapter VIII).

To confirm that the function of each standard-form age parameter and its time-parameter multiplier is the demographically descriptive one intended, we have answered two questions for each set of age standards. What effect does an increment in one time parameter have on the fertility pattern when the other time parameter(s) are held constant? Which age groups are positively affected and which are negatively affected and by how much?

The standard forms of the fits carried forward to Chapters VI–VIII for twelve overall and marital fertility sequences viewed in either cross-sectional or cohort perspective consist of two or three components.

1. The description of each fertility sequence has been simplified in the first component, which expresses a nearly constant underlying pattern of the cumulation of births with age. Major variations in pattern associated with changes in the level of fertility and changes in the timing of childbearing apart from level are described in the other components.
2. The major long-term trend of change, the achievement of a higher proportion of total fertility below age 30, is concentrated in the second component. The portion of this component associated with change in the timing of childbearing apart from the level of fertility will be shown in Chapter VI to be a separable subcomponent when total fertility rate is retained as a separate dimension of the data.
3. The third component, when fitted, expresses some nuances of the change in pattern across ages 20–34—a greater or lesser concentration of childbearing in a narrower age range centered on age group 25–29. This component will be shown in Chapters VI and VIII to have increasing importance in the description of fertility patterns for recent years, not only for Sweden and some other low-fertility European countries, but for some Asian countries as well.

Notes for Chapter V

1. The general case includes variation at either end cut in relation to the other, but in a fertility distribution cumulated to age 45–49 the variation at the last age cut is always small.

2. A linear relation of time parameters is retained in some fertility models, such as the Coale (1971) model of marital fertility (see Fig. 7.2) and the Page (1977) model of fertility by duration of marriage, but it can make interpretation more difficult (see Trussell, 1979, pp. 47–48, and Chapter VII).

3. The "strength" of a constraint may be considered as its relative immunity to sampling–measurement fluctuations as transmitted by the fitting process. It is possible that a different set of constraints with as great or greater overall strength could be chosen. Alternative constraints include fixing one vector exactly instead of as close as possible to linearity, making one vector orthogonal to a fixed vector instead of fixing two vectors, and formal orthogonality with $A_j^{**} \perp B_j^{**}$ and $\alpha_i^{**} \perp \beta_i^{**}$. There is some reason, however, to expect that the demographic interpretation of parameters would be more difficult in many of these cases. Detailed consideration of alternative standard-form re-presentations in the two-way case can be found in Tukey (1976).

4. The very different range of age or time parameter values for a sequence analyzed in 5-year age groups and the corresponding parameter values for a single-year-of-age sequence may seem puzzling. However, there is a simple explanation. The fitting procedure includes this constraint for standardization (see Chapter III):

$$\sum A_j^{*2} = \sum B_j^{*2} = 1.$$

Each age vector has 6 members for a 5-year-age-group sequence and 37 members for a single-year-of-age sequence. Therefore, a 6-member A_j^* vector is equivalent to a 37-member A_j^* vector multiplied by $\sqrt{37/6}$; the same relation holds for the B_j^* vector. To maintain the value of the $\alpha_i^* A_j^*$ component, the α_i^* multiplier of a 37-member A_j^* vector would be divided by $\sqrt{37/6}$ for comparison with the α_i^* multiplier of a 6-member A_j^* vector. The same conversion would be applied to the β_i^* vector. Because the SYAC13 sequence begins with a rate of zero at age 13, however, we should expect the converted value of the nearly constant α_i^* to be slightly higher than that for the same time sequence analyzed by 5-year age groups, with a nonzero rate for age group 15–19. (See later sections of Chapter V on the function of α_i^* as a measure of the degree of concentration of fertility in the central ages of the childbearing age range.)

5. The relation of this EHR component of overall fertility and the Coale–Trussell (1974) model of overall fertility based on the two major determinants of skewness—the age pattern of marriage and the decline of marital fertility at higher ages—will be considered in Chapters VII and VIII.

6. There is the possibility of a bimodal distribution of first births: those that are premaritally conceived and those that are not. However, such a pattern is likely to be missed in aggregate data in which marriages have occurred at various ages.

7. For any one age group, the amount of change in $f_i(a_j)$ on the raw fraction scale varies slightly and systematically over repeated increments in α_i^* or β_i^* to higher levels while holding the other constant. This is a consequence of using a nonlinear re-expression of the data in the fitting procedure. The sign of the change by age group and the age groups emphasized or de-emphasized by the change remain the same, however, over the observed range of values of α_i^* and β_i^*. Similar observations can be made for three-component fits when α_i^*, β_i^*, or γ_i^* is incremented while holding the other two constant.

8. The largest difference between fertility distributions at any age that can be attributed to the difference in α_i^* is .002 (1.7 times the change of .0013 at age 19 for a change of .10 in α_i^*).

9. In each year from 1911 (when recording of births by duration of marriage began) to 1963 (the final year of any marital fertility analyses reported here) approximately 70–80 percent of all legitimate births to women aged 15–19 and approximately 30–40 percent of all legitimate births to women aged 20–24 are reported to have occurred within 8 months after marriage.

VI

Age Patterns of Overall Fertility: Two Centuries of Change

Introduction

Previous chapters have concentrated on procedures, first to achieve closely fitting descriptions of fertility time sequences using a small number of parameters and then to present these fits in a demographically guided standard form so that we can interpret change within a sequence and compare one sequence with another. Now we shall look at the results—the changes in the age pattern of fertility across time. This chapter focuses on two centuries of change in Swedish overall fertility from both cohort and cross-sectional perspectives. Because cohort experience is central to interpretation of the time parameters, for both the country as a whole and the counties of Sweden, we shall present the results of the cohort analyses first.

We begin with the results for the SYAC13 sequence of fertility rates by single year of age of mother for the cohorts aged 15 from 1885/1886 to 1939/1940 and therefore completing their childbearing from 1920/1921 to 1974/1975. This sequence includes the cohorts that carried out the major transition manifested in cross-sectional change from a gradually declining total fertility rate of 4.5 around 1880 and 4.0 around 1900 to a well-below-replacement-level rate of 1.7 in the 1930s. Also included are the cohorts that caused the burst of higher rates between 1942 and 1950 but maintained their level of completed fertility at about 2.0 births per woman on the average—a notable example of the effects of cohort timing of births on cross-sectional levels and age distributions of fertility. The EHR parameters not only provide informative summaries of age variations in fertility but also lead to two summary measures of change in the pace of childbearing apart from the level of fertility. One measure relates change to the EHR age standard pattern B_j^*, the pattern that underlies the shift of the distribution toward ages below 30 as cohorts achieve higher proportions of their total childbearing at young ages. The other measure is expressed in conventional demographic terminology as the mean age of childbearing at a selected standard level of fertility. The relation of these measures to change in the age pattern of marriage for the cohorts and, by extrapolation, to change in the age pattern of entry into childbearing receives attention.

With the results for the 1885/1886 to 1939/1940 cohorts guiding the interpretation of EHR time parameters for all other overall fertility sequences, the second section of the chapter scrutinizes the yearly age-specific fertility data available by 5-year age groups from 1775 onward. Two sets of data are combined in the analysis: data of unusually high quality since 1859—after the establishment of the Central Bureau of Statistics—and 85 years of earlier historical data that were the basis of Sundbärg's (1907) revised rates by 5-year periods and 5-year age groups. Trends and transitions in the age pattern of fertility over 172 cohorts and 202 years are viewed in EHR terms, intersections and divergences of cohort and cross-sectional childbearing experience are examined, and evidence of fertility limitation in the nineteenth century is considered. With these long-term changes as background, attention then focuses on some departures from trend and their relation to either singular historical events that would be expected to disrupt fertility patterns temporarily or certain inaccuracies thought to exist in the data (particularly for the early years).

The cross-sectional EHR description for the country as a whole then becomes the basis for comparison of fertility change in the 25 counties of Sweden over the period 1860–1970. Similarities and differences between counties, which are not apparent in a summary measure such as total fertility rate, are revealed in the EHR time parameters that summarize age patterns of change on the way to the near convergence of pattern across counties in recent decades. Evidence for the influence of migration and changing marriage patterns on fertility change is also presented.

Cohort Fits by Single Year of Age

We shall now consider the 55-cohort, single-year-of-age SYAC13 sequence expressed as

$$\hat{F}_{ij} = \alpha_i^* A_j^* + \beta_i^* B_j^*, \tag{1}$$

where $\hat{F}_{ij}$ is the fitted, cumulated, normalized fertility rate for cohort i and age cut $j = 1, 2, \ldots, n$ expressed on the folded square root scale[1] and $\Sigma A_j^{*2} = \Sigma B_j^{*2} = 1$ for standardization. To discuss the time parameters α_i^* and β_i^* that describe the changes in the sequence, we need to have clearly in mind the characteristics of the age standards A_j^* and B_j^* that underlie these fits.

Age Standards for a Two-Component Fit

The standard-form age parameters (discussed in more detail in Chapter V) can be examined in Fig. 6.1. The smooth, slightly s-shaped curve of the A_j^* vector represents the underlying pattern of the cumulation of births with age centered on a median age of 30.4 years. The $\alpha_i^* A_j^*$ component can be considered almost fixed because the α_i^* multipliers, constrained to be as constant as possible, have the very narrow range 4.16–4.33 in a two-component fit. This means that .002 (or 1.7 times the change of .0013 in $f_i(a_j)$ at age 19 for $\Delta\alpha_i^* = +.10$) is the largest difference between cohort fertility distributions at any age in the fitted schedules that can be attributed to a difference in α_i^* (see Table 5.6).

The B_j^* vector expresses the major underlying pattern of departure from A_j^* in a smooth curve that rises from zero at age cut 13/14 and falls again almost to zero at age cut 49/50. The prominent role played by the $\beta_i^* B_j^*$ component in descriptions of change in the SYAC13 sequence depends on

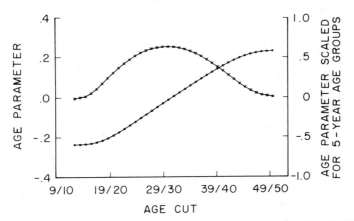

Fig. 6.1 Standard-form age parameters A_j^* (• • •) and B_j^* (× × ×) underlying the SYAC13 sequence for cohorts aged 15 from 1885/1886 to 1939/1940 (values from Table 5.3b).

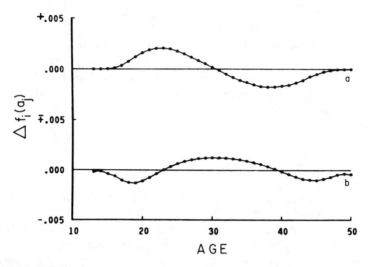

Fig. 6.2   Effect of increments in the time parameters α_i^* and β_i^* on noncumulated fertility distributions (raw fraction scale) constructed from the age parameters A_j^* and B_j^* for double multiplicative fits to the SYAC13 sequence: curve a, change in $\beta_i^* = +.10$; curve b, change in $\alpha_i^* = +.10$ (values from Table 5.6).

the capacity of $\beta_i^* B_j^*$ to express the shift of the age distribution of fertility away from higher ages (particularly ages 35–42) and toward lower ages (particularly ages 20–26) with a positive change in β_i^*.

The effect on the noncumulated fertility distribution when each time parameter α_i^* or β_i^* is changed by $+.10$ while holding the other constant is shown in Fig. 6.2 for easy reference when we study the changes in childbearing patterns over 55 cohorts. We expect positive changes in β_i^* to be associated with decline in childbearing at higher ages and also with decline in the age of entry into childbearing. We expect negative changes in β_i^* to be associated with delay of entry into childbearing.

Time Parameters for a Two-Component Fit

The time parameters α_i^* and β_i^* for the two-component fit to the SYAC13 sequence are shown with the total fertility rate in Fig. 6.3. (See Chapter IV, Note 1 on the designation of these cohorts by year at age 15.) We direct our attention first to the parameter β_i^*. The cohorts aged 15 from 1885/1886 to 1912/1913 show a steady increase in the shift of their age distribution of childbearing away from higher ages and into lower

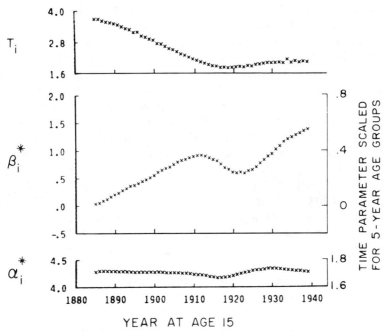

Fig. 6.3 EHR standard-form time parameters α_i^* and β_i^* and total rate of fertility T_i for the SYAC13 sequence, cohorts aged 15 from 1885/1886 to 1939/1940.

ages, as signaled by increasing values of β_i^*. For these cohorts the total rate of fertility simultaneously shows a steady decline. Then, with only the slightest further decline in total fertility, the age distribution of child-bearing steadily shifts toward higher ages again until the cohorts aged 15 from 1921/1922 to 1923/1924 return to a distribution similar to that of the cohort aged 15 in 1901/1902, *but at two-thirds the earlier level of fertility.* The shift toward the younger ages resumes at an accelerated pace with the cohorts aged 15 from 1924/1925 to 1933/1934 and then continues at the pre-1911/1912 cohort pace to the end of the sequence. The cohorts aged 15 after 1929/1930 are the first to have a younger pattern than that achieved by the 1911/1912 to 1912/1913 cohorts. The last 16 cohorts in the sequence provide an example of change in childbearing patterns with little change in the level of completed fertility. These cohorts maintain their total fertility rate quite steadily at the level of the 1911/1912 to 1912/1913 cohorts, only a little above the nadir of the 1917/1918 to 1923/1924 co-horts.

If we direct our attention to the plot of α_i^* in Fig. 6.3, we see in this nearly constant time parameter some small and systematic variations for the cohorts that exhibit major changes in β_i^* with little change in the level of fertility. Recall that lower values of α_i^* denote a slight spreading of the distribution around the median age of A_j^*, whereas higher values of α_i^* denote a slight contraction of the distribution toward the A_j^* median age of 30.4 years (Fig. 6.2). These small variations, which have no obvious relation to change in the total rate of fertility, are of interest in the discussion of fine changes in the distribution. For now, however, we shall concentrate on the major changes in the distribution and their demographic significance, both in cohort perspective and in relation to cross-sectional fertility in the periods the cohorts passed through during their childbearing years. To aid the interpretation of change, we shall consider some of the relations between the two aspects of cohort fertility—timing and level—and carry out some further steps of dissection of the EHR time parameters to construct summary measures of the cohort pace of childbearing, that is, measures of timing standardized for fertility level.

Relations between Cohort Timing of Childbearing
and Cohort Level of Fertility

In the single-year-of-age cohort sequence and all the other Swedish sequences submitted to exploratory data analysis, some shift of the age pattern of fertility to younger ages occurs. In the demographic literature such a change is most commonly summarized as a lower mean age of childbearing. Here it is expressed in the $\beta_i^* B_j^*$ component, which defines not only the degree of shift β_i^* but also an age pattern for the shift B_j^*.

For cohort sequences the two major determinants of a younger fertility pattern have opposite effects on the total rate of fertility expressed as the average number of births per woman: a decline in childbearing at higher ages results in a lower total rate whereas younger entry into childbearing tends to increase the total rate. We have seen that cohort sequences can also exhibit considerable variation in fertility pattern while a steady level of average completed fertility per woman is maintained. Under other circumstances, cohorts within a sequence can achieve higher or lower levels of average completed fertility with little change in the age pattern of childbearing—for example, by having higher or lower proportions of women married across all ages without change in average childbearing behavior per married woman or by an increase or decrease in fecundity that affects all age groups proportionately. Some additional differences in cohort timing or level of fertility occur as disturbances to the long-term trend when period-specific conditions that are favorable or unfavorable to childbearing affect all cohorts passing through that period at various ages.

We saw evidence of such period effects in Chapter IV when we examined the lagged pattern in residuals from the two-component fits to the cohort sequences (Figs. 4.7 and 4.8).

To understand better the observed changes in the age pattern of fertility across a time sequence, we want to separate as completely as we can the influences of cohort timing of childbearing from the influences of change in fertility level. Any separation can only be an approximation (Ryder, 1980) because we lack what Ryder terms the "tempo" and "quantum" inputs to cohort fertility: the age distribution of first births, the lengths of time between births of successive orders, and the parity distribution at the completion of childbearing. Such details of reproductive behavior, however, are frequently unavailable even when quite accurate age-specific fertility rates in time sequence are at hand. We are often forced to work with the aggregate consequences of underlying processes instead of their details and to seek clues to behavioral change without direct information.

To achieve an approximate separation of timing effects and level effects in the EHR time parameters, we standardize for the relation between decline in the level of fertility and shift of the fertility distribution toward younger ages. This establishes a relation of each cohort's pattern of child-bearing to an average tendency for the sequence. We then assess this relation in several ways as an indicator of change in the timing of child-bearing apart from level.

Our procedure responds to Bernhardt's (1971) concern about appropriate measures for comparing the time pattern of childbearing from cohort to cohort in aggregate data. Adopting the cohort approach in her analysis of Swedish reproductive behavior, Bernhardt (p. 22) observes that, "Only when the cumulative fertility rate at age 50 is identical and the mean age at child-bearing for one cohort is lower than for another cohort, is it possible to draw the conclusion that the cohort with the lower mean age at child-bearing has experienced more rapid child-bearing." Her further observation that comparisons of the pace of childbearing without a summary index "is hardly a feasible procedure even if the number of cohorts is small and much less so when you have a long historical series" led her to construct a set of indices for the cumulative exposure to motherhood up to selected ages. The EHR analyses provide two measures of the cohort pace of childbearing (that is, timing standardized for level). One of these measures takes the next step beyond Bernhardt's set of indices and brings into a single index the major temporal differences in cohort childbearing free from association with change in the level of fertility.

The derivation of this first index takes advantage of the fact that the chosen standard form of the EHR-fitted parameters concentrates in the fixed age standard B_j^* and the corresponding variable time parameter β_i^*

almost all the relation between the decline in level of fertility and the shift of the age pattern of fertility from higher to lower ages. By least squares regression of the β_i^* vector on the corresponding time vector of the total rate of fertility, β_i^* is separated into two portions. One portion describes the increase in β_i^* as fertility at ages 30 and higher declines, shifting the fertility distribution toward ages below 30. The other portion, the regression residuals denoted by $\beta_{i\cdot T}^*$, becomes the first index of the cohort pace of childbearing for cohorts $i = 1$ to m. (See Mosteller and Tukey, 1977, pp. 303–304 on the use of this notation to indicate the linear adjustment of the variable on the left of the dot, β_i^*, for the variable on the right, T.) The index describes those changes in β_i^* that are *not* inversely related to change in the total fertility rate across the sequence. The dominant factor underlying cohort-to-cohort differences in this residual portion of β_i^* should be change across time in the age pattern of entry into childbearing. In fact, as we discuss later, these residuals appear to pick up effects of both the later marriage patterns of the cohorts aged 15 from 1909/1910 to 1923/1924 and the increasingly earlier marriage patterns of all subsequent cohorts for which completed childbearing experience was available. Change in the length of interbirth intervals can also influence such a measure of cohort-to-cohort differences in the timing of childbearing. This secondary factor has assumed a growing role in the description of timing change for low-fertility populations like the United States (Ryder, 1980).

The second EHR summary measure of the cohort pace of childbearing, denoted by $\bar{a}_i^s$, is the mean age of childbearing at a standard level of fertility. This index depends on the construction of level-standardized distributions of fertility—the type of distribution that responds to the problem described by Bernhardt in comparisons of the pace of childbearing across cohorts that have different levels of completed fertility. From the EHR parameters, such distributions can be constructed for any selected fertility level—for example, the median or mean level for the sequence could be chosen. One particularly informative choice of fertility level, as we shall see later in this chapter and in Chapter VII, is the relatively high to very high level that would correspond to a predicted value of $\hat{\beta}_i^* = 0$ if all decline in total fertility rate across the sequence were attributed to decline in childbearing at higher ages according to the pattern determined by the B_j^* age standard. The mean age of childbearing for each level-standardized distribution is then calculated by customary procedures. We shall examine the details of the standardization procedures before considering the details of the results.

Compensation of Age Patterns of Fertility for Change in the Level of Fertility   To separate from the time parameters α_i^* and β_i^* the portion of change that is not inversely related to the change in total rate of fertility across the 55 cohorts, we use least squares regression as an exclusion procedure. That is, α_i^* and β_i^* are regressed independently on the time vector $T_i^{1/2}$ so that the time parameters can be expressed as

$$\alpha_i^* = k_1 + k_2 T_i^{1/2} + \alpha_{i \cdot T}^*, \tag{2}$$

$$\beta_i^* = k_3 + k_4 T_i^{1/2} + \beta_{i \cdot T}^*. \tag{3}$$

Any linear association of α_i^* and β_i^* with the change in total rate across the sequence is thus restricted to the terms $k_1 + k_2 T_i^{1/2}$ and $k_3 + k_4 T_i^{1/2}$, where k_2 and k_4 are regression slopes and k_1 and k_3 are intercepts. The regression residuals are referred to as $\alpha_{i \cdot T}^*$ and $\beta_{i \cdot T}^*$ to identify them as time parameters modified by linear compensation for the square root of the total rate of fertility. These are the portions of α_i^* and β_i^* that are free of association with the level of fertility.[2] The two residual time vectors $\alpha_{i \cdot T}^*$ and $\beta_{i \cdot T}^*$ can now be more effectively examined for association with other changes—for example, change in marriage patterns—than could α_i^* and β_i^* before removal of the influence of total fertility change (see Mosteller and Tukey, 1977, pp. 268–270, for additional discussion of this use of regression).

Construction of Level-standardized Distributions of Fertility To construct level-standardized distributions of fertility, we return to Eqs. (2) and (3) and express α_i^* and β_i^* in equivalent forms that incorporate the fertility level selected as the standard T_s:

$$\alpha_i^* = k_1 + k_2(T_i^{1/2} - T_s^{1/2}) + k_2 T_s^{1/2} + \alpha_{i \cdot T}^*, \tag{4}$$

$$\beta_i^* = k_3 + k_4(T_i^{1/2} - T_s^{1/2}) + k_4 T_s^{1/2} + \beta_{i \cdot T}^*. \tag{5}$$

Any relation of α_i^* and β_i^* to the difference between the total rate and the standard level across a time sequence of schedules is described by the terms $k_2(T_i^{1/2} - T_s^{1/2})$ and $k_4(T_i^{1/2} - T_s^{1/2})$. The portions of α_i^* and β_i^* *not* related to the difference between the total rate and the standard level can thus be expressed as

$$\alpha_i^s = k_1 + k_2 T_s^{1/2} + \alpha_{i \cdot T}^*, \tag{6}$$

$$\beta_i^s = k_3 + k_4 T_s^{1/2} + \beta_{i \cdot T}^*. \tag{7}$$

Cumulative fertility distributions standardized to the level T_s are constructed as follows: each element of the level-standardized time vector α_i^s is multiplied by each element of the corresponding age vector A_j^* and each element of the level-standardized time vector β_i^s is multiplied by each element of the corresponding age vector B_j^* to form an $m \times n$ matrix of pairs of components for cohorts $i = 1$ to m at age cuts $j = 1$ to n. For each cohort i and age cut j, the complete level-standardized element at level T_s is

$$F_{ij}^s = \alpha_i^s A_j^* + \beta_i^s B_j^*. \tag{8}$$

Summing the pairs of components within each cell of the matrix then gives a time sequence of level-standardized fertility distributions for the cohorts. The F_{ij}^s expressions on the folded square root scale are then de-transformed to the raw fraction scale (see Chapter VIII for procedure) for comparison of the distributions and calculation of the cohort-specific mean ages of childbearing at the selected standard level of fertility. If the selected standard level is higher or lower than any total rate reported for a sequence, this procedure can be used to identify the age distributions of fertility that would be predicted by that level and the patterns found to underlie the observed distributions.

The special case $T_s = T_m$ occurs when T_s is selected so that

$$k_3 + k_4 T_s^{1/2} = 0,$$

leaving $\beta_i^s = \beta_{i \cdot T}^*$ in Eq. (7). T_m is that "maximum" level of fertility that would correspond to a predicted value of $\hat{\beta}_i^* = 0$ (and therefore the absence of the $\beta_i^* B_j^*$ component from the description) if β_i^* were exactly inversely related to $T_i^{1/2}$ across a sequence and if all decline in the total rate were attributed to decline in fertility at higher ages according to the pattern determined by the B_j^* age standard (Fig. 6.4). The expression of F_{ij}^s, now more clearly called F_{ij}^m, is thus simplified to

$$F_{ij}^m = (k_1 + k_2 T_m^{1/2} + \alpha_{i \cdot T}^*)A_j^* + \beta_{i \cdot T}^* B_j^* = \alpha_i^m A_j^* + \beta_{i \cdot T}^* B_j^*. \tag{9}$$

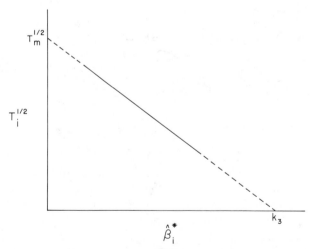

Fig. 6.4 Relation of the standard level of fertility T_m to a predicted linear relation between the EHR time parameter β_i^* and the square root of the sum of age-specific fertility rates T_i.

When we take into consideration the small size of the regression coefficient k_2 for α_i^* regressed on $T_i^{1/2}$ (Table 6.2)—expressing a minimal degree of association between α_i^* and changes in the level of fertility—we see that $k_2 T_{\mathrm{m}}^{1/2}$ is negligible for most purposes and that Eq. (9) can be further simplified to

$$F_{ij}^{\mathrm{m}} = (k_1 + \alpha_{i\cdot\mathrm{T}}^*)A_j^* + \beta_{i\cdot\mathrm{T}}^* B_j^* \tag{10}$$

when we standardize to the specific level of fertility T_{m}.

Calculation of the Mean Age of Childbearing at a Standard Fertility Level   Calculation of the mean age of childbearing $\bar{a}_i^s$ for a level-standardized fertility distribution for cohort $i = 1$ to m is based on the customary procedure for a nonstandardized schedule (Shryock, Siegel, and Associates, 1976):

$$\bar{a} = \sum_a a f_a \Big/ \sum_a f_a,$$

where a is the midpoint of each age (13.5, 14.5, . . . , 49.5) and f_a the fertility rate for each age (13, 14, . . . , 50). However, f_a is more conveniently taken here as the *proportion* of total fertility that occurs at each age (13, 14, . . . , 50).

Temporal Variation in the Swedish Cohort Pace of Childbearing

Both measures of the cohort pace of childbearing defined in the preceding section are based on the EHR time parameters that are freed from association with the square root of the level of fertility by least squares regression. The regression coefficients included in Table 6.2 confirm the visual impression from Fig. 6.5 that little of the variation in α_i^* can be accounted for by change in the total rate of fertility, whereas a considerable amount of the change in β_i^* can be related to change in the level of fertility. At the same time, the portion of change in β_i^* *not* accounted for by change in level has significant features expressed in the regression residuals $\beta_{i\cdot\mathrm{T}}^*$. This is the first index of the cohort pace of childbearing that we shall examine for change across the 55 Swedish cohorts.

The time sequence of $\beta_{i\cdot\mathrm{T}}^*$ should be examined at two levels of detail.

1. For which cohorts is $\beta_{i\cdot\mathrm{T}}^*$ positive? Negative? Zero? The answers relate the pace of childbearing for each cohort to the average pace for the specific sequence.
2. For which cohorts is *change* in $\beta_{i\cdot\mathrm{T}}^*$ ($\Delta\beta_{i\cdot\mathrm{T}}^*$) positive? Negative? Zero? The answers provide clues to behavioral change of which we

observe the aggregate consequences in relating one segment of the sequence to another.

At the first of these levels of detail, the regression residuals $\beta^*_{i\cdot T}$ can be interpreted in the following way:

$\beta^*_{i\cdot T} = 0$ The age distribution of fertility is shifted toward the younger ages to the degree that would be predicted by the observed level of fertility if an inverse relation existed between β^*_i and $T_i^{1/2}$ across the time sequence

$\beta^*_{i\cdot T} > 0$ The age distribution of fertility is shifted more toward the younger ages than would correspond, on the average, to the level of fertility

$\beta^*_{i\cdot T} < 0$ The age distribution of fertility is shifted less toward the younger ages than would correspond, on the average, to the level of fertility

We see in Fig. 6.5 that only for a few cohorts—mainly those aged 15 from 1893/1894 to 1898/1899—is the age pattern of fertility close to the level-predicted pattern. Although the 1885/1886–1892/1893 cohorts had an older-than-level-predicted childbearing pattern, the adoption of a younger-than-level-predicted pattern by the 1900/1901–1912/1913 cohorts makes the rapid transition by subsequent cohorts to a much older pattern all the more noticeable. The following recovery and progression to an increasingly younger-than-level-predicted pattern is equally remarkable.

In the context of these prominent changes, there are three small groups of cohorts for which the level-standardized pattern is quite stable (for which $\Delta\beta^*_{i\cdot T} \simeq 0$)—that is, the relation of the age pattern of fertility expressed by β^*_i to the level of fertility expressed by T_i is unchanged even when both β^*_i and T_i continue to change. For the 1893/1894 to 1898/1899 cohorts, the change toward a younger pattern ($\Delta\beta^*_i > 0$) continues to be that predicted by the decline in the level of fertility ($\Delta T_i < 0$) and both $\beta^*_{i\cdot T}$ and $\Delta\beta^*_{i\cdot T} \simeq 0$. For the 1902/1903 to 1910/1911 cohorts, the pattern described by the increasing value of β^*_i is younger to a consistent degree than the pattern that would correspond, on the average, to the level of fertility as the level continues to decline and $\beta^*_{i\cdot T} > 0$ with $\Delta\beta^*_{i\cdot T} \simeq 0$. The 1920/1921–1923/1924 cohorts with little change in either β^*_i or T_i maintain a consistently older-than-level-predicted pattern and $\beta^*_{i\cdot T} < 0$ with $\Delta\beta^*_{i\cdot T} \simeq 0$.

Difference in the age pattern of entry into childbearing should be the largest single determinant of a younger or older level-standardized pattern of fertility as indicated by $\beta^*_{i\cdot T}$ in conjunction with the age standard B^*_j.

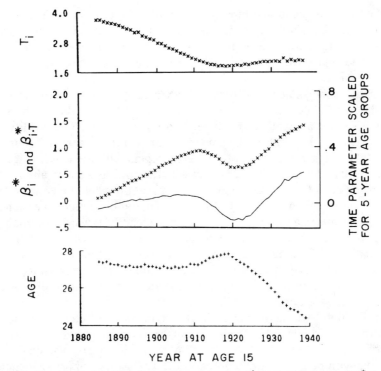

Fig. 6.5 Total rate of fertility T_i and time parameter β_i^* ($\times \times \times$) before and $\beta_{i \cdot T}^*$ (———) after linear compensation for the total rate for the SYAC13 sequence; and mean age at first marriage (data from Ewbank, 1974): cohorts aged 15 from 1885/1886 to 1939/1940.

Because pregnancy has tended to precipitate marriage rather than the other way around in Sweden (Hofsten and Lundstrom, 1976, p. 28), a measure of change in the age pattern of marriage serves as a moderately good proxy for a measure of change in the age pattern of entry into childbearing with which to compare change in $\beta_{i \cdot T}^*$.[3]

It would be convenient to have for marriages an EHR counterpart of the fertility time-sequence description. However, the most coherent description yet developed of change in first marriage patterns for the Swedish cohorts (Ewbank, 1974) is expressed in the convolution of a normal curve and a double exponential curve and is defined by three time parameters. Because these parameters do not provide a ready focus for a comparison involving $\beta_{i \cdot T}^*$ and its associated age-standard pattern B_j^*, we shall substitute a comparison of $\beta_{i \cdot T}^*$ with Ewbank's time sequence of the mean age of first marriage calculated from his three model parameters. Although the nuances of change in marriage pattern are only partially described by this mean age (and its standard deviation, considered later), some prominent similarities are apparent between $\beta^*_{i \cdot T}$ and the mean age of marriage (Fig. 6.5). These similarities appear in mirror-image form because the higher the value of $\beta^*_{i \cdot T}$, the younger the level-standardized fertility pattern.

For the cohorts aged 15 from 1885/1886 to 1892/1893, both the level-standardized childbearing pattern indicated by $\beta^*_{i \cdot T}$ and the mean age of marriage show a slight by steady shift to younger ages. The fertility pattern continues this shift, with some irregularity, for the next 10 cohorts. A reversal to higher ages for both patterns begins with the cohorts aged 15 about 1910 and reaches its maximum with the cohorts aged 15 about 1920. The mean age of marriage begins its recovery toward younger ages a few cohorts sooner than does the fertility pattern, but once recovery is underway, both marriage and fertility progress steadily toward the youngest patterns for the sequence. The similarities and differences between these time patterns of change are examined in more detail in the next section, using the mean age of childbearing at a standard level of fertility as the index of change in pace and bringing the standard deviation of marriage age into consideration.

At this point we have elicited in $\beta^*_{i \cdot T}$ indications of change in the age pattern of entry into childbearing that are consistent with the known marriage experience of the cohorts. Later in this chapter we shall apply the level-compensation procedures to the 1775–1929 cohort sequence to search for evidence of change in marriage pattern and fertility regulation by other means.

Mean Age of Childbearing at a Standard Level of Fertility

The second measure of the cohort pace of childbearing constructed earlier in the chapter, the mean age of childbearing at a standard level of fertility $\bar{a}^s_i$, is better understood after brief consideration of some of the level-standardized distributions from which its values are derived. The effect of level standardization on the cumulative fertility distributions for three cohorts—those aged 15 in 1901/1902, 1920/1921, and 1935/1936—can be examined in Fig. 6.6. Figure 6.6a shows the reported distributions having total rates of 2.76, 1.83, and 2.14, respectively. Figure 6.6b shows the result of standardizing the distributions to the level $T_s = 3.00$. Figure 6.6c shows the result of standardizing the distributions to the level $T_m = 4.31$, at which $\hat{\beta}^*_i = 0$.

In Fig. 6.6a, the true relations of the pace of childbearing for the three cohorts are obscured by the effect of differing levels of total fertility. Both

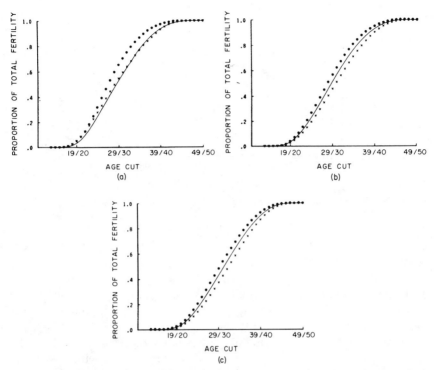

Fig. 6.6 (a) Reported overall fertility distributions and the corresponding level-standardized overall fertility distributions constructed for fertility levels (b) $T_s = 3.00$ and (c) $T_m = 4.31$ from the EHR age standards A_j^* and B_j^* and the level-compensated time parameters $\alpha_{i\cdot T}^*$ and $\beta_{i\cdot T}^*$ from two-component fits to the SYAC13 sequence: selected cohorts by year at age 15, 1901/1902 (——), 1920/1921 (× × ×), and 1935/1936 (• • •).

Figs. 6.6b and 6.6c clarify the variations in pace—the pace is slowest for the 1920/1921 cohort (which had one of the highest mean ages of marriage for any cohort in the sequence) and fastest for the 1935/1936 cohort (which had one of the lowest mean ages of marriage in the sequence). The level of fertility selected for the standardization has made no difference in the relations of the pace of childbearing for the three cohorts to each other. Only the pace itself for all three cohorts together has changed—it is more rapid in Fig. 6.6b with standardization to a level of $T_s = 3.00$ than in Fig. 6.6c with standardization to a level of $T_m = 4.31$.

The mean age of childbearing $\bar{a}_i^s$ calculated from the level-standardized distributions for the two levels $T_s = 3.00$ and $T_m = 4.31$ can be examined in Fig. 6.7 for the 55 cohorts aged 15 from 1885/1886 to 1939/1940. The fact that the time pattern of variation in $\bar{a}_i^s$ is almost identical to that of $\beta_{i\cdot T}^*$

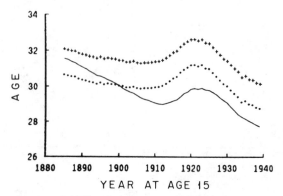

Fig. 6.7   The mean age of childbearing $\bar{a}_i^s$ at selected standard levels of fertility $T_m = 4.31$ (+ + +) and $T_s = 3.00$ (• • •) and the mean age of childbearing $\bar{a}_i$ (——) not compensated for the level of fertility: cohorts aged 15 from 1885/1886 to 1939/1940.

(Fig. 6.5) confirms that $\beta_{i\cdot T}^*$ captures essentially all the change in the age pattern of fertility that is not related to the decline of childbearing at ages above 30.[4] Again, the total rate of fertility selected for the standardization affects only the level of the mean age across all cohorts not the relation of the cohorts to each other.

The mean age of childbearing not compensated for the level of fertility $\bar{a}_i$ is shown in Fig. 6.7 for comparison. Its near identity with the mirror image of β_i^* (Fig. 6.5) provides further confirmation that the EHR-derived β_i^* time parameter, in association with the standard age pattern B_j^*, describes almost all the shift in the age pattern of fertility to younger or older ages. This shift is determined by a combination of factors whose effects we shall try to separate. One advantage of using β_i^*, $\beta_{i\cdot T}^*$, and $\bar{a}_i^s$ is that they *are* associated with standard age patterns that underlie the entire

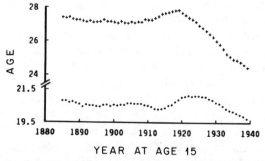

Fig. 6.8   Mean age at first marriage (+ + +) and mean age minus one standard deviation (• • •): cohorts aged 15 from 1885/1886 to 1939/1940 (data from Ewbank, 1974).

time sequence and have demographically meaningful forms. Thus β_i^*, $\beta_{i\cdot T}^*$, and $\bar{a}_i^s$ define change more precisely, age by age, and describe change more completely and with no less parsimony than do the customary statistical measures mean and standard deviation.

The second index of the pace of childbearing $\bar{a}_i^s$, expressed on the same age scale as the mean age of marriage, permits some relations of pace and marriage patterns over time to be discussed in more readily understood terms than when the $\beta_{i\cdot T}^*$ index of pace is used in the comparison. Examining $\bar{a}_i^s$ for the fertility level $T_m = 4.31$ (Fig. 6.7) and the mean age of marriage (Fig. 6.8), we see that the arithmetic difference between the two means has a relatively narrow range for the cohorts aged 15 before 1920/1921—a high of 4.7 years for the 1885/1886 and 1919/1920 cohorts and a low of 4.1 years for the 1910/1911 cohort. The prominent divergence in the time pattern of the two means with the 1920/1921 to 1924/1925 cohorts has already been noted: the decline in the mean age of marriage starts five cohorts earlier while the pace of childbearing exhibits its highest mean age. This difference is not surprising because the mean age of marriage minus one standard deviation is at its highest age for the 1920/1921 to 1927/1928 cohorts, even though the mean age of marriage declines. Such a concentration of the majority of marriages in a narrower age range thus involves a higher age at marriage for some fraction of women in the 1920/1921 to 1927/1928 cohorts in comparison to previous cohorts—a circumstance that would be expected to sustain a later childbearing pattern as measured by $\bar{a}_i^s$. Indeed, the arithmetic difference between $\bar{a}_i^s$ and the mean age of marriage is 5.5 years for the cohort aged 15 in 1925/1926 and continues at approximately this level to the end of the sequence even as both means assume essentially the same rate of decline.

Whether we view $\bar{a}_i^s$ as a useful indicator of change in the age pattern of entry into childbearing for a particular time sequence or as a general measure of change in pace that includes the aggregate consequences of possible changes in the length of interbirth intervals, we may want to relate the observed changes to a constant mean age. For example, all change can be related to the experience of a specific cohort by selecting the cohort's $\bar{a}_i^s$ value at a selected standard level of fertility as the reference mean age.

We shall illustrate such a comparison by first choosing $T_m = 4.31$ as the fertility level used in constructing the level-standardized distributions. We then choose the cohort aged 15 in 1885/1886, with $\bar{a}_i^s = 32.1$ years when $T_m = 4.31$, as a reference cohort and reference mean age of childbearing. These choices enable us to answer two questions about contributions to the unstandardized mean age of fertility $\bar{a}_i$ for a time sequence. How many years has the mean age of childbearing been shifted from the

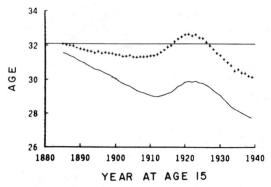

Fig. 6.9 The mean age of childbearing $\bar{a}_i$ (——) not compensated for the level of fertility and the mean age of childbearing $\bar{a}_i^s$ (+ + +) at the standard level $T_m = 4.31$ in relation to a selected reference mean age of 32.1 years: cohorts aged 15 from 1885/1886 to 1939/1940.

selected reference mean age by change in the pace of childbearing? For each cohort in our example (Fig. 6.9), $\Delta\bar{a}_i^s = \bar{a}_i^s - 32.1$ years. What change from the reference mean age of childbearing would have been predicted if all change from the standard level of fertility had been attributable to change in fertility at higher ages, according to the age pattern determined by B_j^*? For each cohort in our example (Fig. 6.9), $\Delta\bar{a}_i = \bar{a}_i - (\bar{a}_i^s$ at level $T_m)$.

We have just considered the extent to which $\bar{a}_i$ falls below 32.1 years for each cohort in terms of the two factors defined by our level compensation procedure: the pace of childbearing at a standard level of fertility and the decline of fertility at higher ages apart from pace. These mean age relations (shown in Fig. 6.9 for all 55 cohorts) are given in Table 6.1 for the reference cohort 1885/1886 and for three cohorts with quite different fertility patterns. Under the specified conditions, one-quarter of the decline in unstandardized mean age of fertility ($\bar{a}_i - 32.1$ years) for the 1907/1908 cohort is accounted for by a more rapid pace of childbearing ($\bar{a}_i^s - 32.1$ years), which we associate here with earlier entry into childbearing, and three-quarters is accounted for by the decline of fertility at higher ages apart from pace ($\bar{a}_i - \bar{a}_i^s$). For the 1939/1940 cohort, a more rapid pace is the principal factor in the further decline in the value of $\bar{a}_i$ and accounts for approximately half the difference from the 1885/1886 reference cohort. In contrast to the $\bar{a}_i$ values for the 1907/1908 and 1939/1940 cohorts, for which both pace and decline of fertility at higher ages contribute to a younger pattern, $\bar{a}_i$ for the 1920/1921 cohort reflects the partially counteracting effect of slower pace (later entry into childbearing). A .6-year greater decline in the value of $\bar{a}_i$ would have been predicted by the observed level of fertility for the 1920/1921 cohort if all decline from the

TABLE 6.1

Relations between a Reference Mean Age of Childbearing
(32.1 Years), the Mean Age of Childbearing ($\bar{a}_i$) Not
Compensated for the Level of Fertility, and the Mean Age ($\bar{a}_i^s$)
at the Standard Level $T_m = 4.31$: Selected Cohorts by Year at
Age 15

Cohort by year at age 15	Difference in mean age		
	$\bar{a}_i^s - 32.1$	$\bar{a}_i - \bar{a}_i^s$	$\bar{a}_i - 32.1$
1885/1886	0	−.5	−.5
1907/1908	−.7	−2.1	−2.8
1920/1921	.6	−2.8	−2.2
1939/1940	−1.9	−2.4	−4.3

standard level of fertility had been attributable to decline in childbearing at higher ages.

In assessing the indicators of change in the relative importance of the major factors underlying cohort age patterns of fertility, remember that we see only the aggregate consequences of underlying behavioral change. It is entirely possible, for example, that counterbalancing changes occur in the timing of childbearing by subpopulations while the aggregate measures are relatively unchanged. If data for subpopulations were available, these circumstances could be detected and related to aggregate population patterns by the procedures used later in this chapter for the counties of Sweden.

Two Centuries of Overall Fertility: Cohort and Cross-sectional Perspectives

We shall now extend our view of Swedish fertility history back to 1775 using the same exploratory steps that effectively described the nature of change in childbearing behavior by 55 of the most recent cohorts with completed childbearing experience. We shall focus our attention at two levels of detail: one, the characterization of trends and transitions in overall fertility patterns, both in cohort perspective and as cohort childbearing experience is manifested in cross-sectional fertility patterns; two, the nature of some short-term variations in the trend over two centuries in relation to unusual events or possible errors in the data.

Discussion centers on two-component fits to cohort and cross-sectional sequences by 5-year age groups from 1775 to 1959 for all childbearing ages

15–49 and for childbearing at ages 20–49 only. These sequences are designated C15, C20, X15, and X20 to distinguish cohort from cross-sectional perspectives and indicate the youngest age included in the analysis. Supplementary information comes from two sources: a three-component fit to the *X202* sequence, which is the X15 sequence extended to 1976, and the two-component fit to the single-year-of-age cohort sequence SYAC13 (examined in a previous section of this chapter), which is composed of cohorts that completed their childbearing at age 50 between 1920/1921 and 1974/1975.

The data for the basic cohort and cross-sectional analyses are the 185 years of age-specific fertility rates described in Chapter III. These data are submitted to EHR analysis in cross section by year from 1775 to 1959 and on the diagonal by cohort aged 15–19 from 1775 to 1929. The 185 years of data provide complete information for 155 cohorts. Two triangles of incomplete cohort experience are omitted, one at the beginning of the sequence and one at the end. However, we do not have true cohort data for these analyses. Instead, we have approximations of cohort experience constructed from data that relate childbearing to a woman's age at the time of confinement but not to her year of birth and that aggregate confinements by 5-year age groups on a cross-sectional basis. We must accept "cohort by year at age 15–19" as the closest designation we can give, but one that does not apply precisely.

Proceeding to a dual perspective on this fertility data set, we expect to transmit in the fitted descriptions two basic cohort and cross-sectional interrelations: one, each cross-sectional slice of fertility is the composite of a small portion of the childbearing experience of many cohorts whose diverse histories influence their behavior at any given period; two, the period in which the cross-sectional slice is taken then has its own influence on the experience of all the cohorts of women passing through the period at various ages. Three possible outcomes for the EHR fitting of these intersecting sequences would be the following.

1. The underlying similarities of the data in cohort and cross-sectional forms may dominate the fitted parameters, leaving most of the divergence of the two forms in the residuals.
2. The systematic differences may be well described by the separate sets of fitted parameters for the cohort and cross-sectional sequences.
3. Either "true" similarities or "true" differences between cohort and cross-sectional underlying regularities may be obscured by diffusion through the fitted parameters and residuals for one or both sequences.

We already have some evidence about the outcome under the set of fitting conditions selected for the EHR analysis. For two-component fits, we found in Chapter V that a given combination of the time parameters α_i^* and β_i^* generated very close to the same fertility distribution with both the cross-sectional and the cohort A_j^* and B_j^* age standards. We also found that varying a cross-sectional $\alpha_i^* A_j^*$ or $\beta_i^* B_j^*$ component in even increments while holding the other component constant had essentially the same effect on the magnitude and direction of change in the fertility distribution as did varying a cohort $\alpha_i^* A_j^*$ or $\beta_i^* B_j^*$ component in the same even increments. Change in the two sequences can therefore be compared by means of the time parameters α_i^* and β_i^*.

Regarding differences not captured in the fitted parameters, we found in Chapter IV that EHR analysis of overall fertility for two components gave closely fitted descriptions to the cohort sequences and even more closely fitted descriptions to the cross-sectional sequences. However, a different type of regularity remained in the residuals from the cohort analysis than in the residuals from the cross-sectional analysis. We also found in Chapter IV that most of the remaining regularity for a cross-sectional sequence could be expressed in a third fitted component. Under these circumstances, looking for systematic differences in cohort and cross-sectional fitted parameters should be more profitable after fine-tuning the data re-expression and carrying out further three-component fitting of the comparable 202-year and 172-cohort sequences. We shall now concentrate on the similarities of the pairs of the $\alpha_i^* A_j^*$ and $\beta_i^* B_j^*$ components derived in two-component analyses using the folded square root re-expression.

Trends and Transitions

We shall consider first the EHR evidence for the occurrence of change over two centuries before turning to an interpretation of the changes in the time parameters. The α_i^* pairs and β_i^* pairs for the C15 and C20 sequences and the X15 and X20 sequences differ principally in level (Figs. 6.10 and 6.11), giving evidence for the small part that age group 15–19 has played in change in the age pattern of fertility over these time sequences. The narrow range of departure of α_i^* from a constant value is similar in all the sequences when some of the post-1914 cohorts are excluded. Fitting a third component to the $X202$ sequence does not change the time pattern of α_i^* from 1775 to 1959, only its level (compare α_i^* in Figs. 6.11 and 6.12). Systematic variations, however, are worth noting even in a near constant.

A gradual rise in the value of α_i^* over the first 60 years of the cross-sectional sequences (Figs. 6.11 and 6.12, or Fig. 6.13 where the scale for

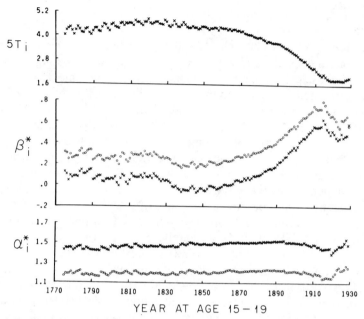

Fig. 6.10 EHR standard-form time parameters α_i^* and β_i^* for the C15 ($\times\times\times$) and C20 ($\circ\circ\circ$) sequences and total rate of fertility $5T_i$ for the C15 sequence: cohorts aged 15–19 from 1775 to 1929.

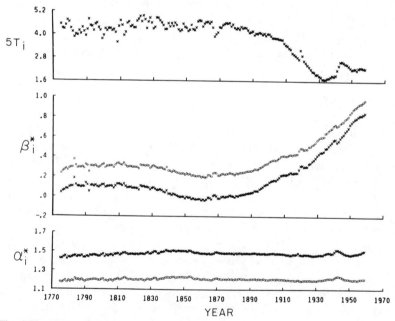

Fig. 6.11 EHR standard-form time parameters α_i^* and β_i^* for the X15 ($\times\times\times$) and X20 ($\circ\circ\circ$) sequences and total rate of fertility $5T_i$ for the X15 sequence: 1775–1959.

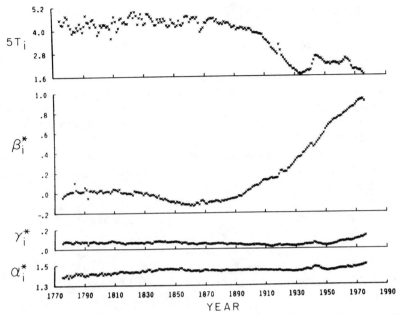

Fig. 6.12   EHR standard-form time parameters α_i^*, β_i^*, and γ_i^* and total rate of fertility $5T_i$ for the *X202* sequence: 1775–1976.

α_i^* and γ_i^* is expanded) indicates that a slightly increasing proportion of total childbearing occurs in the 25–40 age range over these years (see Table 5.8 and the discussion in Chapter V). The 1942–1945 aberration in cross-sectional α_i^* values, which indicates a higher proportion of total fertility concentrated in ages 25–40 than has occurred previously, has been related in the first section of this chapter to unusual cohort childbearing behavior and is examined in Chapter VII in relation to cross-sectional marital fertility patterns.

   The post-1950 rise in α_i^* values for the X15 but not the X20 sequence (Fig. 6.11) is found from analysis of the *X202* sequence to continue to 1976

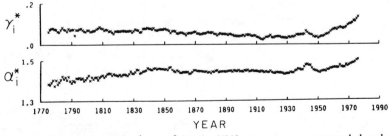

Fig. 6.13   Time parameters α_i^* and γ_i^* for the *X202* sequence on an expanded scale.

and to be accompanied by a pronounced rise in the third time parameter γ_i^* (Figs. 6.12 and 6.13). Up to this point in the time sequence, γ_i^* has been nearly constant. The change in γ_i^* signals that the most recent transition in the age pattern of fertility began in the early 1950s and also suggests that the transition reflects new patterns of behavior. The extent to which this change involves the concentration of childbearing in an increasingly narrow age range centered on age group 25–29 is shown in Table 5.8. The EHR evidence for this type of transition in other countries is considered in Chapter VIII.

Until the post-1950 period, however, the principal evidence for transitions in both cohort and cross-sectional sequences appears in the second time parameter β_i^*, the measure of the extent to which the age distribution of fertility is shifted from ages 30 and above to ages below 30 (Figs. 6.10 and 6.11, and Fig. 6.12 where the plot of β_i^* is seen to differ from that in Fig. 6.11 only in level, not in time pattern). On the basis of the behavior of β_i^* shown in Fig. 6.10, the cohorts designated by year at age 15–19 can be divided into 6 groups: pre-1825, 1825–1838, 1838–1850, 1850–1885, 1885–1910, and post-1910. The terminal cohorts assigned to these groups should be considered approximate choices among several transition cohorts.

pre-1825   Fluctuations occur around a fairly steady age distribution of fertility; greater variability for the pre-1811 cohorts is possibly due both to specific events, such as the 1808–1809 war, and to the lesser accuracy of the data for the early years (see discussion at the end of this section)

1825–1838   An increasingly older age pattern of fertility develops

1838–1850   Fluctuations occur around the older fertility pattern that was developed by the preceding 13 cohorts

1850–1885   A reversal to an increasingly younger age pattern of fertility occurs, with the 1880 cohort recapturing the pattern of the pre-1825 cohorts, but at a lower level of fertility

1885–1910   The shift toward a younger childbearing pattern accelerates

post-1910   A brief, sharp reversal to an older pattern occurs and is then reversed again by post-1924 cohorts to the continued development of an increasingly younger pattern (see also Fig. 6.3, which shows β_i^* for the 1929–1939 cohorts by single year of age)

How is this evidence of changing cohort experience reflected in cross-sectional fertility changes? We can gain a quite vivid impression by superimposing the cohort sequence of β_i^* values on the cross-sectional se-

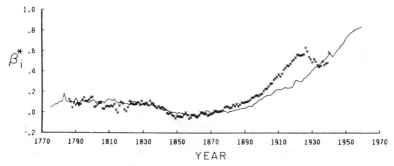

Fig. 6.14 Time parameter β_i^* for the C15 ($\times \times \times$) and X15 (——) sequences, 1775–1959, with β_i^* for the C15 sequence centered on year at age 26–30.

quence of β_i^* values in several ways. We shall then gain some understanding of the points of divergence of the cohort and cross-sectional experience by examining $\beta_{i \cdot T}^*$, the measure of cohort timing of childbearing at a standard level of fertility, for the C15 sequence.

In Fig. 6.14 β_i^* for the C15 sequence is moved forward 11 years on the time line so that cohort values are centered on year at age 26–30. Before 1877, and again during the period 1933–1940, the extent to which the cross-sectional age distribution of fertility changes in degree and direction of shift toward older or younger ages is very similar to the extent to which cohorts then aged 26–30 shift their age pattern of childbearing to older or younger ages. In the nineteenth-century period of change, however, β_i^* for the X15 sequence exhibits a more gradual decline than does that for the C15 sequence because the effects of the precipitous change by 13 cohorts are spread over a number of years. The 1933–1940 period of change is shown in Chapter VII to coincide with notable increases in the proportion of women married at ages 20 and higher.

Before 1877 and in the brief period in the 1930s, the cross-sectional age distribution of fertility thus appears to reflect a prominent influence of change in the age pattern of entry into childbearing. The divergence beginning in 1877, with β_i^* for the X15 sequence lagging behind that for the C15 sequence, indicates a transition to greater dependence of the cross-sectional fertility distribution on the changing behavior of women above age 30. When we move β_i^* for the C15 sequence forward another 7 years on the time line so that cohort values are centered on year at age 33–37 (Fig. 6.15), this relation is confirmed in the similarity in the rates of change of β_i^* for the C15 and X15 sequences until another divergence beginning in 1910. The β_i^* values for the years 1851–1877, shown in Fig. 6.14 superimposed by β_i^* for the cohorts then aged 26–30 and in Fig. 15 superimposed by β_i^* for the cohorts then aged 33–37, represent the influence of both the younger pattern of childbearing developing in cohorts

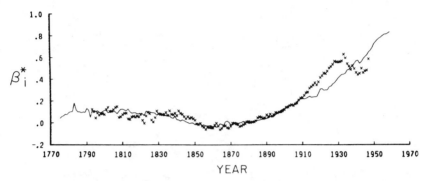

Fig. 6.15   Time parameter β_i^* for the C15 ($\times \times \times$) and X15 (——) sequences, 1775–1959, with β_i^* for the C15 sequence centered on year at age 33–37.

aged 15–19 after 1850 and the older pattern for the last of the cohorts aged 15–19 before 1850. In contrast, the 1910 divergence of β_i^* for the X15 sequence results from a tempering of the influence of the increasingly younger childbearing pattern of cohorts then above age 30 by the increasingly older pattern of cohorts then at lower ages.

If we move the post-1910 β_i^* values for the C15 sequence forward another 13 years on the time line so that these cohort values are superimposed on the β_i^* values for the X15 sequence for the years 1924 and after— that is, the cohorts are centered on year at age 46–50—a further similarity, lasting about 20 years, becomes apparent before divergence beginning in 1945 (Fig. 6.16). The extent to which the cross-sectional age distribution of fertility shifts steadily toward younger ages in these two decades approximates the extent to which cohorts then at the end of childbearing (and therefore little involved in the cross-sectional distribution during these years) have shifted fertility increasingly toward younger ages. Total

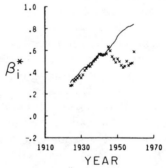

Fig. 6.16   Segments of time parameter β_i^* for the C15 ($\times \times \times$) and X15 (——) sequences, 1775–1959, with β_i^* for the C15 sequence centered on year at age 46–50.

fertility rates exhibit quite different changes, however: cross-sectional total rate expressed as the mean number of births per woman drops from 2.43 to 1.70 and then rises again to 2.60; total rate for the 21 cohorts aged 46–50 from 1924 to 1944 declines steadily from 3.43 to 2.06 (Figs. 6.10 and 6.11). If β_i^* for the C15 sequence is standardized for level of fertility—that is, if we consider only the portion of β_i^* that is associated with change in the timing of childbearing apart from change in the level of fertility—we can interpret further the trends and divergences in β_i^* for the C15 and X15 sequences.

Transitions and Cohort Timing of Childbearing

In the first section of this chapter, we constructed for the 55-cohort SYAC13 sequence two related measures of the cohort pace of childbearing apart from the level of completed fertility: $\beta_{i\cdot T}^*$, the portion of change in β_i^* that is not inversely related to the change in total rate across the sequence; and $\bar{a}_i^s$, the cohort-specific mean age of childbearing at a selected standard level of fertility across the sequence. Our proposal that differences in the age pattern of entry into childbearing should be the largest determinant of differences in pace was highly consistent with the prominent variations reported in the age pattern of marriage for the SYAC13 cohorts. In that example, we worked with the cohorts aged 15 from 1885/1886 to 1939/1940, for which we had single-year-of-age data on both fertility and marriage. We now propose that the same relations exist between the measures of pace and the age pattern of entry into childbearing for the 1775–1884 cohorts, for which we have the EHR-derived fertility parameters by 5-year age groups, but less detailed and less certain information about marriage patterns.

The coefficients from the independent regression of α_i^* and β_i^* for the C15 sequence on $T_i^{1/2}$ confirm the minimal association of change in α_i^* and the high association of change in β_i^* with the change in total rate (Table 6.2). The systematic variations in $\beta_{i\cdot T}^*$ over time reveal changes in β_i^* that are *not* inversely related to the change in total rate (Fig. 6.17). The cohorts with positive $\beta_{i\cdot T}^*$ values are those whose age pattern of fertility is shifted more toward ages below 30 than would correspond on the average to the level of fertility; the cohorts with negative $\beta_{i\cdot T}^*$ values are those with older age patterns of fertility than would correspond on the average to the level.

When level-standardized distributions of fertility are constructed from $\alpha_{i\cdot T}^*$ and $\beta_{i\cdot T}^*$ for the C15 sequence at a selected standard fertility level T_s or T_m, as in the preceding section for the single-year-of-age cohorts, the mean age of childbearing $\bar{a}_i^s$ at that standard level can be calculated for

TABLE 6.2

Regression Coefficients and Constants in the Linear
Compensation of EHR Time Parameters for the Level of
Fertility, Total Fertility Rate Implied by $\hat{\beta}_i^* = 0$: Selected Overall
Fertility Sequences 1775–1976

Parameter[a]	Regression coefficient	Constant	$5T_{\mathrm{m}}$
Two-component fit			
SYAC13 α_i^*	.059	4.171	—
β_i^*	−1.350	2.803	4.31[b]
C15 α_i^*	−.014	1.491	—
β_i^*	−1.602	1.552	4.69
County α_i^*	−.040	1.516	—
β_i^*	−2.012	1.968	4.78
Three-component fit			
X202 α_i^*	−.072	1,501	—
β_i^*	−2.061	1.902	4.26
γ_i^*	.029	.035	—

[a] All parameters are compensated for the time vector of $T_i^{1/2}$ for the particular sequence involved.
[b] The total fertility level shown for the SYAC13 sequence is T_{m}, *not* $5T_{\mathrm{m}}$.

each of the 155 cohorts.[5] This summary measure is shown in Fig. 6.17 for the level $T_{\mathrm{m}} = 4.69$, at which β_i^* would equal zero if $T_i^{1/2}$ and β_i^* varied exactly inversely across the sequence. The mean age $\bar{a}_i^{\mathrm{s}}$ for the C15 sequence exhibits the same time course of variation as does $\beta_{i\cdot\mathrm{T}}^*$, but in mirror image. An increase of .10 in $\beta_{i\cdot\mathrm{T}}^*$ for the C15 sequence is equivalent to a .6-year decline in the mean age of childbearing at a standard level of fertility. This relation is independent of the level used for standardization because the mean age $\bar{a}_i^{\mathrm{s}}$ would have the same spread and the same time course at any standard level selected (see Fig. 6.7). To bring together the evidence of the onset of changes in the age pattern of entry into childbearing, the evidence of cohort fertility decline at higher ages, and the manifestations of these changes in cross-sectional patterns, we shall return to the earliest cohorts and move through the time sequence systematically by the groups of cohorts that can be identified in Fig. 6.17.

Cohorts Aged 15–19 before 1805   The fluctuation of $\beta_{i\cdot\mathrm{T}}^*$ around a fairly constant value (zero, in this case) indicates that these cohorts differ from each other very little in the timing of entry into childbearing. The regularity emerges even though the cohorts exhibit greater fluctuation in β_i^* and T_i than do subsequent cohorts. The variability is thus described by a

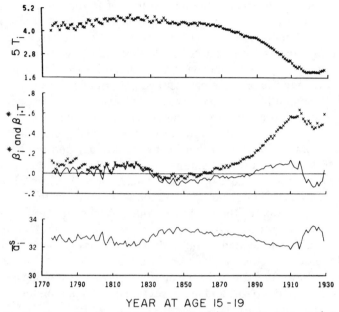

Fig. 6.17 Total rate of fertility $5T_i$, time parameter β_i^* ($\times \times \times$) before and $\beta_{i\cdot T}^*$ (———) after linear compensation for the total rate, and mean age of childbearing, $\bar{a}_i^s$ at the standard level of fertility $T_m = 4.69$ for the C15 sequence: cohorts aged 15–19 from 1775 to 1929.

generally inverse, level-predicted relation between change in β_i^* and change in the level of fertility: the higher β_i^* value of a younger childbearing pattern is associated with lower fertility and the lower β_i^* value of an older pattern is associated with higher fertility. This variability could be caused by errors that have commonly been assumed to exist in the early "Grunddragen" data, particularly in the eighteenth century. These include errors in population totals, omission of births that did not occur in the parish where the mother was registered, and misplacement of births in time or by age of mother (see Chapter II and the discussion later in this chapter). If it is not due to errors in the data, variation of the type observed must be assigned to considerable cohort-to-cohort variation in childbearing at ages 30 and higher.

Cohorts Aged 15–19 from 1805 to 1825 For these cohorts the mean number of births per woman is the highest in the sequence and has relatively small fluctuations. Their younger-than-level-predicted fertility pattern ($\beta_{i\cdot T}^* \simeq .07$) shows only small variations except for the 1808–1810 cohorts, which are composed of women who entered childbearing ages during the time of the Russian war. The change from the pattern of the preceding cohorts, for which the age pattern of fertility is generally the level-predicted one ($\beta^*_{i \cdot T} \simeq 0$), represents a decline of about .4 of a year in the mean age of childbearing at a standard level of fertility (see Fig. 6.17). For these 21 cohorts we might conclude that the higher total rate is accounted for by an earlier age pattern of entry into childbearing—that these cohorts experienced the earliest age pattern of marriage before the end of the nineteenth century. We would then ask how this happened at a time of increasing pressure for further restriction on marriage (see Chapter II). Alternatively, we could adopt Quensel's view (cited in Hofsten and Lundstrom, 1976, p. 154) that births were underreported before the reporting requirements were tightened in 1801. We would then conclude that the total rates for most of the pre-1805 cohorts were too low. The more that a cohort's childbearing years fell within the eighteenth century the more underestimated the total rate would be. Higher rates, if applicable to all ages proportionately, would tend to raise the level of $\beta^*_{i \cdot T}$ and therefore modify the evidence that indicates a later age pattern of entry into childbearing for the pre-1805 cohorts than for the 1805 to 1825 cohorts. Procedures for examining the alternatives and estimating data revisions based on both cohort and cross-sectional EHR parameters are considered later in this chapter.

Cohorts Aged 15–19 from 1825 to 1836   These cohorts carry out a transition from a younger-than-level-predicted fertility pattern ($\beta^*_{i \cdot T} > 0$) to an older-than-level-predicted pattern ($\beta^*_{i \cdot T} < 0$), a transition we interpret as a change to an increasingly later age pattern of entry into marriage and childbearing.

Cohorts Aged 15–19 from 1837 to 1851   For these 15 cohorts the older fertility pattern indicated by $\beta^*_i < 0$ and the later pattern of entry into childbearing indicated by $\beta^*_{i \cdot T} < 0$ continue with only small fluctuations in pattern and total fertility rate.

Cohorts Aged 15–19 from 1852 to 1866   Following the cohorts with the oldest childbearing patterns in the sequence (lowest β^*_i values) and the oldest level-standardized patterns (most negative $\beta^*_{i \cdot T}$ values), these cohorts begin a transition to a younger pattern and earlier marriage. The total rate, however, remains relatively unchanged ($\Delta T_i \simeq 0$). This is the expected outcome from an increase in childbearing at younger ages that is fully offset by a decline at higher ages so that the average number of births per woman remains the same, the difference being one of timing. We therefore have a new basis on which to speculate with Hofsten and Lundstrom (1976) and Eriksson and Rogers (1978) that the total fertility rate, never high in Sweden, may reflect fertility limitation by means in addition to nonmarriage well before the sustained decline in fertility generally considered to start about 1880 with the cohorts aged 15 after 1865. In the last section of this chapter we shall consider evidence for regional differences in fertility limitation that may be obscured in national averages.

Cohorts Aged 15–19 from 1867 to 1890   The stable level-standardized pattern of fertility ($\Delta\beta^*_{i\cdot T} \simeq 0$) suggests that the age pattern of entry into childbearing is not changing for these cohorts and that the continued change toward a younger age pattern of fertility ($\Delta\beta^*_i > 0$) is attributable to the decline of childbearing at higher ages. The fact that $\beta^*_{i\cdot T}$ remains slightly negative indicates that the increasing values of β^*_i describe consistently slightly older age patterns of fertility than would correspond, on the average, to the declining level of fertility. The first cohort in this group, the cohort aged 15–19 in 1867 and therefore aged 26–30 in 1878, marks the first divergence of β^*_i values for the C15 and X15 sequences (see Fig. 6.14).

Post-1890 Cohorts   The second divergence of β^*_i values for the C15 and X15 sequences (Fig. 6.15) begins with the cohort aged 15–19 in 1891 and therefore aged 33–37 in 1909. This is the first of a group of cohorts that adopted a younger-than-level-predicted pattern of fertility ($\beta^*_{i\cdot T} > 0$ in Fig. 6.17) combined with slightly earlier marriage (Figs. 6.5 and 6.8). The similarity of change in independent cohort and cross-sectional experience as shown in Fig. 6.16 involves the cohorts aged 15–19 from 1895 to 1915— all cohorts having the younger-than-level-predicted pattern.

The evidence revealed by $\beta^*_{i\cdot T}$ for the C15 sequence on cohort stability and cohort transitions in the timing of childbearing apart from the level of fertility has made two contributions to our analysis of two centuries of Swedish fertility experience. One, it has aided interpretation of the nature of cohort effects on cross-sectional fertility patterns in various periods, including the pre-1860 periods of flawed data. Two, it has provided an indicator of change in the age pattern of entry into childbearing that is particularly useful in examining the eighteenth- and nineteenth-century periods of less detailed and less certain information on the marital status of women by age.

Fertility Patterns during Periods
of High Emigration

One of the purposes of our EHR analysis is to develop sufficiently stable and close-fitting descriptions of fertility trends so that brief departures from trend due to unusual circumstances can be identified, either in the fitted parameters or the residuals. Such departures in overall fertility have already been noted for the World War I period and the early 1940s. These departures are discussed in Chapter VII in relation to marital fertility and in Chapter VIII in comparison with U.S. fertility experience.

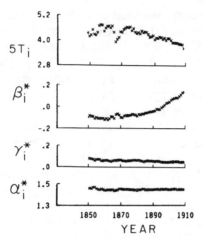

Fig. 6.18   EHR time parameters α_i^*, β_i^*, and γ_i^* and total fertility rate $5T_i$ across periods of high emigration from 1850 to 1910 (segment of Fig. 6.12).

Departures from trend in the age pattern of fertility might also be expected during the periods of high emigration in the latter half of the nineteenth century. Thomas (1941, p. 90) observes that this "movement did not progress evenly to a maximum nor having spent its strength, decline gradually to a minimum, but proceeded rather in a series of great waves." The first, rapidly building crest appeared in 1868–1869 when more than 65,000 people are reported to have left the country. Subsequent crests appeared in 1881–1882, 1887–1888, and 1891–1893, with annual population losses of about 50,000 in 1882, 1887, and 1888. Noting that emigration was highly concentrated in the 15–29 age range for all these periods, Hofsten and Lundstrom (1976) cite official reports of 1877 and 1879 on the changing composition of the emigrant group: from 1860 onward the proportion of family groups decreased, the proportion of single adult males increased, and the number of males who left their wife and children in Sweden increased.

To focus on fertility patterns for the high emigration periods in their nineteenth-century context, we examine in Fig. 6.18 the 1850–1910 segment of Fig. 6.12. The oldest age patterns of childbearing identified for Sweden—$\beta_i^* = -.10$ to $-.12$ from 1854 to 1866—precede the first wave of emigration by only a few years. The trend across all the periods of high emigration is for the development of a younger childbearing pattern than in the preceding decades.

The only prominent departure from trend begins slightly *before* the 1868–1869 wave of emigration. As measured by an increase in β_i^*, the age pattern of fertility becomes suddenly younger in 1867–1869 (that is, for conceptions occurring between April 1866 and March 1869) and reverts to an older pattern in 1870–1871 (that is, for conceptions occurring between April 1869 and March 1871). The total fertility rate begins falling in 1867 (the result of fewer conceptions occurring between April 1866 and March 1867), reaches its lowest level in 1868, and recovers only slightly before 1871. The concurrent decline in fertility level and change to a younger fertility pattern in 1867–1869 suggest a disproportionately greater reduction of childbearing at ages 30 and higher than ages lower than 30 during those years. Unless there are data errors that distort the age pattern and level of fertility for this period, we can claim evidence for the limitation of fertility at higher ages in response to circumstances that also led to a period of high emigration. In the age pattern of fertility for the nonemigrants, the subsequent periods of high emigration—1881–1882, 1887–1888, and 1891–1893—are identified only by brief pauses ($\Delta\beta_i^* \leq 0$) in the development of a younger childbearing pattern.

The view that the period associated with the 1868–1869 wave of emigration was the only high emigration period with a pronounced effect on the age pattern of fertility is supported by the cohort residuals from EHR fits to the C15 sequence. A diagonal segment of these residuals taken from Fig. 4.7 is shown in Fig. 6.19 to emphasize period effects on cohort patterns (see Fig. 4.9 for background information). Note first the prominent positive residuals associated with the years 1862–1866. The effects are apparent at all age cuts above 19/20: at age cut 24/25 for the cohorts aged 15–19 in 1857–1861, at age cut 29/30 for the cohorts aged 15–19 in 1852–1856, and similarly for earlier cohorts at higher age cuts. Then note the negative residuals associated with the following years, particularly 1868–1870 at age cut 34/35 for the cohorts aged 15–19 from 1853 to 1855 and at age cut 39/40 for the cohorts aged 15–19 from 1848 to 1850. No similarly prominent positive or negative residuals are associated with the periods of high emigration in the 1880s.

Cohort versus Cross-sectional Evidence for Data Points of Lesser Accuracy

We have examined the well-defined trends and transitions in the age pattern of fertility revealed by the EHR parameters. We have also considered some period-specific departures from trend and some effects that data errors may have on the interpretation of change or difference. We shall now ask two, more general questions. One, what is the evidence for errors in the pre-1860 data from "Grunddragen"? Two, what procedures

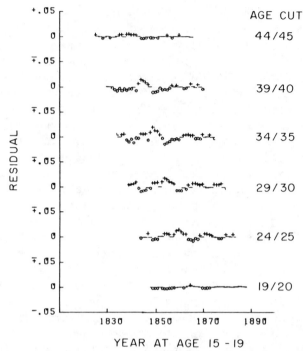

RESIDUAL

YEAR AT AGE 15 - 19

Fig. 6.19   Effect of high emigration periods on the age pattern of fertility: evidence in cohort residuals (diagonal segment of Fig. 4.7).

for revision of the single-year historical data are suggested by the exploratory analysis results? We have both cross-sectional and cohort indications of error. These indications appear in both the fitted parameters and the residuals.

In a cross-sectional perspective, we observe that the calculated total fertility rate varies widely from year to year before 1870 (Fig. 6.11). In contrast, the time parameters α_i^* and β_i^* for the X15 and X20 sequences are characterized by small year-to-year irregularity (Fig. 6.11), particularly for α_i^* after 1815 and β_i^* after 1822. The only pre-1860 singular departures are the high β_i^* value in 1783, the change from a high to a very low β_i^* value in 1790–1792, and the 1822–1823 discontinuity in the value of β_i^*. The more detailed fits developed for the *X202* sequence do not alter the identification of these years as aberrant (Fig. 6.12).[6] The years 1783 and 1792 also stand out in the residuals (see Figs. 4.5 and 4.6). Other irregular but lesser departures from fit before about 1815 are more apparent in the *X202* residuals (see Fig. 4.6)—that is, after additional pattern has been removed in the third component $\gamma_i^* C_j^*$—than in the X15 residuals (see Fig. 4.5).

A surprisingly stable picture of pre-1860 age patterns of fertility emerges from the age-specific rates that are based on the "Grunddragen" birth and population data. This suggests that nonsystematic error in the "Grunddragen" data may be less than what it is generally thought to be (see Chapter II). With minor revisions, these data could provide a fairly accurate representation of eighteenth- and early nineteenth-century *age patterns* of fertility even though the *level* of fertility may be in error for many of the years.[7]

The cohort sequences constructed from the cross-sectional, age-specific rates should reflect any year-specific errors in level in two ways. First, the less accurate rates for a specific year would be disseminated across seven cohorts at one 5-year age group in each cohort. Thus the age pattern of births in each cohort would be distorted in a different way. Second, the cohort total rate, which is the sum of the sometimes more, sometimes less accurate age-specific rates across the seven age groups for a cohort, would serve to average errors in the cross-sectional total rate. Cohort total rate should thus follow a smoother course than does cross-sectional total rate.[8]

The results of the EHR cohort analyses are consistent with such a dissemination of cross-sectional errors. For the C15 and C20 sequences, jumpiness is evident in the plots of both α_i^* and β_i^* at about 5-year intervals for the cohorts aged 15–19 before 1815 (Fig. 6.10). Cohort total rates are much less irregular than cross-sectional total rates, but they are less stable for cohorts aged 15–19 before 1840 than for later cohorts. In the cohort residuals (see Fig. 4.7), the backward diagonal of period effects on cohort fertility patterns, although apparent for the pre-1850 cohorts, is less clearly defined for these early cohorts than for later cohorts.

With two perspectives on the data in hand, we now ask what procedures would identify "true" differences in cross-sectional patterns and total rates and would estimate revisions for spurious differences? We propose to work backward, reconstructing cross-sectional rates from cohort rates after fine tuning the cohort fits. This will again be an iterative, data-guided process. The following six steps provide one possible procedure for beginning the revisions.

1. Assume that the α_i^* and β_i^* parameters for the late eighteenth- and early nineteenth-century cohorts should have no more cohort-to-cohort variation than do those for later nineteenth-century cohorts and apply to both α_i^* and β_i^* an appropriate compound, nonlinear smoothing procedure

(see Tukey, 1977, pp. 205–264 and 523–542). This would de-emphasize irregular fluctuations while retaining systematic variations in the revised parameters. Parameters revised in this manner will be termed α_i' and β_i'.

2. Construct a first revision to the age distributions of cohort fertility

$$\hat{F}_{ij} = \alpha_i' A_j^* + \beta_i' B_j^*$$

for cohorts $i = 1, 2, \ldots, m$ and age cuts $j = 1, 2, \ldots, n$ and obtain a set of additional residuals

$$z_{ij}' = (\alpha_i^* A_j^* + \beta_i^* B_j^*) - (\alpha_i' A_j^* + \beta_i' B_j^*)$$

to supplement the residuals z_{ij} obtained in the original fitting procedure.

3. Submit the revised set of residuals

$$\hat{z}_{ij} = z_{ij} + z_{ij}'$$

by age cut $j = 1, 2, \ldots, n$ to the nonlinear smoothing procedures to bring out more clearly the systematic variations that reflect "true" period effects on cohort patterns while separating out the "true" error terms. That is, for each age cut $j = 1, 2, \ldots, n$, separate $\hat{z}_{ij}$ into two vectors

$$\hat{z}_{ij} = \hat{z}_{ij}(\text{smooth}) + \hat{z}_{ij}(\text{rough}).$$

4. Update the revised cohort cumulative fertility distributions as

$$\hat{F}_{ij} = \alpha_i' A_j^* + \beta_i' B_j^* + \hat{z}_{ij}(\text{smooth}).$$

De-transform these distributions from the folded square root scale to the raw fraction scale (see Chapter VIII for the procedure) and de-cumulate them to yield for each cohort a revised proportion of total fertility accounted for by each 5-year age group.

5. Submit the cohort total rates T_i to nonlinear smoothing to yield two vectors

$$T_i = T_i(\text{smooth}) + T_i(\text{rough}).$$

Obtain estimates of cohort age-specific rates by multiplying the age distributions of fertility from step 4 by the corresponding values of $T_i(\text{smooth})$.

6. Assemble revised cross-sectional, age-specific fertility schedules from the revised cohort, age-specific schedules.[9]

In the search for coherent revisions, the analyst should be prepared to adjust the conditions for fine tuning the cohort fits several times. The time parameters α_i^* and β_i^* and the total rates T_i for the full sequence should be retained throughout the revision as a check on the procedures. The following questions could be used to test the appropriateness of any tentative set of revised schedules.

1. Have the age-specific rates for the portions of cohort experience that occurred in the latter half of the nineteenth century undergone relatively little change in the revision process?
2. Have the results achieved greater stability in the pre-1860, cross-sectional total fertility rates while diminishing (or at least not increasing) the year-to-year variability in the cross-sectional *age pattern* of fertility expressed in normalized age-specific rates?
3. Have period effects on cohort fertility patterns been sharpened in the revised and smoothed set of residuals?
4. Have any demographically inconsistent changes been introduced in the revised rates?

Clearly, a broad understanding of fertility data and a knowledge of Sweden's social history will continue to be important guides in further steps of exploratory analysis. Several examples of the revision or estimation of marital fertility rates on the basis of intersequence relations of EHR parameters will be reported in Chapter VII.

Fertility Change in the Counties of Sweden from 1860 to 1970

This section illustrates the use of national EHR fertility standards to reveal subpopulation similarities and differences that are not apparent in total fertility rates. We shall look for evidence of periods of regional change in the age pattern of fertility to use in more detailed study of relations between fertility and the complex history of social and economic change in the counties of Sweden. Previous studies have used more general measures of fertility: births per thousand total population (the crude birth rate) or births to married and unmarried women in the broad age group 15–50 (Friedlander, 1969; Hyrenius, 1946; Institute for Social Sciences, 1941; Mosher, 1980; Thomas, 1941). Comparisons between fertility change and social change have been hampered by the lack of better fertility measures for small geographic areas, as Thomas, Friedlander, and Mosher all point out.

The EHR measures, which incorporate the more detailed county fertility data now available, provide a new set of appropriate descriptions of fertility change for the extension of previous studies. The insights on modernization and migration recently articulated by Anderson (1982) provide a basis for further assessment of the abundant data on Swedish social and economic change.[10] In particular, the relation between fertility

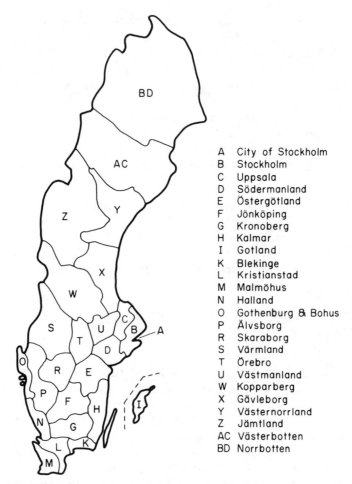

A   City of Stockholm
B   Stockholm
C   Uppsala
D   Södermanland
E   Östergötland
F   Jönköping
G   Kronoberg
H   Kalmar
I   Gotland
K   Blekinge
L   Kristianstad
M   Malmöhus
N   Halland
O   Gothenburg & Bohus
P   Älvsborg
R   Skaraborg
S   Värmland
T   Örebro
U   Västmanland
W   Kopparberg
X   Gävleborg
Y   Västernorrland
Z   Jämtland
AC Västerbotten
BD Norrbotten

Fig. 6.20   The counties of Sweden. County outlines and letter designations are taken from Hofsten and Lundstrom (1976).

change and timing and types of migration, urban and rural industrialization, and the changing social structure of the agricultural population merit
further detailed analysis for all regions of the country. We shall concentrate on the identification of periods of change in the fertility patterns and
comment only briefly on their possible relations to social change. It is the
Hofsten and Lundstrom (1976) calculated fertility rates for the counties of
Sweden that we shall examine in EHR terms (see Chapter III for a description of these county sequences of age-specific rates centered on cen-

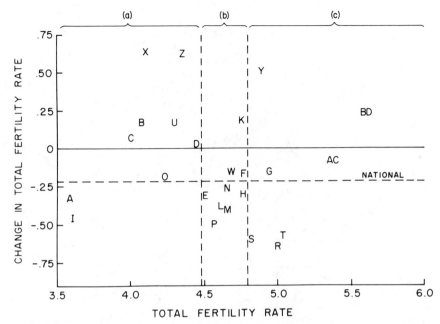

Fig. 6.21 Changes in county and national total fertility rates between 1860 and 1880 in relation to 1860 rates: (a) total fertility $<(M - \frac{1}{4}I)$, (b) total fertility from $(M - \frac{1}{4}I)$ to $(M + \frac{1}{4}I)$, and (c) total fertility $>(M + \frac{1}{4}I)$.

sus years). The Hofsten and Lundstrom county outlines and letter designations (Fig. 6.20) have been adopted for the maps and discussion.

The Route from Diversity to Similarity
in Rate and Pattern

In 1970 the city of Stockholm (classified as a separate county until 1968), with a total fertility rate of 1.4 births per woman, was the only one of Sweden's 25 counties to have a rate outside the range 1.9–2.1. In contrast, the diversity of the counties in 1860 is apparent in rates ranging from 3.6 for the city of Stockholm (A) and the island of Gotland (I) to levels between 5.0 and 5.5 for the two most northern counties, Västerbotten (AC) and Norrbotten (BD), and two of the central counties. Örebro (T) and Skaraborg (R). With a median county rate $M = 4.6$ (also the national rate) and an interquartile range of rates $I = .6$, nine counties had 1860 rates in the range $M - \frac{1}{4}I$ to $M + \frac{1}{4}I$, nine were below this range, and seven were above this range (Fig. 6.21).

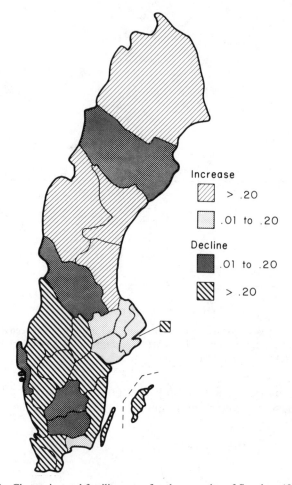

Fig. 6.22 Change in total fertility rates for the counties of Sweden, 1860–1880.

The diversity of the counties is further apparent in the changes in total rates between 1860 and 1880. For the country as a whole, the small difference (about $-.22$) between the total rate in 1860 and the total rate in 1880 obscures the fact that 9 counties experienced an *increase* in rate during this period and 11 counties experienced a greater decrease than the national average (Figs. 6.21 and 6.22). Six of the counties with an increase had lower rates and three had higher rates in 1860 than did the country as a whole; two of the counties with a decrease greater than the national average were the lowest-fertility counties in the country in 1860 and three were among the highest-fertility counties (Fig. 6.21).

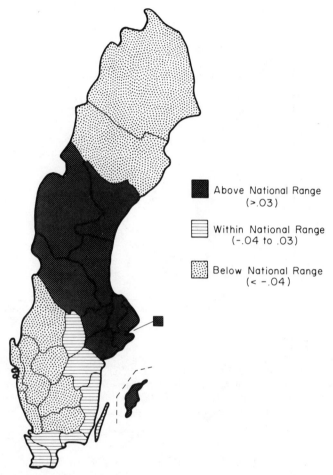

Fig. 6.23   EHR time parameter β_i^* for the counties of Sweden in relation to the national value of β_i^*, 1860–1880.

To discover the patterns that underlie the geographic and numeric diversity of total fertility rates at the beginning of the county sequences and the near convergence of the rates at the end, EHR descriptions of the cumulated, normalized age-specific rates are developed for each county at 15 time periods, using A_j^* and B_j^* for the X15 sequence as the age standards in the least squares regressions[11] (see Chapter VIII for procedure). This permits, first, a comparison of the change in the fertility patterns of the counties over time in relation to the national pattern of change. Linear compensation of the second time parameter β_i^* for change in the total fertility rate across all counties and all time periods then permits direct

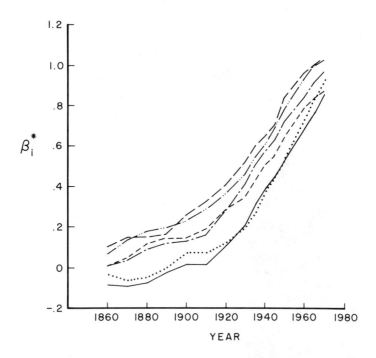

Fig. 6.24   Time parameter β_i^* from the regression of age-specific fertility sequences for the counties of Sweden (1860–1970) on the A_j^* and B_j^* age vectors for the X15 sequence: counties with rising values of β_i^* followed by a plateau in the period 1860–1900 [Väst-manland (U, — —), Gävleborg (X, — · · —), Västernorrland (Y, — — —), and Jämtland (Z, – – –)] and the counties of Västerbotten (AC, ——) and Norrbotten (BD, · · ·).

comparisons of county fertility patterns at a standard fertility level without reference to the national pattern.

The first time parameter α_i^* varies over a narrow range for the counties, essentially the same range as that for the country as a whole. The second time parameter β_i^*, which expresses most of the differences between counties and between periods, is used to group counties by similar time courses of change in the extent to which the age distribution of childbearing is shifted from ages 30 and higher to ages lower than 30 according to the pattern determined by B_j^*. In Fig. 6.23 counties are grouped by their starting point: whether the value of β_i^* is greater than, less than, or approximately equal to the national level from 1860 to 1880. Recall that a higher value of β_i^* corresponds to a younger age pattern of fertility. Essentially the same geographic groupings are identified (with a few exceptions) when the criteria given in Fig. 6.23 are related to the behavior of β_i^*

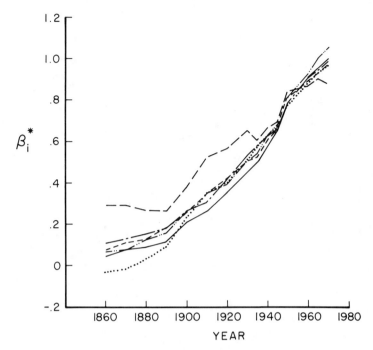

Fig. 6.25 Time parameter β_i^* from the regression of age-specific fertility sequences for the counties of Sweden (1860–1970) on the A_j^* and B_j^* age vectors for the X15 sequence: counties with gradually rising values of β_i^* from 1860 to 1900 [Stockholm (B, – – –), Uppsala (C, — – —), Södermanland (D, — · · —), Malmöhus (M, · · ·), and Kopparberg (W, ——)] and the city of Stockholm (A, — —).

between 1860 and 1900. Four groups that include 21 counties can be distinguished on this basis (Figs. 6.24–6.27). Sequences of β_i^* values for the four remaining counties are sufficiently distinctive that they have been included in whichever figure allows their variation to be examined most easily, even though the sequences may meet some of the criteria for a different group.

The first two groups, taken together, comprise nine counties that have a rising β_i^* value from the beginning of the sequence. This suggests that the shift of these distributions toward younger ages began before 1860. For all of these counties but Malmöhus (M), β_i^* is positive from 1860 onward, whereas in 1860 the national value of β_i^* is at its lowest point (−.04) for the two centuries analyzed (Fig. 6.11). Two possible explanations for the higher 1860 value of β_i^* for counties such as Stockholm (B), Uppsala (C), and Södermanland (D) are: one, they experienced to a relatively lesser extent the shift toward later childbearing that began about 1830 at the

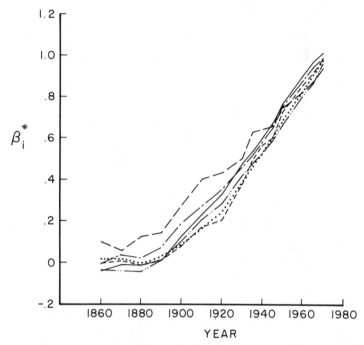

Fig. 6.26 Time parameter β_i^* from the regression of age-specific fertility sequences for the counties of Sweden (1860–1970) on the A_j^* and B_j^* age vectors for the X15 sequence: counties with values of β_i^* near the national level from 1860 to 1880 [Östergötland (E, — — —), Kalmar (H, · · ·), Blekinge (K, – – –), Kristianstad (L, — · · —), and Örebro (T, ——)] and the county of Gotland (I, — —).

national level or, two, they had a younger fertility pattern before 1830 than did the majority of counties.

Four of the nine counties—Västmanland (U), Gävleborg (X), Västernorrland (Y), and Jämtland (Z)—exhibit a pronounced rise in the value of β_i^* and then a deceleration or a plateau before resuming the trend toward an increasingly younger pattern (Fig. 6.24). Two factors suggest that change in the composition of the population may underlie these changes in the age distribution of fertility: one, the concomitant rise in the total rate of all four counties—enough in Gävleborg and Jämtland to carry them into the group of highest fertility counties, which already includes Västernorrland (Fig. 6.21) and, two, the fact that these four counties are among the few reported to have positive net migration during this period (Hofsten and Lundstrom, 1976).

Västerbotten (AC) and Norrbotten (BD), the two most northern counties, are included in Fig. 6.24 to make the distinctively different progres-

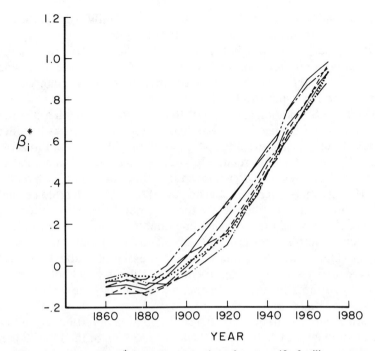

Fig. 6.27 Time parameter β_i^* from the regression of age-specific fertility sequences for the counties of Sweden (1860–1970) on the A_j^* and B_j^* age vectors for the X15 sequence: counties with values of β_i^* below the national level from 1860 to 1880 [Jönköping (F, $\cdots$), Kronoberg (G, $-\cdot\cdot-$), Halland (N, $-\ -$), Gothenburg and Bohus (O, $-\ -\ -\ -$), Älvsborg (P, $---$), Skaraborg (R, $---$), and Värmland (S, $-$)].

sion of change in their fertility patterns more apparent. A plateau also occurs in the plot of β_i^* for these counties, but it begins several decades later than for the other counties in Fig. 6.24. Because of their older-than-average fertility pattern from 1860 to 1880, Västerbotten and Norrbotten belong with the counties in Fig. 6.27 in the early decades. They then change to a younger pattern from 1880 to 1900 at the same rate as do the southeastern counties in Fig. 6.26 until this progression is interrupted by a plateau. Västerbotten never regains as young a pattern as exhibited by the other counties and Norrbotten does so only in the last decade of the sequence. When the level-compensated changes expressed by $\beta_{i\cdot T}^*$ are considered, the relations between fertility change and migration for all the northern counties will emerge more clearly.

Of the five counties that exhibit a more gradual but continued rise in the level of β_i^* during the first decades of the sequence (Fig. 6.25), Stockholm (B), Uppsala (C), and Södermanland (D) cluster closely throughout the sequence, while Kopparberg (W) maintains its slightly older pattern until 1935. Malmöhus (M) accelerates rapidly from 1890 to 1910 toward adoption of the youngest pattern in the group. This change could reasonably be examined not only in relation to the growth of Malmö (one of Sweden's major urban centers) and the growth of other towns in the county but also in relation to rural industrialization.

The city of Stockholm (A), one of the four counties with a distinctive time sequence of change in the age distribution of fertility, is included in Fig. 6.25 to emphasize the differences in its β_i^* pattern from those of the surrounding counties. Its relatively younger pattern is maintained from 1860 to 1890 at a level of β_i^* achieved by other counties only by 1900 or later. The city then enters a 4-decade period of change at a rate not unlike that of some other counties. Only for the brief 1945–1950 period, however, are the city and the surrounding counties similar in both regards: how young a fertility pattern they have and how rapidly the pattern is changing. Only when the changes are expressed at a standard level of fertility can we see the similarity of the city of Stockholm's fertility pattern to patterns in the rest of the country across the whole time sequence.

A third group of counties has an age distribution of fertility close to that for the country as a whole in the 1860–1880 section of the time sequence (Figs. 6.23 and 6.26). In the crescent-shaped area formed by the counties of Örebro (T), Östergötland (E), Kalmar (H), Blekinge (K), and Kristianstad (L), a shift toward a younger pattern indicated by an increase in β_i^* begins about 1890 and then accelerates. Between 1890 and 1920, the acceleration of change for Örebro is sufficient for it to join Östergötland at the forefront of the group. Gotland (I), the island county off the southeastern coast of Sweden, is included in Fig. 6.26 to allow examination of its distinctively irregular progression of change in β_i^*. In all periods up to 1940, Gotland presents an overall younger childbearing pattern than those for the other five counties shown in Fig. 6.26—a pattern more like those for some of the mainland counties to the north (see Fig. 6.25).

Of the seven counties beside Västerbotten (AC) and Norrbotten (BD) with β_i^* values below the national level from 1860 to 1880 (Fig. 6.27), all but Jönköping (F) and Kronoberg (G) begin the shift to a younger childbearing pattern by 1890. Gothenburg and Bohus (O), which contains one of Sweden's major urban centers, quickly changes to the pattern of the group in Fig. 6.26 that started with β_i^* near the national level and by 1920 Värmland (S) has also joined this group. In contrast, the pace of change for Halland (N) slows noticeably between 1900 and 1920 and the pattern for this county then becomes similar to that for Jönköping and Kronoberg, which delayed the development of a younger pattern until 1900. The pace of change for Kronoberg lags behind the pace for the rest of this group of counties until 1930.

The plots of β_i^* against time provide clues to periods of broader change in the counties when similar fertility patterns diverge or dissimilar patterns converge. The level-compensated parameter $\beta_{i\cdot T}^*$ which allows us to view β_i^* across all counties and in all 15 periods at a standard level of fertility, suggests more about what factors may underlie the county fertility patterns and provides a few surprises.

Change in Level-standardized Fertility Patterns

The multiple regressions of the 25 × 15 matrices of county α_i^* and β_i^* time parameters independently on the matrix of county $T_i^{1/2}$ values confirm that change in α_i^* is little related to change in the total rate of fertility, whereas change in β_i^* is highly related to change in the total rate (Table 6.2). Interpretation of the resulting level-compensated parameter $\beta_{i\cdot T}^*$ for cross-sectional data across many counties differs from the interpretation of $\beta_{i\cdot T}^*$ for cohorts that was described earlier in this chapter. There, with the childbearing experience of all cohorts translated to a standard level of fertility, we related the experience of women at lower ages to that of the survivors at higher ages across all cohorts in a single time sequence. Here, with childbearing experience at all points in time and in all 25 counties translated to a standard level of fertility, we shall relate the experience of younger women to that of women who are older during the same time period in comparisons across time both within and between counties. We shall therefore interpret the regression residuals $\beta_{i\cdot T}^*$ in the following way.

$\beta_{i\cdot T}^* > 0$ Women below age 30 account for a disproportionately larger fraction of a county's total fertility during a particular time period (and women aged 30 and above account for a correspondingly smaller fraction) than would be predicted from relating the age distribution of fertility to the total rate across all counties and all time periods

$\beta_{i\cdot T}^* < 0$ Women aged 30 and above account for a disproportionately larger fraction of a county's total fertility during a particular time period than would be predicted in a comparison across all counties and all time periods

The $\beta_{i\cdot T}^*$ time sequences guide division of the counties into two major groups: those that experience a period of disproportionately higher childbearing for ages lower than 30 at some time before 1920 (Fig. 6.28 and the counties of Gotland (I) and Malmöhus (M) in Fig. 6.29) and those for

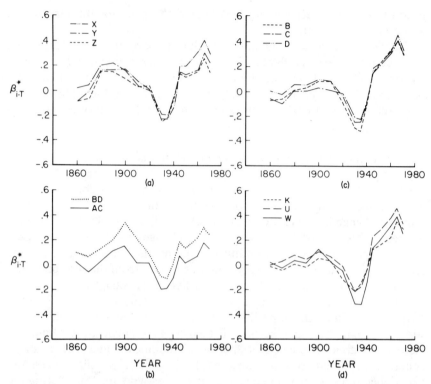

Fig. 6.28   Level-compensated time parameter $\beta^*_{i \cdot T}$ for the counties of Sweden 1860–1970: counties with a younger-than-level-predicted pattern of childbearing at some time before 1920 [(a), Gävleborg (X), Västernorrland (Y), and Jämtland (Z); (b), Norrbotten (BD) and Västerbotten (AC); (c), Stockholm (B), Uppsala (C), and Södermanland (D); (d), Blekinge (K), Västmanland (U), and Kopparberg (W)].

which $\beta^*_{i \cdot T}$ does not rise above zero until the general transition in 1945 to a younger-than-level-predicted childbearing pattern (the remaining counties in Fig. 6.29). The pre-1920 periods of positive $\beta^*_{i \cdot T}$ values, most prominent for the five northern counties, reach their peak in Gävleborg (X), Västernorrland (Y), and Jämtland (Z) a decade before they peak in Västerbotten (AC) and very prominently in Norrbotten (BD) (Fig. 6.28a,b). For all of these five counties except Västerbotten, these periods of younger-than-level-predicted age distributions of fertility coincide with periods of reported net in-migration as first the sawmill industry and then the mining industry expanded. Such distributions provide clues about changes in the composition of the population. The similar fertility pattern for Västerbotten indicates that in-migration may have played a more important role in this county than the reported net migration figures suggest. Composite

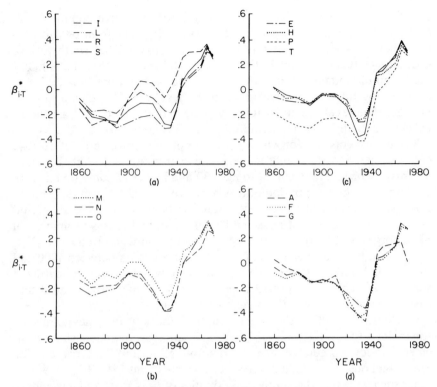

Fig. 6.29   Level-compensated time parameter $\beta^*_{i \cdot T}$ for the counties of Sweden, 1860–1970: counties with an older-than-level-predicted pattern of childbearing until 1945 [(a), Kristianstad (L), Skaraborg (R), and Värmland (S); (b), Halland (N) and Gothenburg and Bohus (O); (c), Östergötland (E), Kalmar (H), Älvsborg (P), and Örebro (T); (d), city of Stockholm (A), Jönköping (F), and Kronoberg (G)] and the counties of Gotland (I) and Malmöhus (M).

measures of migration, however, can obscure differences in the age and sex composition of the in-migrants and out-migrants that would be significant for fertility rates.

In the five counties immediately south and east of the five northern counties, a pre-1920 period of disproportionately early childbearing is much less prominent and tends to be highest from 1900 to 1910 (Fig. 6.28c,d). Even for these lower positive $\beta^*_{i \cdot T}$ levels, however, differences between counties can be noted: the earlier start of the period in Västmanland (U), for which clues have already been noted in β^*_i, and the tendency in Uppsala (C) for an age distribution of fertility very close to the level-predicted distribution from 1880 to 1920.

Elsewhere in the country, only the southeastern county of Blekinge (K) exhibits a level-standardized time sequence of change in the fertility distribution up to 1920 similar to the changes for these five counties (Fig. 6.28c,d). Malmöhus (M) has a slightly positive $\beta_{i\cdot T}^*$ value from 1900 to 1910 but otherwise its time course resembles that of two other southwestern counties, Gothenburg and Bohus (O) and Halland (N) (Fig. 6.29b). For the island of Gotland (I), a 1910–1920 period of disproportionately early childbearing following a sharp rise in the level of $\beta_{i\cdot T}^*$ begins a unique, younger-than-level-predicted fertility pattern that covers half a century except for the brief period centered on 1930 (Fig. 6.29a).

The twelve counties for which $\beta_{i\cdot T}^*$ does not rise above zero before 1945 can be grouped by the extent to which the distribution of fertility becomes less disproportionately shifted to ages 30 and higher at some time before 1945 and by when the period of less negative $\beta_{i\cdot T}^*$ values occurs, if at all. For Värmland (S), Skaraborg (R), and Kristianstad (L), such a period begins by 1900, does not peak until 1910–1920, and is less prominent in Skaraborg (Fig. 6.29a). For Halland (N), Gothenburg and Bohus (O) (Fig. 6.29b), and the counties in Fig. 6.29c, the peak occurs between 1900 and 1910, with Älvsborg (P) maintaining a noticeably older level-standardized pattern throughout the pre-1925 period than do the three central and eastern counties or even the neighboring counties in the west.

In contrast to all of the other counties, the city of Stockholm (A), Jönköping (F), and Kronoberg (G) experience a continued shift to an older-than-level-predicted age distribution of fertility, interrupted for Stockholm only by a slight reversal that occurs about 1910 (Fig. 6.29d). It is not surprising that the contiguous counties of Jönköping and Kronoberg should have this similarity. They are two of the counties that maintained levels of fertility above the national level during the period 1860–1880; they are the only two counties to show no evidence in β_i^* of a shift toward a younger childbearing pattern before 1900 (Fig. 6.27); they are among the counties that experienced the highest net out-migration throughout the 1860–1900 period. It *is* surprising that the fertility pattern for the city of Stockholm should reveal any similarity to the patterns for Jönköping and Kronoberg in view of Stockholm's lower total fertility rates than those for all other counties at each period in the time sequence, its younger age distribution of fertility (Fig. 6.25) than those for all other counties at each period through 1950 (as expressed by β_i^*), and its history of high net in-migration. The $\beta_{i\cdot T}^*$ parameter tells us that from 1880 to 1945 Stockholm's age distribution of fertility is not shifted as much toward ages below 30 as would be predicted from the level of fertility. In other words, the persistently lower total fertility rate for the city of Stockholm is attributable not only to the fertility-limiting behavior (including nonmarriage) of women aged 30 and higher but also to a lower than level-predicted contribution by women below age 30.

For a short period beginning about 1900, the tendency in about two-thirds of the counties for some shift toward a younger level-standardized fertility pattern—expressed by either a positive or a less negative value of $\beta_{i\cdot T}^*$—seems logically associated with the shift to a slightly earlier age pattern of marriage that is documented for the country as a whole for cohorts aged 15 from 1890 to 1910. The subsequent reversal to an older level-standardized fertility pattern in all counties appears to be highly associated with a prominent change to a later age pattern of marriage by the cohorts aged 15 from 1910 to 1924 (Figs. 6.5 and 6.8). Period-specific differences that underlie the general shift of the age distribution of childbearing toward younger ages (the shift expressed in the parameter β_i^*, Figs. 6.24–6.27) are even more apparent in the changes occurring in $\beta_{i\cdot T}^*$ between 1910 and 1945. In 1910, 12 counties have a long-standing, older-than-level-predicted pattern; by 1920, 19 counties have an older pattern; by 1930, all the counties have entered this category. Gotland (I, 1935) and Norrbotten (BD, 1940) are the first counties to regain a positive value of $\beta_{i\cdot T}^*$. By 1945 every county but Älvsborg (P) has attained a younger-than-level-predicted pattern, and some degree of disproportionately early childbearing continues for all 25 counties to the end of the sequence, falling back slightly in the last decade. For all but four counties, the negative $\beta_{i\cdot T}^*$ values during the 1930–1935 period represent the oldest level-standardized age distribution of fertility in the counties' recorded fertility history. The remaining four counties—Värmland (S), Skaraborg (R), Kristianstad (L), and Gotland (I)—experience as old or older a distribution in the period before 1900. The generality of the 1930–1935 low in the level of $\beta_{i\cdot T}^*$ should not obscure county differences in the date at which the decline in $\beta_{i\cdot T}^*$ begins, the magnitude of the decline, or the pace of adoption of the post-1945 pattern of disproportionately early childbearing.

The range of level-standardized patterns associated with similar levels of fertility in 1930 should be noted (Fig. 6.30). For example, Älvsborg (P) and Jönköping (F), which have two of the oldest patterns, and Uppsala (C) and Västmanland (U), which are among the counties with the youngest patterns, have almost the same total fertility rate, slightly below the median rate for all counties $M = 1.97$. Five other counties—Gävleborg (X), Östergötland (E), Värmland (S), Skaraborg (R), and Halland (N)—with intermediate patterns had rates in the range $M - \frac{1}{4}I$ to $M + \frac{1}{4}I$, where the interquartile range of rates $I = .52$.

The range of fertility rates associated with similar level-standardized patterns in 1930 should also be noted (Fig. 6.30). The younger patterns of Uppsala (C) and Västmanland (U) are matched in the southeastern county of Blekinge (K) and the two northern counties of Västernorrland (Y) and Västerbotten (AC) but with fertility rates ranging from below replacement

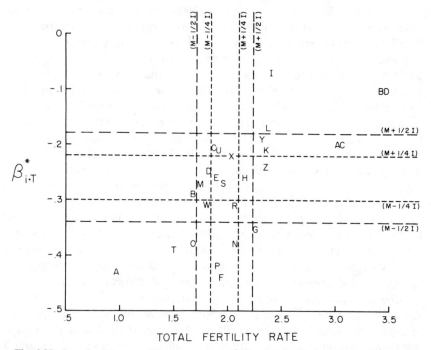

Fig. 6.30   Level-compensated time parameter $\beta_{i\cdot T}^{*}$ for 1930 in relation to 1930 total fertility rates for the counties of Sweden.

level to 3.0. At the extreme of the oldest level-standardized patterns, we have already commented on the similarity of the city of Stockholm (A), with its fertility rate below 1.0, and Jönköping (F). Figure 6.31 shows the geographic location of counties having a 1930 $\beta_{i\cdot T}^{*}$ value above, within, or below the range $M - \frac{1}{4}I$ to $M + \frac{1}{4}I$, where the median $\beta_{i\cdot T}^{*}$ value for all counties in 1930 $M = -.26$ and the interquartile range of $\beta_{i\cdot T}^{*}$ values $I =$ .14. We suggest that the counties with the lowest values of $\beta_{i\cdot T}^{*}$ are those in which the fertility pattern was the most affected at that time by the limitation of childbearing at younger ages through delay of marriage or by other means. Glass (1967, p. 324) has noted the probable role of abortion in the low fertility rates during the 1930s. He cites estimates that as many as a third of all illegitimate pregnancies and a sixth of all legitimate pregnancies were aborted.

The new information about changing age patterns of overall fertility contained in the EHR time parameters for 110 years—including both the similarities and the differences between counties—should now be supple-

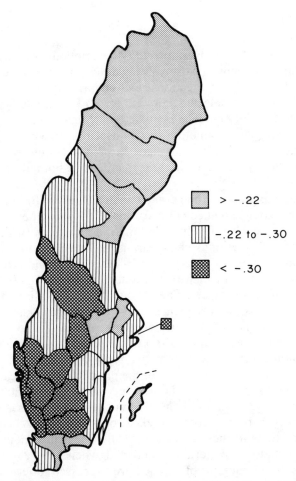

Fig. 6.31 Counties of Sweden by level-compensated fertility pattern in 1930 as indicated by the value of the $\beta^*_{i\text{-}T}$ parameter.

mented by EHR descriptions of the changing age distributions of marital fertility in the counties. Together these analyses can provide more detailed summary measures than do the total rates of overall and marital fertility. These new summary measures would aid in exploring the associations between fertility change, the age–sex–marital-status composition of the population as influenced by migration, and the progress of urban and rural industrialization over decades of significant change in Sweden.

Summary

This chapter begins with overall fertility descriptions that meet our first goal of fertility modeling: a closely fitting description in a small number of parameters for each cross-sectional and cohort sequence. This chapter demonstrates that the selected standard form of the close fits meets our second goal of fertility modeling: stable, interpretable descriptions of the age pattern of fertility in all of its variations across two centuries. Trends and transitions are clearly identified. Brief departures from trend are therefore profitably examined in some detail, using both fitted parameters and residuals.

The value of expressing the parameters in a standard form is illustrated in a series of cross-sequence comparisons. Relations among the derived parameters, the level of fertility, and marriage patterns (which approximate patterns of entry into childbearing) are revealed for cohorts in a detailed examination of the fertility parameters by single year of age for the 55 cohorts that completed their childbearing from 1920/1921 to 1974/1975 (the SYAC13 sequence). The validity of extrapolating this information to the 155-cohort C15 sequence for 5-year age groups is supported by the 45-cohort overlap of the standard-form parameters for the two sequences. Cohort effects on cross-sectional patterns are identified in superimposed time parameters for the two types of sequence. Evidence for the nature and magnitude of errors in the pre-1860, single-year data from "Grunddragen" is revealed in the two sets of standard-form parameters that give cross-sectional and cohort perspectives on the same data set. These parameters then become the basis of a proposed scheme for estimating corrections to these early data. Differences in regional contributions to the national pattern are detected when 110-year fertility sequences for the 25 counties of Sweden are expressed in terms of the age standards derived for the country as a whole.

Two factors in particular are shown to enhance the interpretability of the time parameters for all the sequences: one, the choice of a standard form that concentrates in one standard age pattern and the corresponding variable time parameter the major, long-term trend of change—the shift of a higher or lower proportion of total childbearing to ages below 30; two, the retention of total fertility rate as one dimension of the data. Both decline of fertility at higher ages and younger entry into childbearing contribute to a younger fertility pattern but tend to have opposite effects on the total fertility rate. We have standardized for the relation between decline in the level of fertility and shift of the distribution toward younger ages. The direct outcome is an additional indicator of change—an indicator of the pace or timing of childbearing apart from the level of fertility. For the 55 single-year-of-age cohorts, the revealed transitions in timing at the aggregate level are shown to follow closely the cohorts' changes in the age pattern of marriage (and by implication, the age pattern of entry into child-bearing). A further step uses the age standards and level-compensated time parameters to construct level-standardized distributions of childbearing and calculate the mean age of fertility of the distributions in time sequence. This step translates the relative change expressed by the timing parameter into years of change in the mean age of childbearing attributable to change in timing at the aggregate level. By extrapolation from the 55 more recent cohorts, the indicators of timing apart from level then reveal evidence of change in the age pattern of entry into childbearing for the pre-1885 cohorts as well—cohorts for which we have fertility descriptions by 5-year age groups but less certain or less detailed information about the marital status of women by age.

The closely fitting, stable descriptions of overall fertility yield several unexpected results.

1. The pre-1860, single-year data from "Grunddragen" have surprising year-to-year stability in pattern despite wide fluctuations in the total fertility rate. This suggests that there may be less nonsystematic error in these early data than is commonly thought.
2. Clues for fertility limitation (or increased limitation) by means other than nonmarriage appear earlier in the nineteenth century than is usually reported.
3. Except for a prominent deviation from trend in fertility pattern beginning slightly before the 1868–1869 wave of emigration, only brief pauses in the trend toward a younger pattern are associated with years of high emigration.
4. Recent low-fertility variations on fertility patterns can be brought into a well-fitted, interpretable description by fitting and standardizing one additional age parameter and its variable time parameter.

Notes for Chapter VI

1. Recall that this is a linearizing re-expression of the cumulative distribution of fertility f_{ij} as $F_{ij} = (f_{ij})^{1/2} - (1 - f_{ij})^{1/2}$ so that the distribution is centered on its median age and both tails of the sigmoid configuration are stretched and straightened (see Chapter III).

2. To understand the choice of $T_i^{1/2}$ in the linear compensation of α_i^* and β_i^* for the total rate of fertility, recall from Chapter III the relation between the cumulative rates and the cumulative, normalized rates of fertility for cohort i. With no linearizing re-expression of the data

$$f'_{ij} = T_i f_{ij},$$

where f'_{ij} is the schedule of cumulative rates for cohort i and age cuts $j = 1$ to n without normalization, f_{ij} the schedule of cumulative, normalized rates for cohort i and age cuts $j = 1$ to n, and $T_i = \Sigma_{j=1}^{n} f_i(a_j)$ the total fertility rate across age groups $j = 1$ to n. On the folded square root scale used in the EHR analyses, however,

$$F'_{ij} = T_i^{1/2} F_{ij},$$

where F'_{ij} is the re-expressed schedule of cumulative fertility rates for cohort i and age cuts $j = 1$ to n without normalization and F_{ij} the re-expressed schedule of cumulative, normalized rates for cohort i and age cuts $j = 1$ to n. Therefore, the cumulative rates approximated from the fitted cumulative distribution $\hat{F}_{ij}$ are expressed as

$$T_i^{1/2} \hat{F}_{ij} = T_i^{1/2} (\alpha_i^* A_j^* + \beta_i^* B_j^*).$$

The square root is therefore shown to be the form of the total rate that is on the same scale as the EHR parameters.

3. The fertility variations expressed in $\alpha_{i\cdot T}^*$ and $\beta_{i\cdot T}^*$ also reflect the influence of illegitimate fertility, most prominently at ages lower than 25. A parallel EHR analysis of the corresponding legitimate overall fertility sequence would refine the examination of relations between fertility patterns and marriage changes. Even if exposure to the possibility of a first pregnancy occurred mainly within marriage, the comparison between change in $\beta_{i\cdot T}^*$ and a measure of change in marriage pattern would still be of interest as an indicator of change in the time lag between marriage and entry into childbearing.

4. This index of the pace of childbearing is also reported in a later section of this chapter for the 155 cohorts aged 15–19 from 1775 to 1929 (see Fig. 6.17).

5. Calculation of this summary measure is based on the standard procedure for data by 5-year age groups (Shryock et al., 1976):

$$\bar{a} = \sum_a a f_a \bigg/ \sum_a f_a,$$

where a is the midpoint of each age interval (17.5, 22.5, . . . , 47.5) and f_a the age-specific birth rate for each 5-year age group (15–19, 20–24, . . . , 45–49). As Bernhardt (1971, p. 182) points out, however, true "central points" obtained from single-year rates would differ from the midpoints of the 5-year intervals, particularly for age groups 15–19 and 45–49.

6. The years 1790–1792 fall in a period of political unrest leading to the 1792 assassination of King Gustavus III. Severe famine is variously recorded for the years from 1780 to 1785. Thomas (1941, pp. 81–88, 102–108) identifies 1780–1783 and 1785 as years of major crop failures. Utterstrom (1954) questions the harvest index that was Thomas's criterion and identifies 1783–1785 as the famine years.

7. Systematic errors, such as the pre-1895 practice of recording births by the mother's age at a near birthday, go undetected unless corrective measures are reflected by a sudden change in pattern. See the discussion in Chapter VII on the 1894–1895 disjunction in marital fertility patterns and rates and the use of relations between cohort and cross-sectional EHR parameters to estimate pre-1895 corrections.

8. Cohort total rates can be more stable than cross-sectional total rates in the absence of date errors as well. When volition has a prominent role in determining pregnancy, cohort-to-cohort variation in the timing of births over the reproductive span leads to irregularity in the cross-sectional total rates even when differences in the average number of births per woman between cohorts are small.

9. Only partial schedules of revised cross-sectional rates are obtained for years before 1810 by this procedure because a triangle of higher ages in the earliest years of the cross-

sectional sequence was omitted in the original construction of the cohort schedules for EHR analysis (see Chapter III).

10. Anderson's consideration of the characteristics of areas from which migration occurs, the characteristics of people who migrate, and the kinds of migration alternatives other than permanent rural–urban migration or emigration, available to rural people during modernization appears to be very pertinent to the Swedish experience. Eriksson and Rogers (1978), in their thorough study of two nineteenth-century cohorts selected from parish registers for a district in the county of Uppsala, have already provided evidence for the importance of circular migration of the short-term, rural–rural type.

11. A_j^*, B_j^*, and C_j^* for the $X202$ sequence can also be used for a more detailed description. They should be used for the closest fits from 1960 to 1970, when the greater degree of concentration of fertility in age group 25–29 begins to appear in all counties, but more strongly in some than in others.

VII

Age Patterns of Marital Fertility: Seven Decades of Change

Introduction

The examination of age patterns of marital fertility has traditionally focused on evidence of parity-dependent control as a signal of a population's stage of transition from high to low fertility. Births at ages 15–19 or for marriage durations of less than 2 years are usually omitted to lessen the effect of premarital pregnancy on the analyses. The EHR analyses of marital fertility reported here have a broader focus. Emphasis is placed on developing a close-fitting, coherent description of the changes in aggregate fertility experience across the full range of childbearing ages and across an extended period of time. This brings under scrutiny not only the results of efforts to terminate childbearing but also the aggregate effects of such diverse factors as premarital pregnancy, spacing of births, subfecundity, and subpopulations with different childbearing patterns. The EHR analyses seek evidence for transitions in fertility patterns whatever their cause. Therefore, they naturally include further dissection of time parameters to examine variation in the age pattern of fertility apart from change in the level of fertility. Time-sequence relations established in the fitted parameters then provide a powerful means of estimating missing values and identifying and correcting errors in marital fertility data.

The logical start for the discussion of EHR descriptions of marital fertility is the traditional question about the decline of marital fertility with age. This will be accomplished by a fairly detailed comparison with one established model of cross-sectional marital fertility (Coale, 1971) that incorporates the concepts of "natural fertility" and "degree of parity-dependent control."

Discussion then moves to a broader examination of change in both cross-sectional and cohort perspectives. We consider the analyses of the complete marital fertility sequences, which are highly influenced by premarital pregnancy not only in age group 15–19 but also in age group 20–24 in this late-marriage population, and the parallel analysis of the NX15 sequence for childbearing occurring 9 months or more after marriage, which takes advantage of the large amount of detail in the available data. Observed intersequence relations of EHR time parameters and level compensation of the time parameters then permit estimations that extend the shorter NX15 sequence backward in time.

The value of level-compensated time parameters and level-standardized distributions is again demonstrated in relating marital fertility change to overall fertility change and detecting the effects of cohort behavior in cross-sectional patterns. Examination of residuals again aids the identification of period effects on cohort behavior. By bringing all births under consideration, the analyses provide a methodological basis for extracting from aggregate data more information about societal changes over time, not only in the incidence of nonmarital conception leading to birth of a child, but also in the decision to marry or not marry before giving birth to a nonmaritally conceived child.

Comparison of the EHR and Coale Descriptions of Marital Fertility

To confirm the demographic significance of the parameters of the EHR-derived marital fertility model

$$F_{ij} = \alpha_i^* A_j^* + \beta_i^* B_j^*,$$

one appropriate step is comparison with an earlier model (Coale, 1971),

$$f(a) = M \cdot n(a) \exp[m \cdot v(a)],$$

whose parameters are considered to have demographic meaning.

The structural similarity of the two marital fertility descriptions is more apparent when we take the logarithm of the Coale equation and insert subscripts to indicate that it, too, describes a series of schedules and age groups:

$$\ln f_i(a_j) = \ln M_i \cdot n(a_j) + m_i \cdot v(a_j).$$

Both the EHR (folded square root scale) and Coale (logarithmic scale) expressions are thus of the form

$$y_{ij} = K_i L_j + M_i N_j.$$

By stated intent, each description focuses on the age pattern of fertility apart from level, although the Coale model is concerned only with the pattern after age 24. The parameters can be compared as follows:

$f_i(a_j)$ The fertility rate for women within an age group $j = 1, 2,$ . . . , n for age groups 20–24, 25–29, . . . , 45–49

F_{ij} The proportion of total fertility (using the normalized, cumulative distribution) achieved by an age cut $j = 1, 2, . . . , n$ with cuts at 19/20, 24/25, . . . , 44/45 for a full age 15–49 distribution or at 24/25, . . . , 44/45 for a truncated age 20–49 distribution

Each model relates its own expression of the observed fertility schedule to a standard schedule:

$n(a_j)$ For each age group, an arithmetic mean of ten of the schedules identified by Henry (1961) as having a "natural" marital fertility pattern

A_j^* A central, cumulative marital fertility pattern extracted from a time sequence of schedules (in this chapter, the 68-year, 50-year, or 42-cohort Swedish sequences) and presented in a standard form[1]

Each model has a multiplier of its standard schedule:

M_i A variable scale factor

α_i^* A positive-valued near constant that measures the extent to which the cumulation of births expressed by A_j^* accelerates toward the median age of A_j^* and then decelerates over higher ages

Each model expresses deviations from its first component—$M_i \cdot n(a_j)$ or $\alpha_i^* A_j^*$—in terms of a standard pattern of departure with age:

$v(a_j)$ An average logarithmic departure after age 24 based on recent schedules for 43 countries and interpreted to reflect the age pattern of conscious behavior to control fertility after some desired number of children is reached[2]

B_j^* An age vector derived from analysis of the selected time sequence of schedules (in this chapter, the 68-year, 50-year, or 42-cohort Swedish sequences) and including all of the age cuts for the sequence

Each model provides a measure of the degree of this deviation from the first component:

m_i The extent to which the marital fertility distribution after age 24 is positively (and sometimes negatively) skewed according to the age pattern of $v(a_j)$, interpreted as a measure of the "degree of parity-dependent control" of fertility at higher ages

β_i^* The extent to which the entire age distribution of marital fertility is skewed according to the age pattern determined by B_j^*

Testing the parameters of the two models for comparability, we obtain the following results.

1. The $\alpha_i^* A_j^*$ component for either the 68-year MX20 sequence or the 50-year NX15 sequence provides a standard age pattern of fertility that differs only slightly from the pattern exhibited by several of the natural fertility schedules that were averaged to arrive at the $n(a_j)$ standard.
2. The β_i^* time parameter for both the MX15 and MX20 sequences has very close to the same pattern of variation over time as does the Coale measure of the "degree of control," m_i, when m_i is calculated by either of two methods for Swedish age 20–49 cross-sectional schedules from 1890 to 1960.
3. The parameters of the EHR model bring the variability of the data more fully into the fitted description than the Coale model parameters do.

We shall examine the evidence for each of these statements and then briefly discuss some other similarities and differences in the two models.

The EHR $\alpha_i^* A_j^*$ Component and Natural Fertility

Henry (1961) applied the term "natural fertility" to a type of age pattern of marital fertility characteristic of populations in which couples' behavior affecting fertility is not influenced by the number of children already born to them. He originally observed the similarity of pattern in 13 schedules of age 20–49 marital fertility[3] with total fertility rates ranging from 10.9 to 6.2 births per married woman. He considered the relatively small variations in pattern between the schedules, as well as the differences in level of fertility, to reflect population cultural and biological differences that are independent of the conscious control of fertility related to parity. The population differences that he emphasized were the varied customs on the duration of breast feeding and postpartum sexual abstinence that affect the length of interbirth intervals (see Page and

Lesthaeghe, 1981, for recently assembled evidence on such effects.) Under natural fertility conditions as defined by Henry, many other factors may also contribute to population variations in the age pattern and level of marital fertility: the incidence of diseases that affect fecundity, age differences between spouses (Anderson, 1975; Smith, 1972), the frequency and duration of separation of spouses (Menken, 1979; Van de Walle, F., 1975), the age pattern of marriage (see Charbonneau, 1979, and Dupâquier, 1979, for summaries of evidence from various sources), and possibly nutritional status (for example, Anderson and McCabe, 1977).

The close relation between the EHR-derived $\alpha_i^* A_j^*$ standards and the cluster of marital fertility patterns identified with the term "natural fertility" will be demonstrated in two ways: one, direct comparisons of the distributions expressed by $\alpha_i^* A_j^*$ for the MX20 and NX15 sequences with natural fertility distributions and with the $n(a_j)$ average of distributions adopted by Coale (1971) and Coale and Trussell (1974) for modeling purposes; two, indirect comparisons by regression of natural fertility distributions on the A_j^* and B_j^* pairs of age standards derived from the MX20 and NX15 sequences so that schedule-specific α_i^* values can be compared with α_i^* values for the Swedish sequences and schedule-specific departures from $\alpha_i^* A_j^*$ are expressed by $\beta_i^* B_j^*$ and a set of residuals.

Direct Comparisons with Natural Fertility   De-transforming the $\alpha_i^* A_j^*$ components for the MX20 and NX15 sequences from the folded square root scale used in the fitting gives the implied cumulated, normalized fertility distributions (see Chapter VIII for procedure). De-cumulation gives the proportion of total fertility attributed to each 5-year age group from 20–24 to 45–49 by $\alpha_i^* A_j^*$ for the MX20 sequence and from 15–19 to 45–49 by $\alpha_i^* A_j^*$ for the NX15 sequence. The age-specific fertility patterns implied by $\alpha_i^* A_j^*$ for the NX15 sequence are examined in two forms: as originally derived, with $\Sigma_{15-19}^{45-49} f_i(a_j) = 1$, and further normalized to see the pattern across ages 20–49 only, with $\Sigma_{20-24}^{45-49} f_i(a_j) = 1$. The natural fertility schedules and the $n(a_j)$ standard schedule are also normalized (divided by their sum of age-specific fertility rates) to reveal the patterns for comparison with the $\alpha_i^* A_j^*$ distributions.

First, the similarity of the two differently derived sets of age 20–49 $\alpha_i^* A_j^*$ distributions should be noted (upper section of Table 7.1). Then the pattern similarity of these distributions to the natural fertility distributions for the earlier and later Hutterites, Canada, Norway, Europeans of Tunis, and earlier Greenland can be examined in Tables 7.1 and 7.5 (both tables relate mainly to analyses in later sections of the chapter). In fact, the EHR-derived $\alpha_i^* A_j^*$ distributions, characterized by a slow fertility decline between ages 25 and 40, are more similar to these natural fertility distributions than all of Henry's natural fertility distributions shown in Table 7.1

are similar to each other or to the Coale model $n(a_j)$. In a late-marriage population such as Sweden's, low-order births well beyond age 25 should contribute to this pattern of slow decline. The occurrence of such a pattern for the Hutterites and eighteenth-century Canadians, with their high levels of fertility, prompts the following question: Is this the pattern that would typify a late average decline in fecundity combined with continued high exposure to the possibility of pregnancy?

For the age range 15–49, we can compare the age pattern of fertility determined by the complete $\alpha_i^* A_j^*$ component for the NX15 sequence with the age pattern of the $n(a_j)$ standard incorporated in the Coale–Trussell model fertility schedules. The close relation of the normalized $n(a_j)$ standard and the de-transformed and decumulated (median α_i^*)A_j^* component can be examined in Table 7.2. This similarity provides evidence that the $n(a_j)$ standard, with its averaged values for $n(20$–$24)$ to $n(45$–$49)$ and its estimated value for $n(15$–$19)$, closely expresses a pattern found empirically to underlie a 50-year time sequence of fertility schedules that excludes most premaritally conceived births. Viewed another way, the similarity provides further evidence that a pattern that demographers have considered to be demographically meaningful can be derived empirically.

Indirect Comparisons with Natural Fertility To approximate a natural fertility schedule by a weighted sum of EHR-derived A_j^* and B_j^* vectors, the schedule in cumulated, normalized form is first re-expressed on the folded square root scale. An age 20–49 schedule is then regressed on A_j^* and B_j^* for the MX20 sequence; an age 15–49 schedule is regressed on A_j^* and B_j^* for the NX15 sequence.[4]

For Henry's thirteen schedules (Table 7.1) the first regression coefficient α_i^*, the degree of central concentration, ranges from 1.083 to 1.20, much like the range of 1.080 to 1.138 for the MX20 sequence. The second regression coefficient β_i^*, the measure of shift of the fertility distribution away from higher ages, ranges from .035 to .240 for the natural fertility schedules, compared to a low of .204 for the MX20 sequence. The closeness of fit of these EHR approximations to the reported natural fertility distributions is shown in raw-scale, noncumulated form. For two schedules, the Hutterites before 1921 and the Europeans of Tunis, 1840–1859, differences between reported and fitted distributions are no greater than in the third decimal place for any age group. For five other schedules— Canada, Crulai, Taiwan, Sotteville-lès-Rouen, and Iran—no departure of the fitted from the reported distributions exceeds .015 for any age group. The schedules for India and Guinea, which Henry considered to be less reliable than the others, are also the schedules least well fit by A_j^* and B_j^*.

TABLE 7.1

Fertility Distributions $f(a)$ Implied by EHR Standard $\alpha_i^* A_j^*$ and Coale Model Standard $n(a)$: Age 20–49 Distributions of Natural Fertility Reported and Fitted as Weighted Sums of the Age Standards A_j^* and B_j^* Derived from EHR Analysis of the MX20 Sequence, 1892–1959

	EHR time parameter		Age group						
Distribution[a]	α_i^*	β_i^*	20–24	25–29	30–34	35–39	40–44	45–49	$5 \sum f(a)$
MX20 $\alpha_i^* A_j^*$									
with lowest α_i^*	1.080	0	.2473	.2110	.2001	.1891	.1284	.0241	
with highest α_i^*	1.138	0	.2348	.2212	.2107	.1961	.1238	.0134	
Renormalized NX15 $\alpha_i^* A_j^*$									
with lowest α_i^*	—	—	.2465	.2183	.2154	.1839	.1133	.0224	
with highest α_i^*	—	—	.2548	.2294	.2249	.1854	.0988	.0067	
Normalized $n(a)$	—	—	.2557	.2396	.2201	.1784	.0928	.0133	9.0
Hutterites, marriages 1921–1930									
Reported			.2514	.2294	.2043	.1856	.1015	.0279	10.9
Fitted	1.083	.058	.2633	.2177	.1990	.1807	.1180	.0213	
Residual			−.0119	.0117	.0053	.0049	−.0175	.0066	
Canada, marriages 1700–1730									
Reported			.2358	.2293	.2242	.1899	.1070	.0139	10.8
Fitted	1.151	.035	.2422	.2274	.2119	.1920	.1161	.0105	
Residual			−.0064	.0019	.0123	−.0021	−.0091	.0034	

188

Hutterites, marriages before 1921									
Reported	1.141	.050	.2425	.2302	.2169	.1909	.1046	.0148	9.8
Fitted			.2482	.2274	.2098	.1887	.1145	.0114	
Residual			-.0057	.0028	.0071	.0022	-.0099	.0034	
Bourgeoisie of Geneva, wives of men born 1600-1649									
Reported	1.163	.218	.2788	.2576	.2278	.1524	.0749	.0085	9.4
Fitted			.2928	.2490	.2065	.1636	.0833	.0048	
Residual			-.0140	.0086	.0213	-.0112	-.0084	.0037	
Europeans of Tunis, marriages 1840-1859									
Reported	1.165	.095	.2562	.2354	.2200	.1773	.1040	.0071	9.2
Fitted			.2561	.2365	.2123	.1840	.1039	.0071	
Residual			.0001	-.0009	.0077	-.0067	.0001	.0000	
Sotteville-lès-Rouen, marriages and births 1760-1790									
Reported	1.200	.185	.2682	.2514	.2291	.1760	.0698	.0056	9.0
Fitted			.2744	.2526	.2147	.1725	.0837	.0021	
Residual			-.0062	-.0012	.0144	.0035	-.0139	.0035	
Crulai, marriages 1674-1742									
Reported	1.182	.165	.2643	.2523	.2252	.1682	.0841	.0060	8.3
Fitted			.2727	.2472	.2125	.1742	.0896	.0039	
Residual			-.0084	.0051	.0127	-.0060	-.0055	.0021	
Norway, marriages 1874-1876									
Reported	1.091	.045	.2434	.2336	.2096	.1776	.1106	.0252	8.1
Fitted			.2577	.2179	.2009	.1836	.1197	.0201	
Residual			-.0143	.0157	.0087	-.0060	-.0091	.0051	

(*table continues*)

189

TABLE 7.1 (*continued*)

Distribution[a]	EHR time parameter		Age group						$5\,\Sigma\,f(a)$
	α_i^*	β_i^*	20–24	25–29	30–34	35–39	40–44	45–49	
Bourgeoisie of Geneva, wives of men born before 1600									
Reported	1.155		.2602	.2421	.2187	.1839	.0823	.0127	7.5
Fitted		.130	.2683	.2385	.2092	.1773	.0991	.0075	
Residual			–.0081	.0036	.0095	.0066	–.0168	.0052	
Iran, marriages 1940–1950									
Reported	1.141		.2642	.2475	.2174	.1706	.0870	.0134	7.5
Fitted		.146	.2762	.2377	.2061	.1733	.0978	.0089	
Residual			–.0120	.0098	.0113	–.0027	–.0108	.0045	
Taiwan, women born c.1900									
Reported	1.174		.2626	.2403	.2201	.1892	.0820	.0058	7.0
Fitted		.129	.2639	.2419	.2126	.1794	.0969	.0053	
Residual			–.0013	–.0016	.0075	.0098	–.0149	.0005	
India, marriages 1945–1946									
Reported	1.101		.2609	.2326	.2278	.1712	.0808	.0267	6.2
Fitted		.118	.2769	.2274	.2001	.1735	.1063	.0158	
Residual			–.0160	.0052	.0277	–.0023	–.0255	.0109	
Guinea, marriages 1954–1955									
Reported	1.093		.2881	.2583	.2203	.1477	.0597	.0258	6.2
Fitted		.240	.3149	.2380	.1936	.1537	.0867	.0132	
Residual			–.0268	.0203	.0267	–.0060	–.0270	.0126	

[a] Sources: $\alpha_i^* A_j^*$ for the MX20 sequence is de-transformed from the folded square root scale and de-cumulated; $\alpha_i^* A_j^*$ for the NX15 sequence is de-transformed to the raw fraction scale, de-cumulated, and normalized for ages 20–49 only so that $\Sigma_{20-24}^{45-49} f(a) = 1$ (see Table 5.9 for the $\alpha_i^* A_j^*$ values used in these calculations); $n(a)$ for normalization to $\Sigma f(a) = 1$ is taken from Coale (1971); natural fertility schedules for normalization to $\Sigma f(a) = 1$ are taken from Henry (1961).

The capacity of the EHR age standards to describe the fertility distributions of actual populations considered to have a natural fertility pattern is further demonstrated in Table 7.2 with several of the age 15–49 distributions cited by Hansen (1979). These distributions are very closely approximated by a weighted sum of the A_j^* and B_j^* vectors for the NX15 sequence. The values of α_i^* and β_i^* for Iceland, 1891–1900, are almost identical to those reported in a later section of this chapter to describe the age pattern of confinements occurring 9 months or more after marriage in Sweden from 1911 to 1913. The values for Greenland, 1901–1930, are very similar to those estimated for Sweden from 1892 to 1896 in an extension of the NX15 sequence (Fig. 7.11).[5]

The relation between natural fertility distributions and EHR-derived age patterns can be more fully examined when the A_j^* and B_j^* vectors have been refined through additional analyses of a full range of fertility schedules representing a variety of populations and periods (see the discussion in Chapter VIII). The first component of a marital fertility description derived solely from time sequences of Swedish data, however, comes remarkably close to the pattern that appears to underlie a series of schedules drawn from different time periods and geographic locations and identified as having a natural fertility pattern with some population-specific variations.

The EHR Time Parameter β_i^* and the Coale "Control" Parameter m_i

We shall now examine the similarity of the 1892–1959 sequences of the EHR-derived β_i^* parameter and calculated m_i parameter (the Coale model "degree of parity-dependent control"). Both of these parameters are measures of the extent to which the age distribution of marital fertility is shifted away from the higher ages and toward the lower ages. The results of two different methods of calculating m_i are shown for comparison.

In an earlier comparison of m_i with β_i (Breckenridge, 1976), m_{ij} for each age group in all of the 1892–1959 Swedish schedules was calculated by the expression

$$m_{ij} = \frac{\ln[f_i(a_j)/M_i \cdot n(a_j)]}{v(a_j)}$$

using the values of $n(a_j)$ and $v(a_j)$ that underlie the Coale–Trussell (1974) model schedules and the equation $M_i = f_i(20\text{–}24)/n(20\text{–}24)$ from the Coale (1971) model of marital fertility. If the Coale model fit a schedule perfectly, the value of m_{ij} calculated in this way would be the same for all age

TABLE 7.2

Fertility Distributions $f(a)$ Implied by $\alpha_i^* A_j^*$ for the NX15 Sequence and Coale–Trussell Model $n(a)$; Age 15–49 Distributions of Natural Fertility Reported and Fitted as Weighted Sums of the Age Standards A_j^* and B_j^* Derived from EHR Analysis of the NX15 Sequence, 1911–1963

Distribution[a]	EHR time parameter		Age group							$5\,\Sigma f(a)$
	α_i^*	β_i^*	15–19	20–24	25–29	30–34	35–39	40–44	45–49	
Normalized $n(a)$	—	—	.186	.208	.195	.179	.146	.076	.011	
NX15 (median α_i^*)A_j^*	1.257	0	.1720	.2068	.1844	.1814	.1550	.0898	.0127	
Iceland 1891–1900										
Reported			.195	.210	.204	.177	.130	.076	.008	10.2
Fitted	1.258	.116	.1884	.2232	.1962	.1762	.1350	.0716	.0093	
Residual			.0066	−.0132	.0078	.0008	−.0050	.0044	−.0013	
Greenland 1901–1930										
Reported			.172	.224	.190	.173	.140	.086	.015	9.5
Fitted	1.241	.045	.1821	.2111	.1867	.1774	.1451	.0840	.0137	
Residual			−.0101	.0129	.0033	−.0044	−.0051	.0020	.0013	
Geneva 1600–1649										
Reported			.182	.228	.211	.186	.125	.061	.007	11.5
Fitted	1.290	.147	.1856	.2318	.2037	.1784	.1314	.0638	.0052	
Residual			−.0036	−.0038	.0073	.0076	−.0064	−.0028	.0018	

[a] Sources: $n(a)$ for normalization to $\Sigma f(a) = 1$ is taken from Coale and Trussell (1974); the distributions for Iceland, Greenland, and Geneva are taken from Hansen (1979).

groups, indicating that the population follows the standard pattern of age-related decline of fertility with a uniform intensity. The calculated values of m_{ij} for the Swedish schedules show considerable variability with age for any given year, however, and they vary in different ways in different periods. For example, consider the accompanying tabulation of m_{ij} values. According to Coale, this variability is probably due in part to the effect that changing age patterns of marriage and of entry into childbearing have had on the cross-sectional schedules. An additional factor in the late-marriage Swedish population is that low-order births have influenced the distribution well beyond age 25 for much of the 1892–1959 period. Page (1977) reports similar variability in m_{ij} across age for other populations.

	Age group				
Year	*25–29*	*30–34*	*35–39*	*40–44*	*45–49*
1894	.598	.323	.278	.142	.108
1924	1.06	.675	.628	.476	.471
1932	1.21	.811	.839	.697	.751
1944	.952	.662	.786	.848	1.08
1959	1.21	1.07	1.33	1.36	1.49

To obtain for each year a single value of m_i to compare with β_i^*, a weighted average of m_{ij} ($\bar{m}_i$) was calculated, weighting the m_{ij} for each age group by the proportion of the year's births occurring in the age group. This emphasizes the shape of the schedule over the central ages of childbearing, the portion of the schedule that Coale and Trussell (1978) consider to be of primary importance in estimating the "degree of parity-dependent control". The difference $(m_{ij} - \bar{m}_i) \cdot v(a_j)$ at each age for schedule i then becomes a residual—the departure from fit.

When the values of β_i^* for the MX15 and MX20 sequences are rescaled by a linear function and superimposed on the sequence of $\bar{m}_i$ values[6], the similarity of variations in these three measures across time becomes apparent (Fig. 7.1). β_i' for the MX15 sequence and $\bar{m}_i$ are particularly close, except for a short period in the mid-1940s.

Another procedure for determining a single value of m_i regresses $\ln[f_i(a_j)/n(a_j)]$ on $v(a_j)$, omitting some higher ages from the regression (Coale and Trussell, 1978). This procedure emphasizes the shape of the schedule over the central ages of childbearing and systematically leaves departures from fit in the residuals although, as Coale and Trussell point out, it may not provide the best fit to a schedule. Because the slope is a measure of m_i and the regression constant is a measure of $\ln M_i$, the

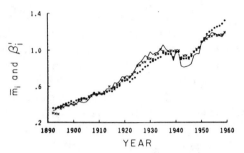

Fig. 7.1   Coale model "parity-dependent control" parameter $\bar{m}_i$ (weighted average, ——) and EHR time parameter β_i^* for the MX15 ($\times\times\times$) and MX20 ($\cdot\cdot\cdot$) sequences on the scale of $\bar{m}_i$: cross-sectional marital fertility schedules from 1892 to 1959.

procedure removes a troubling dependence of M_i on age group 20–24 but maintains the dependence of $v(a_j)$ on that age group. As reported by Trussell (1979) for Swedish decennial and quinquennial schedules, this procedure provides a time sequence of m_i values with the same general pattern of variation as the sequences in Fig. 7.1 but with values of m_i ranging from .2 to 1.8 instead of .3 to 1.2 for the period 1890–1960 (Fig. 7.2).

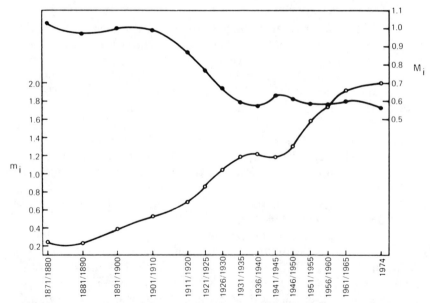

Fig. 7.2   Values of m_i (o——o) and M_i (●——●) derived from regression fitting of the Coale marital fertility model to Swedish decennial and quinquennial fertility schedules from 1871/1880 to 1961/1965 (from Trussell, 1979).

All of these procedures leading to values of β_i^* or m_i appear to pick up the same time pattern for one type of change in the Swedish schedules. This outcome demonstrates that any one of a number of similar sets of age standards—even age standards that do not optimally capture the underlying systematic variability in the data—can be used to detect a single *major* difference between fertility schedules. When it is useful to know about smaller or more subtle differences or when several types of difference are of interest the benefits of the EHR approach become apparent in the closer fits achieved in a small number of parameters and the better separation of effects achieved by a standard form of the fitted parameters. As discussed in the next section, the EHR standard-form parameter β_i^* appears to register more fully in a single parameter the change in the age distribution of fertility associated with limitation of births at higher ages than do the Coale–Trussell procedures and their analogs.

Other Similarities and Some Differences between the EHR and Coale Model Parameters

Because the Coale model age standards $n(a_j)$ and $v(a_j)$ and the variable parameter m_i are given causal interpretations, the fact that this model was also empirically derived may be obscured. Coale, however, has made its empirical nature clear. The model grew from Henry's (1961) recognition of the similarity of configurations in a group of marital fertility schedules for populations not considered to practice parity-dependent control of fertility and his further observation that a selected schedule for a population practicing such control had a different configuration. The arithmetic mean of 10 schedules from the "non-control" group provided the $n(a_j)$ standard. An expression of the differences for age groups 25–29 to 45–49 between $n(a_j)$ and each of 43 schedules from the U.N. "Demographic Yearbook 1965" led to 43 estimates of $v_i(a_j)$, which were then averaged to provide a single departure pattern $v(a_j)$. Based on visual pattern recognition and demographic intuition, the model thus developed as a description of a particular type of difference in aggregate fertility distributions—the steepness of the decline of marital fertility with age.

The EHR approach builds on the insights of Henry and Coale and extends them through the methods of exploratory data analysis. The EHR descriptions of marital fertility result from a systematic search for the patterns that underlie changing age distributions of fertility in a long time sequence. They concentrate on capturing in a small number of fitted parameters as much as possible of the regularity in diverse schedules and present these closely fitting descriptions in a standard form that enhances comparisons across time and place.

The emphasis of the EHR descriptions has been broadened from the age 25–40 focus of the Coale model. Thus the EHR analyses are concerned not only with describing the decline of fertility at higher ages but also with describing other differences in aggregate fertility experience across the full range of childbearing ages, including variations associated with the timing of childbearing apart from level. These more comprehensive descriptions are important to identify different types of transitions in time-sequence data and permit similar schedules to be grouped on the basis of more than one type of difference in the distributions (see Chapter VIII on cross-population comparisons using the EHR age standards derived from the Swedish data). For marital fertility, the contributions of EHR analyses thus lie in both expanded focus and procedure.

Specific procedural contributions that the EHR approach makes by using normalized distributions in the fitting and introducing standard-form re-presentation of fitted parameters are brought out clearly by Trussell's (1979) discussion of the problems of interpreting M_i, the second parameter needed to describe a marital fertility schedule with the Coale equation. Originally M_i was viewed as the fertility level at which a population experienced "natural fertility". The considerable change in M_i over time for a given population (Fig. 7.2 shows the change for Sweden in the decades after 1870) led Trussell to comment, however, that M_i appears to be a "composite of several factors": not only the level of underlying natural fertility but also functions of the degree of control m_i and variations in the distribution due to the spacing of births. He noted the same problem of interpretation in one parameter of Page's (1977) related model of marital fertility by duration of marriage and concluded that further separation could not be accomplished with marital fertility models of the Coale–Page type.[7]

Expanded Focus on Cross-sectional Marital Fertility Change

The preceding section presented a relatively narrow view of an EHR description of change in marital fertility by relating the demographic significance of this description to the parameters of a previously established cross-sectional model of the decline of marital fertility with age. We shall now expand our focus to consider evidence of several types of transition in marital fertility patterns and their relation to overall fertility patterns in both cross-sectional and cohort perspectives. This broader view is made possible by the close fits achieved with a small number of parameters by

the EHR approach to time-sequence change and the re-presentation of
fitted parameters in a standard form before comparison of change in the
various sequences.

We shall concentrate first on five related cross-sectional sequences—
MX20, MX15, NX15, XX20, and XX15—that cover approximately the
same time period. Figure 7.3 summarizes in 5-year averages the changes
in age-specific marital fertility rates that underlie our analysis of change in
the age pattern of fertility by single year across seven decades. The comparable summary of overall fertility rates for the same period is shown in
Fig. 2.1. That *all* age groups contributed to the decline in the total marital
fertility rate should be kept in mind as we analyze the normalized, cumulative rates, the proportion of the total rate in each year that is accounted
for by women a given age and younger, and then relate the observed
changes in pattern to changes in the level of total fertility across the
sequence.

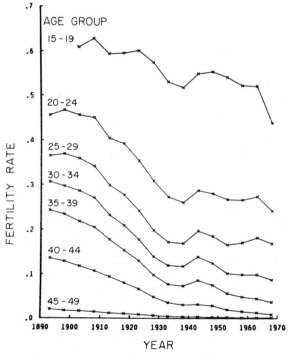

Fig. 7.3 Quinquennial age-specific marital fertility rates for Sweden from 1891/1895 to
1966/1970 (data from Hofsten and Lundstrom, 1976).

Sample Distributions with Increasing β_i^* Values

A set of sample fertility distributions for the five cross-sectional sequences is shown in Table 7.3 for reference as we consider actual values of the time parameters α_i^* and β_i^* across seven decades. Based on the sequence-specific age standards A_j^* and B_j^*, these distributions are constructed from the $\alpha_i^* A_j^*$ component, with α_i^* equal to the mean of its nearly constant value for the sequence, and the $\beta_i^* B_j^*$ component, with increasing values of β_i^*. The distributions are expressed in three forms that are useful for comparison: the cumulated form on the folded square root scale that was used in the fitting and both the cumulated and noncumulated forms on the raw fraction scale.

The raw fraction scale noncumulated distributions implied by $\alpha_i^* A_j^*$ with no $\beta_i^* B_j^*$ component added reveal the extent to which the age pattern of fertility for each sequence shows some underlying concentration in the central portion of the reproductive ages. The decline in the median age of childbearing upon addition of the $\beta_i^* B_j^*$ component is clearly shown in the cumulative distributions on either scale.[8] The contribution of $\beta_i^* B_j^*$ to the description of both marital and overall fertility will receive particular attention. In a later section of the chapter we shall see that this component expresses not only essentially all of the association with change in the level of fertility but also important aspects of change in the pattern that are *not* associated with change in level. These latter aspects will be examined separately by linear adjustment of the β_i^* time sequence for change in the level of fertility. With the functions of α_i^* and β_i^* in mind, we shall turn to the seven-decade sequence of each EHR time parameter.

Change in α_i^*

The limited year-to-year variations in the first time parameter α_i^* can be examined in Figs. 7.4 and 7.5 for the three cross-sectional marital fertility sequences—MX20, MX15, and NX15—and in Fig. 7.6 for the related overall fertility sequences—XX20 and XX15. Although the α_i^* values differ in level by sequence, the small departures of α_i^* from constancy are similar in extent for all sequences. The most prominent variations are the temporary peak at 1942–1945 for all sequences, which is related mainly to a brief disproportionate increase in childbearing at ages 30–39, and the post-1955 rise in α_i^* for the MX15 and XX15 sequences. The post-1955 rise, shown in Chapter VI to continue for overall fertility at least until the end of the *X202* sequence in 1976, indicates a new variation on fertility patterns that is related at least partially to marital fertility.

TABLE 7.3

Fertility Distributions Constructed from the $\alpha_i^* A_j^*$ and $\beta_i^* B_j^*$ Components for the MX15, MX20, NX15, XX15, and XX20 Sequences, 1892–1963

Components[a]	Age cut					
	19/20	24/25	29/30	34/35	39/40	44/45
MX15 Sequence						
Folded square root scale						
1.226 A_j^*	−.5903	−.2743	−.0071	.2565	.5477	.8442
1.226 A_j^* + .2 B_j^*	−.4892	−.1715	.0886	.3374	.6028	.8657
1.226 A_j^* + .6 B_j^*	−.2869	.0341	.2802	.4990	.7130	.9088
1.226 A_j^* + 1.0 B_j^*	−.0847	.2397	.4717	.6607	.8233	.9518
Raw fraction scale, cumulated						
1.226 A_j^*	.1207	.3097	.4950	.6784	.8570	.9789
1.226 A_j^* + .2 B_j^*	.1755	.3797	.5626	.7317	.8856	.9841
1.226 A_j^* + .6 B_j^*	.3013	.5241	.6942	.8302	.9354	.9924
1.226 A_j^* + 1.0 B_j^*	.4402	.6671	.8144	.9131	.9733	.9978

	Age group						
	15–19	20–24	25–29	30–34	35–39	40–44	45–49
Raw fraction scale, non-cumulated							
1.226 A_j^*	.1207	.1890	.1853	.1834	.1786	.1219	.0211
1.226 A_j^* + .2 B_j^*	.1755	.2042	.1829	.1691	.1539	.0985	.0159
1.226 A_j^* + .6 B_j^*	.3013	.2228	.1701	.1360	.1052	.0570	.0076
1.226 A_j^* + 1.0 B_j^*	.4402	.2269	.1473	.0987	.0602	.0245	.0022

	Age cut				
	24/25	29/30	34/35	39/40	44/45
MX20 Sequence					
Folded square root scale					
1.106 A_j^*	−.3791	−.0605	.2325	.5428	.8528
1.106 A_j^* + .2 B_j^*	−.2887	.0519	.3415	.6230	.8823
1.106 A_j^* + .6 B_j^*	−.1079	.2768	.5595	.7833	.9413
1.106 A_j^* + 1.0 B_j^*	.0730	.5017	.7766	.9436	1.0002
Raw fraction scale, cumulated					
1.106 A_j^*	.2417	.4573	.6622	.8544	.9811
1.106 A_j^* + .2 B_j^*	.3002	.5367	.7343	.8955	.9876
1.106 A_j^* + .6 B_j^*	.4329	.6920	.8634	.9612	.9967
1.106 A_j^* + 1.0 B_j^*	.5515	.8317	.9593	.9970	1.0000

(*table continues*)

TABLE 7.3 (*continued*)

Components[a]	Age group					
	20–24	25–29	30–34	35–39	40–44	45–49
MX20 Sequence						
Raw fraction scale, non-cumulated						
$1.106\ A_j^*$	.2417	.2155	.2049	.1923	.1266	.0189
$1.106\ A_j^* + .2\ B_j^*$	.3002	.2366	.1976	.1611	.0921	.0124
$1.106\ A_j^* + .6\ B_j^*$	.4239	.2680	.1714	.0978	.0356	.0033
$1.106\ A_j^* + 1.0\ B_j^*$	.5515	.2802	.1276	.0377	.0030	.0000

	Age cut					
	19/20	24/25	29/30	34/35	39/40	44/45
NX15 Sequence						
Folded square root scale						
$1.260\ A_j^*$	−.4966	−.1732	.0898	.3584	.6290	.8831
$1.260\ A_j^* + .2\ B_j^*$	−.4470	−.0918	.1993	.4666	.7086	.9126
$1.260\ A_j^* + .6\ B_j^*$	−.3479	.0709	.4185	.6831	.8678	.9717
$1.260\ A_j^* + 1.0\ B_j^*$	−.2487	.2336	.6376	.8995	1.0270	1.0307
Raw fraction scale, cumulated						
$1.260\ A_j^*$	.1712	.3785	.5633	.7452	.8983	.9877
$1.260\ A_j^* + .2\ B_j^*$	.2001	.4352	.6395	.8115	.9336	.9930
$1.260\ A_j^* + .6\ B_j^*$	.2616	.5501	.7827	.9229	.9845	.9992
$1.260\ A_j^* + 1.0\ B_j^*$	.3269	.6629	.9024	.9908	.9993	.9990

	Age group						
	15–19	20–24	25–29	30–34	35–39	40–44	45–49
Raw fraction scale, non-cumulated							
$1.260\ A_j^*$	.1712	.2073	.1849	.1818	.1532	.0894	.0123
$1.260\ A_j^* + .2\ B_j^*$	.2001	.2351	.2043	.1719	.1221	.0594	.0070
$1.260\ A_j^* + .6\ B_j^*$	.2616	.2885	.2326	.1403	.0616	.0147	.0008
$1.260\ A_j^* + 1.0\ B_j^*$	.3269	.3361	.2395	.0884	.0085	.0000	.0000

	Age cut					
	19/20	24/25	29/30	34/35	39/40	44/45
XX15 Sequence						
Folded square root scale						
$1.468\ A_j^*$	−.8792	−.5544	−.1897	.1701	.5289	.8546
$1.468\ A_j^* + .2\ B_j^*$	−.8232	−.4575	−.0797	.2697	.5983	.8795
$1.468\ A_j^* + .6\ B_j^*$	−.7112	−.2637	.1404	.4690	.7370	.9293
$1.468\ A_j^* + 1.0\ B_j^*$	−.5991	−.0698	.3605	.6683	.8757	.9791

TABLE 7.3 (*continued*)

	Age cut					
Components[a]	19/20	24/25	29/30	34/35	39/40	44/45
XX15 Sequence						
Raw fraction scale, cumulated						
1.468 A_j^*	.0131	.1394	.3671	.6194	.8469	.9815
1.468 A_j^* + .2 B_j^*	.0267	.1939	.4438	.6872	.8833	.9870
1.468 A_j^* + .6 B_j^*	.0653	.3168	.5988	.8129	.9448	.9953
1.468 A_j^* + 1.0 B_j^*	.1163	.4507	.7465	.9165	.9862	.9996

	Age group						
	15–19	20–24	25–29	30–34	35–39	40–44	45–49
Raw fraction scale, non-cumulated							
1.468 A_j^*	.0131	.1263	.2277	.2523	.2275	.1346	.0185
1.468 A_j^* + .2 B_j^*	.0267	.1672	.2499	.2434	.1961	.1037	.0130
1.468 A_j^* + .6 B_j^*	.0653	.2515	.2820	.2141	.1319	.0505	.0047
1.468 A_j^* + 1.0 B_j^*	.1163	.3344	.2958	.1700	.0697	.0134	.0004

	Age cut				
	24/25	29/30	34/35	39/40	44/45
XX20 Sequence					
Folded square root scale					
1.187 A_j^*	−.6232	−.2619	.1066	.4851	.8398
1.187 A_j^* + .2 B_j^*	−.5317	−.1467	.2148	.5618	.8678
1.187 A_j^* + .6 B_j^*	−.3487	.0836	.4311	.7152	.9239
1.187 A_j^* + 1.0 B_j^*	−.1657	.3140	.6474	.8685	.9800
Raw fraction scale, cumulated					
1.187 A_j^*	.1044	.3180	.5752	.8222	.9778
1.187 A_j^* + .2 B_j^*	.1516	.3968	.6501	.8646	.9845
1.187 A_j^* + .6 B_j^*	.2611	.5590	.7903	.9363	.9946
1.187 A_j^* + 1.0 B_j^*	.3837	.7165	.9070	.9847	.9996

	Age group					
	20–24	25–29	30–34	35–39	40–44	45–49
Raw fraction scale, non-cumulated						
1.187 A_j^*	.1044	.2136	.2571	.2471	.1556	.0222
1.187 A_j^* + .2 B_j^*	.1516	.2452	.2533	.2145	.1200	.0155
1.187 A_j^* + .6 B_j^*	.2611	.2980	.2313	.1460	.0583	.0054
1.187 A_j^* + 1.0 B_j^*	.3837	.3328	.1905	.0777	.0149	.0004

[a] See Table 5.2 for the values of the members of the A_j^* and B_j^* vectors. For each sequence, α_i^* is set at its mean value shown in Table 5.2.

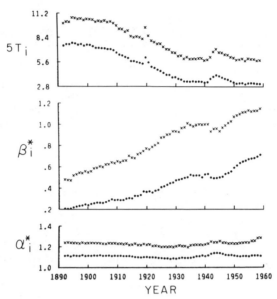

Fig. 7.4   EHR standard-form time parameters α_i^* and β_i^* and total rate of fertility $5T_i$ for the MX15 (×××) and MX20 (· · ·) sequences from 1892 to 1959.

Change in β_i^*

The second time parameter β_i^* exhibits distinct period-specific variations in its generally ascending course (Figs. 7.4–7.6). The slow but steady shift of the distribution toward younger ages through the early portion of these time sequences accelerates around 1920 for all but the

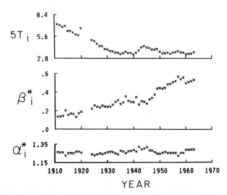

Fig. 7.5   EHR standard-form time parameters α_i^* and β_i^* and total rate of fertility $5T_i$ for the NX15 sequence from 1911 to 1963, with 1921–1923 missing.

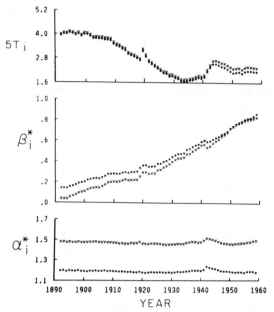

Fig. 7.6 EHR standard-form time parameters α_i^* and β_i^* and total rate of fertility $5T_i$ for the XX15 ($\times\times\times$) and XX20 ($\cdot\cdot$) sequences from 1892 to 1959.

NX15 sequence, which continues its earlier pace of change until a 1935–1945 period of fluctuation. Although reported data for the NX15 sequence begin with 1911, a method of extending the sequence by estimating the β_i^* values back to 1892, as well as filling in the missing 1921–1923 data, is presented in a later section of this chapter. Estimated EHR parameters for these years are included in Fig. 7.11.

For the MX20 and MX15 sequences, the post-1919 accelerated pace of change is interrupted by a 1934–1941 period of stability and a brief 1942–1945 reversal before resumption of the previous pace of change toward a younger age pattern of fertility. The temporary reversal toward later ages in the early 1940s reflects again (as did α_i^*) the prominent short-term increase in childbearing at ages 30–39 that accompanied the more prolonged period of increase for ages less than 30.

Because β_i^* for the NX15 sequence shows no evidence of acceleration until after 1945, the 1920–1934 increases in β_i^* for the MX20 and MX15 sequences seem to require a revised interpretation. Traditionally viewed as expressing an accelerated rate of control of fertility at higher ages in the 1920–1934 period, they appear instead to express an increased relative importance of premarital pregnancy leading to marriage, not only at ages 15–19 but also at ages 20–24, at a time when conceptions within marriage continue to change toward a younger age pattern at their previous steady pace.

About 1935 the rate of change in overall fertility diverges noticeably from that of marital fertility as the β_i^* values for the XX20 and XX15 sequences continue to rise.[9] Recall that the degree to which the overall fertility distribution is shifted away from higher ages depends on both the age distribution of marital fertility and the age distribution of entry into childbearing. The divergence of β_i^* for the cross-sectional overall and marital fertility sequences appears to have picked up the prominent increase that occurred between 1935 and 1950 in the proportion of women married at all childbearing ages greater than 19. The extent to which such changes in marriage patterns are captured intact in the standard-form EHR parameters and transmitted through further steps of dissection of the fitted parameters will be demonstrated more systematically in a later section of this chapter. We turn first to the steps of dissection that separate from α_i^* and β_i^* the portion of each that is not associated with change in the level of fertility.

Change in Marital Fertility Distributions Not Accounted for by Change in the Level of Marital Fertility

The concept of linear compensation of EHR time parameters for change in the level of fertility was introduced in Chapter VI, which includes a detailed consideration of the procedure applied to cohort overall fertility time sequences. Level-compensated variations in α_i^* and β_i^* for the MX20 and MX15 sequences are the focus of this section. Similar variations in the NX15 sequence for confinements occurring 9 months or more after marriage and the MC15 cohort sequence receive attention later in the chapter.

To summarize the procedure briefly: least squares regressions of α_i^* and β_i^* independently on $T_i^{1/2}$ for the MX20 and MX15 sequences provide the following expressions of the α_i^* and β_i^* vectors:

$$\alpha_i^* = k_1 + k_2\, T_i^{1/2} + \alpha_{i \cdot T}^*,$$
$$\beta_i^* = k_3 + k_4\, T_i^{1/2} + \beta_{i \cdot T}^*.$$

The residuals $\alpha_{i \cdot T}^*$ and $\beta_{i \cdot T}^*$ are the portions of the time parameters not linearly related to change in the total rate of fertility over the 68 years. The regression coefficients (Table 7.4) from these linear adjustments confirm that very little of the small amount of variation in the first parameter

TABLE 7.4

Regression Coefficients and Constants in the Linear Compensation of
EHR Time Parameters α_i^* and β_i^* for the Level of Fertility; Total Fertility
Rate $5T_m$ Implied by $\hat{\beta}_i^* = 0$: Selected Marital and Overall Fertility
Sequences, 1892–1963

Parameter[a]	Sequence	Regression coefficient	Constant	$5T_m$
α_i^*	MX15	.002	1.223	
	MX20	.007	1.099	
	NX15	−.045	1.302	
	MC15	−.009	1.375	
	XX15	.027	1.448	
	XX20	.013	1.178	
β_i^*	MX15	−1.354	2.507	17.14
	MX20	−.813	1.218	11.22
	NX15	−.807	1.068	8.76
	MC15	−1.335	2.415	16.36
	XX15	−1.630	1.583	4.72
	XX20	−1.419	1.461	5.30

[a] All parameters are compensated for the time vector of $T_i^{1/2}$ for the particular sequence involved.

α_i^* over the 68 years of the MX15 and MX20 sequences can be accounted
for by change in the level of fertility but that change in the second time
parameter β_i^* is highly related to the change in total rate.

At the same time, the portion of change in β_i^* for the MX20 sequence
not accounted for by the change in total rate has some prominent features
that are expressed by $\beta_{i \cdot T}^*$ (Fig. 7.7): the transition from positive to negative at 1910, the long, largely negative stretch from 1911 to 1942 (with one
notable exception, the post-war peak in 1920–1921), and the increasingly
positive values after 1950. The corresponding sequence of $\beta_{i \cdot T}^*$ values for

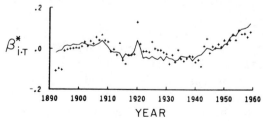

Fig. 7.7 Level-compensated time parameter $\beta_{i \cdot T}^*$ for the MX20 (———) and MX15 (+ + +)
sequences from 1892 to 1959.

the MX15 sequence is more irregular, particularly during the 1911–1914 period, but presents the same general picture.

The $\beta^*_{i\cdot T}$ regression residuals can be interpreted in the following way:

$\beta^*_{i\cdot T} = 0$ The age distribution of marital fertility is shifted toward the younger ages to the degree that would be predicted by the level of fertility if an inverse relation existed between β^*_i and $T_i^{1/2}$ across the time sequence

$\beta^*_{i\cdot T} > 0$ The age distribution of marital fertility is shifted *more* toward the younger ages (according to the pattern determined by B^*_j) than would be predicted by the level of fertility if β^*_i and $T_i^{1/2}$ were inversely related across the time sequence—women at ages 30 and higher are limiting their fertility disproportionately more than are younger women

$\beta^*_{i\cdot T} < 0$ The age distribution of marital fertility is shifted *less* toward the younger ages (according to the pattern determined by B^*_j) than would correspond, on the average, to the level of fertility

Figure 7.7 demonstrates that more systematic variation can occur in marital fertility than is described by a measure of the decline of marital fertility with age. We shall now examine these variations in more detail.

Trends in $\beta^*_{i\cdot T}$ for Cross-sectional Marital Fertility

The transition from a younger-than-level-predicted pattern of childbearing to an increasingly older-than-level-predicted pattern occurs over the 7 years from 1908 to 1914 (Fig. 7.7).[10] The negative change in $\beta^*_{i\cdot T}$ indicates that an increasing proportion of the decline in total fertility shown in Fig. 7.4 can be accounted for by limitation of fertility at ages lower than 30, supplementing limitation at ages 30 and higher. Following a prominent 1920–1921 post-war fertility response, the consistently negative $\beta^*_{i\cdot T}$ values for the MX20 sequence and the variably negative $\beta^*_{i\cdot T}$ values for the MX15 sequence (Fig. 7.7) indicate that a continued greater-than-level-predicted role in fertility limitation is played by ages lower than 30 in the further decline of total fertility from 1922 to 1932 and then in the maintenance of a steady, low level of total fertility from 1932 to 1941.

In the post-1941 transition from the older-than-level-predicted pattern to the increasingly younger-than-level-predicted pattern, $\beta^*_{i\cdot T}$ for the MX20 sequence approximately equals zero from 1943 to 1949. These years of moderate "baby boom" (see $5T_i$ in Fig. 7.4) are among the few years in which the distribution is shifted toward the younger ages to the level-predicted degree for the seven-decade sequence of marital fertility. The increasingly positive $\beta^*_{i,T}$ values from 1950 onward (Fig. 7.7), when total fertility fluctuates around a level that is slightly below the low levels of the 1930s, describe the extent to which married women above age 30 were limiting their fertility disproportionately more than were younger married women.

In the broader focus of the EHR analyses, we not only have evidence for the systematic variation in fertility limitation at ages 30 and higher, we also have evidence for the systematic contribution of fertility limitation below age 30 to change in the age pattern and total rate of marital fertility from at least 1908 onward. We need to consider the relative importance of at least two factors that could account for the apparent regulation of fertility at younger ages: one, control of conception at younger ages within marriage; two, change in the occurrence of nonmarital conceptions legitimated by marriage before the birth of the child. The EHR analysis of the NX15 sequence for confinements occurring 9 months or more after marriage indicates the presence of some control at younger ages within marriage. Level-compensated change, expressed in the $\beta^*_{i,T}$ values for the NX15 sequence, suggests variations in the contribution of such control that are not predicted by the total rate of fertility: with a time pattern similar to that found in $\beta^*_{i,T}$ for the MX15 and MX20 sequences, $\beta^*_{i,T}$ for the NX15 sequence declines from its 1911 level as total fertility declines, is at its most negative between 1926 and 1942, and shows a post-1942 transition from the older-than-level-predicted pattern to an increasingly younger-than-level-predicted pattern until 1960 (Figs. 7.10 and 7.11). The additional EHR analyses proposed at the end of the chapter should identify time-sequence trends in the variable border between illegitimate and marital fertility, thus clarifying the role of legitimated conceptions in the observed marital fertility pattern variations. The EHR perspective on twentieth-century Swedish fertility patterns challenges the conventional wisdom that measures of the decline of marital fertility with age or marriage duration are sufficient indicators of the extent of marital fertility control in a population either during or after a transition from higher to lower fertility.

Departures from Trend in $\beta^*_{i,T}$ for Cross-sectional Marital Fertility

Example 1   The prominent 1920–1921 departure of $\beta^*_{i,T}$ from trend (Fig. 7.7) is an indicator of postwar fertility response—a disproportionately high fertility rate for the extent to which the age pattern of fertility is shifted toward younger ages as registered by β_i^* (Fig. 7.4). This departure is also an example of a brief aberration in fertility brought quite well into the fitted parameters for all four types of sequence analyzed, leaving no outstanding departures from fit in either cross-sectional or cohort residuals for overall or marital fertility (see Figs. 4.5, 4.10, and 7.13). It is, in addition, an aberration that would have been obscured had we used 5-year averages (Fig. 7.3) instead of single-year schedules. For overall fertility, this period will be considered in Chapter VIII in relation to U.S. fertility experience in the years immediately following World War I.

Example 2   The abnormally low $\beta_{i\cdot T}^*$ values for the MX15 sequence from 1892 to 1894, derived from the depressed total rate of age 15–49 marital fertility and the low β_i^* values for those years (Fig. 7.4), should be viewed in relation to the 1895 change from the practice of recording the mother's reported age at confinement to the practice of recording her exact age as calculated from her birth date. The 1894–1895 discontinuity in the fertility data that results from this change is noted by Hofsten and Lundstrom (1976) and, in the EHR analyses, was first detected in the α_i^* time parameter for the cohort overall fertility sequences by 5-year age groups (see Fig. 6.10). Not surprisingly, the discontinuity is more evident in the EHR descriptions of marital fertility, both in the MX15 cross-sectional sequence parameters examined here and the MC15 cohort sequence parameters shown in Fig. 7.12. A simplified example comparable to Swedish data will serve now to illustrate the magnitude of the effect on marital fertility rates of relatively small numerical errors in the age classification of births between age groups 15–19 and 20–24.

We first assume 1500 births to 3000 married women aged 15–19 and 20,000 births to 45,000 married women aged 20–24. If 300 births to women aged 19 but close to age 20 were recorded as occurring at age 20, the rate for age group 20–24 would be only .003 too high, but the rate for age group 15–19 would be .05 too low. The sum T_i of the age-specific rates of marital fertility for the year would be underestimated by .047 and the total fertility rate $5T_i$ would be underestimated by .235. These calculations assume that the 300 women were included as age 20 in the denominator as well as the numerator in the rate calculations. If, instead, the population figures retained these women in age group 15–19 but placed their births in age group 20–24, the rate for age group 15–19 would be underestimated by .10, T_i would be underestimated by .094, and the total fertility rate $5T_i$ would be underestimated by .47. This is approximately the amount by which the total rate from 1892 to 1894 for the MX15 sequence differs from the total rate for the immediately following years.

Based on both cross-sectional and cohort EHR parameters—α_i^*, $\alpha_{i\cdot T}^*$, β_i^*, and $\beta_{i\cdot T}^*$—revisions to the reported age-specific marital fertility rates for the years 1892–1894 are proposed in a later section of this chapter. We shall first consider another use of the level-compensated time parameters: the construction of level-standardized distributions of marital fertility.

Change in Age-specific Proportions Married: Approximation from EHR Fertility Parameters

In Chapter VI we constructed level-standardized distributions of cohort overall fertility using the level-compensated time parameters $\alpha_{i\cdot T}^*$ and $\beta_{i\cdot T}^*$ and selected standard levels of total fertility. A particularly informative choice of level was the high level—T_m for single-year-of-age schedules, $5T_m$ for schedules by 5-year age groups—that would be achieved at $\hat{\beta}_i^* = 0$ if β_i^* were inversely related to $T_i^{1/2}$ across the time sequence. For cohort overall fertility our interest was change in the mean age of childbearing at a standard fertility level considered as an index of change in the timing of childbearing apart from level. We shall now follow the same procedures to construct level-standardized distributions of both marital and overall fertility in a cross-sectional perspective.

The reader may want to review the discussion of the procedures in Chapter VI at this point. In this section we shall:

1. summarize procedures for the construction of MX20 distributions at $5T_m = 11.22$ and XX20 distributions at $5T_m = 5.30$;
2. briefly consider examples of MX20 level-standardized distributions in relation to some "natural fertility" distributions;
3. concentrate on the time sequence of approximations of age-specific proportions married that is constructed from the level-compensated EHR parameters and the sums of age-specific fertility rates for the MX20 and XX20 sequences.

The effect of illegitimate fertility on such approximations will be discussed briefly in this section, but will be considered again at the end of the chapter in relation to possible extensions of the EHR analysis of fertility distributions.

Construction of Level-standardized Marital and Overall Fertility Distributions

We begin with the least squares regression of the α_i^* and β_i^* vectors for the MX20 sequence independently on the vector of $T_i^{1/2}$ and the regression of the α_i^* and β_i^* vectors for the XX20 sequence independently on the corresponding vector of $T_i^{1/2}$ to separate from each time parameter the portion of change that is not linearly related to change in the total rate of fertility over the 68 years considered. To form the pairs of $\alpha_i^s A_j^*$ and $\beta_i^s B_j^*$ components for each year at each age cut for the MX20 marital fertility sequence, first, the level-compensated time vector $\alpha_{i\cdot T}^*$ is centered on the regression constant k_1 and each element of the resulting vector $k_1 + \alpha_{i\cdot T}^*$ is multiplied by each element of the age vector A_j^*. Second, each element of the level-compensated time vector $\beta_{i\cdot T}^*$ (Fig. 7.7) is multiplied by each element of the age vector B_j^* so that the sequence is compensated to the standard level of fertility ($5T_m = 11.22$) at which $\hat{\beta}_i^* = 0$. For each year i and age cut j the complete level-compensated element for the MX20 sequence is given by

$$M_{ij} = (k_1 + \alpha_{i\cdot T}^*)A_j^* + \beta_{i\cdot T}^* B_j^*,$$

where $\alpha_{i\cdot T}^*$ and $\beta_{i\cdot T}^*$ are the α_i^* and β_i^* parameters linearly compensated for $T_i^{1/2}$ and k_1 the constant from the regression of α_i^* on $T_i^{1/2}$.

The corresponding sequence of cumulative distributions of overall fertility standardized to the level $5T_m = 5.30$ is constructed in the same way from the $\alpha_{i\cdot T}^*$ values and the $\beta_{i\cdot T}^*$ values (Fig. 7.8) for the XX20 sequence so that for each year i and age cut j the complete level-compensated element for the XX20 sequence is given by

$$X_{ij} = (k_1 + \alpha_{i\cdot T}^*)A_j^* + \beta_{i\cdot T}^* B_j^*,$$

where $\alpha_{i\cdot T}^*$ and $\beta_{i\cdot T}^*$ are the α_i^* and β_i^* parameters linearly compensated for $T_i^{1/2}$ and k_1 the constant from the regression of α_i^* on $T_i^{1/2}$. The expressions M_{ij} and X_{ij} on the folded square root scale used in the analysis are then de-transformed to the raw fraction scale (see Chapter VIII for the procedure) and de-cumulated to give the level-standardized, age-specific marital and overall fertility distributions M_{ij}' and X_{ij}'.

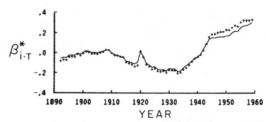

Fig. 7.8 Level-compensated time parameter $\beta_{i\cdot T}^*$ for the XX20 (——) and XX15 (+++) sequences from 1892 to 1959.

Level-standardized and "Natural" Marital
Fertility Patterns

The $\alpha_i^* A_j^*$ component for the MX20 sequence has been shown to describe, by itself, an age pattern of marital fertility very close to some patterns identified with the term "natural fertility". Because the level-standardized MX20 distributions at $5T_m = 11.22$ represent age 20–49 marital fertility patterns that would have resulted if all the relation between change in pattern and decline of marital fertility with age were excluded across the sequence, they should resemble but differ slightly from the pattern described by $\alpha_i^* A_j^*$ alone. At the high fertility level $5T_m = 11.22$ with $\hat{\beta}_i^* = 0$, these distributions should also resemble some distributions with a natural fertility pattern.

Inspection of Table 7.5 reveals both similarities—Greenland 1901–1930 and Sweden 1958, Hutterites 1921–1930 and Sweden 1951, Canada 1700–1730 and Sweden 1944—and some small but distinct differences. The differences include the lower proportion of fertility in age group 25–29 and the higher proportion in age group 40–44 for the earlier Swedish schedules than for all others, even the later Swedish schedules. The level-standardized and natural fertility distributions can be described as a close family of patterns that reflect small time- or culture-specific variations of a more general underlying pattern on which the age pattern of decline of marital fertility is imposed with varying intensity.

Examples of the level-standardized distributions X'_{ij} for overall fertility are shown in Table 7.5. Free of linear association between change in pattern and change in level of fertility across the sequence, these distributions represent the remaining systematic variations in cross-sectional overall fertility, including the contributions of level-standardized variations in marital fertility.

Approximation of Age-specific
Proportions Married

The age-specific proportions of women married in year i can be approximated from the level-standardized distributions of overall and marital fertility in the following way. The summed rates of overall fertility T_i^X and marital fertility T_i^M for each year are allocated to the age groups proportionately, according to the corresponding level-compensated patterns X'_{ij} and M'_{ij} derived for that year. This provides a pattern-standardized overall fertility rate (births per woman) and a pattern-standardized marital fertil-

TABLE 7.5

EHR Standard Fertility Distributions, Reported Natural Fertility Distributions, and EHR Level-standardized Distributions of Marital and Overall Fertility, Selected Examples

Distribution	Age group						
	20–24	25–29	30–34	35–39	40–44	45–49	5 $\Sigma f(a)$
EHR standard distributions							
MX20 $\alpha_i^* A_j^*$							
lowest $\alpha_i^* = 1.080$	.2473	.2110	.2001	.1891	.1284	.0241	
highest $\alpha_i^* = 1.138$	.2348	.2212	.2107	.1961	.1238	.0134	
Reported natural fertility distributions[a]							
Hutterites							
Marriages 1921–1930	.2514	.2294	.2043	.1856	.1015	.0279	10.9
Marriages before 1921	.2425	.2302	.2169	.1909	.1046	.0148	9.8
Canada, marriages 1700–1730	.2358	.2293	.2242	.1899	.1070	.0139	10.8
Norway, marriages 1874–1876	.2434	.2336	.2096	.1776	.1106	.0252	8.1
Greenland							
1851–1900	.246	.230	.223	.189	.098	.015	7.7
1901–1930	.271	.229	.208	.169	.104	.018	7.8
Europeans of Tunis, marriages 1840–1859	.2562	.2354	.2200	.1773	.1040	.0071	9.2

EHR level-standardized distributions

MX20 $f(A_j^*, B_j^*)^b$

Year						
1898	.2477	.2181	.2044	.1891	.1227	.0180
1924	.2330	.2059	.2018	.1967	.1371	.0255
1934	.2313	.2055	.2022	.1976	.1380	.0254
1944	.2378	.2207	.2094	.1945	.1233	.0142
1951	.2513	.2182	.2033	.1871	.1215	.0186
1958	.2732	.2276	.2016	.1754	.1072	.0151

XX20 $f(A_j^*, B_j^*)^c$

Year						
1898	.1039	.2125	.2566	.2475	.1567	.0229
1924	.0788	.1875	.2528	.2658	.1835	.0317
1934	.0696	.1812	.2537	.2729	.1908	.0318
1944	.1308	.2380	.2592	.2280	.1296	.0144
1951	.1491	.2389	.2507	.2167	.1256	.0190
1958	.1767	.2559	.2477	.1986	.1064	.0147

[a] Sources: data for the Hutterites, Canada, Norway, and Tunis were taken from Henry (1961); data for Greenland were taken from Hansen (1979).
[b] MX20 fits are standardized to a total fertility rate of $5T_m = 11.2$.
[c] XX20 fits are standardized to a total fertility rate of $5T_m = 5.3$.

ity rate (births per married woman) for each age group in each year. An approximation of the proportion of all women in age group j that are married in year i is then given by

$$P_{ij} = (X'_{ij}T^X_i)/(M'_{ij}T^M_i).\text{[11]}$$

Time sequences of such approximations based on the EHR parameters for the MX20 and XX20 sequences are shown in Fig. 7.9 for three age groups that experienced notable alterations in marriage pattern over the 68 years analyzed. The prominent increase in age-specific proportions married beginning in 1935 and the deceleration in change after 1945 are clearly transmitted by the EHR parameters. If all childbearing occurred within marriage, these approximations would differ from the actual proportions married only to the extent that small variations are left in the residuals by the original fitting procedures for both overall and marital fertility sequences. In the present case, significant illegitimate fertility (as high as 30 percent and no less than 12 percent of all births at ages 20–24 in the years 1892–1959) is represented in T^X_i and the parameters used to construct X'_{ij} but is excluded from T^M_i and the parameters used to construct M'_{ij}. Accepting the existence of premarital pregnancy and illegitimacy (or nonmarital childbearing) in most populations, later in the chapter we shall propose extensions of the EHR analyses to extract from

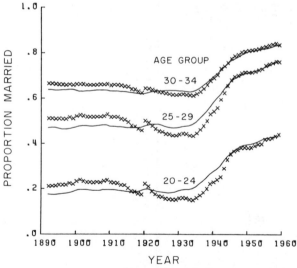

Fig. 7.9   Age-specific proportions of women married, reported (——) and approximated ($\times\times\times$) from EHR-derived level-standardized distributions of overall and marital fertility and sums of age-specific rates of overall and marital fertility from 1892 to 1959.

aggregate fertility data a description of any systematic change over time in the tendency to marry or not marry before giving birth to a nonmaritally conceived child.

Use of Intersequence EHR Relations to Detect the Unusual and Estimate Missing Data

The NX15 sequence for confinements occurring 9 months or more after marriage includes the years 1911–1920 and 1924–1963. Some important aspects of this sequence, as viewed through EHR time parameters, were discussed earlier in this chapter. Now we shall use the NX15 sequence in conjunction with its parent sequence, the MX15 sequence for all confinements occurring within marriage, to detect unusual years and estimate missing values.

Departures from Trend in Childbearing Occurring
9 Months or More after Marriage

The NX15 residuals (see Fig. 4.11) suggest individual years to investigate for unusual circumstances: particularly the years 1937, 1949, and 1960–1963—or rather, 1936/1937, 1948/1949, and 1959/1960–1962/1963 if we are looking for relations to time of conception. For the years 1937 and 1949, the large positive residuals ($>.03$) at age cut 19/20 indicate that even a higher proportion of confinements occurred at ages 15–19 than was accommodated by the sharp increase in the value of β_i^* observed in Fig. 7.5 (indicating a shift toward younger ages according to the pattern of B_j^*). For the years 1960–1963, the large negative residuals at age cut 19/20 accompanied by positive residuals at age cut 29/30 indicate that even a smaller proportion of confinements occurred at ages 15–19 and even a larger proportion was attributable to ages 25–29 than the decline in the value of β_i^* (indicating a shift toward older ages according to the pattern of B_j^*) would have predicted. Because the total rate of fertility for the NX15 sequence rose slightly for 1937 and 1949 and declined slightly for 1960 to 1962, linearly adjusting β_i^* for change in total rate makes these years stand out even more in the value of $\beta_{i \cdot T}^*$ as having noticeably different patterns from those for the adjacent years (Fig. 7.11).

Viewed through EHR fits to the MX15 sequence for all legitimate births, the years 1937 and 1949 do not show evidence of unusual circumstances in the residuals (see Fig. 4.10), the fitted parameters, or the total rates (Fig. 7.4). The large NX15 residuals for these two years therefore suggest either: one, an unusual division of the total age 15–19 confinements for legitimate births between the categories "occurring 9 months or more after marriage" and "occurring less than 9 months after marriage"; or two, a need to attribute to a larger number of women aged 15–19 the possibility of having a confinement occurring 9 months or more after marriage. Did some circumstance encourage an unusually high number of imminent marriages to occur in these years at ages 15–19 before conception? Did some circumstance lead to the recording of a number of premaritally conceived births as occurring 9 months or more after marriage? Did an unusually large number of women aged 15–19 who gave birth to one child in those years less than 9 months after marriage (and who were therefore omitted from the number of married women having the possibility of a birth occurring 9 months or more after marriage in those years in calculating the NX15 rates) have a second child in the same year? The exploratory analyses can reveal unusual observations and suggest directions in which to look for the causes, but they cannot confirm which of the possible causes is responsible for an aberration.

The 1960–1963 departures from fit that occur near the end of the NX15 sequence present a different set of considerations than do the 1937 and 1949 singular departures from fit that occur in the middle of the sequence. Are they brief departures from trend or do they presage new variations in marital fertility patterns? Two sources of evidence suggest that the 1960–1963 departures represent a new trend. The EHR fits to the MX15 sequence for all legitimate births reveal similar departures from previous patterns during the late 1950s: negative residuals at age cut 19/20 and increasingly positive residuals at age cut 29/30 (see Fig. 4.10) as well as an increasingly positive value of α_i^* (Fig. 7.4). When later Swedish marital fertility schedules are expressed as weighted sums of the A_j^* and B_j^* vectors for the MX15 sequence, this type of change in pattern is found to intensify in the 1970s (see Chapter VIII on cross-population comparisons for recent decades). We also know from the EHR analysis of the overall fertility sequence $X202$ in Chapter VI that a transition in overall fertility patterns had already begun in the late 1950s (Fig. 6.12). This transition became more pronounced in the 1960s and 1970s in concurrence with several social changes: family formation and legal marriage became increasingly dissociated from the mid-1960s onward, new contraceptives became available (the pill in 1964, the IUD in 1966) and increased in popularity in the 1970s (Gendell, 1980), and the incidence of divorce increased. Although we see in the EHR parameters and residuals only the aggregate consequences of behavioral change, the evidence of a post-1955 transition in fertility patterns leads to a first expectation about the NX15 patterns: EHR fitting of an NX15 sequence extended to the most recent years should largely bring the 1960–1963 departures from fit into a new set of fitted parameters to reveal a transition in the age pattern of confinements occurring 9 months or more after marriage.

The EHR analysis of the *X202* sequence also discloses evidence for a brief departure superimposed on the apparent new trend in overall fertility. The 1964–1968 high positive residuals for age group 15–19 (see Fig. 4.6) coincide with a short-term elevation in the total rates of overall fertility (see Fig. 6.12) and marital fertility. This observation leads to a second expectation about marital fertility patterns in the 1960s and 1970s: EHR fits to the NX15 and MX15 sequences extended to the most recent years are likely to reveal a brief variation in pattern in the mid-1960s. Whether this variation is largely brought into the fitted parameters, as occurred with the 1920–1921 and 1942–1948 variations, or whether it is left in the residuals will depend not only on whether childbearing experience in these years is a real departure from previous patterns but also on how well we have captured the "true" systematic variability in the fitted parameters and left the "true" irregularity in the residuals. Different fitting conditions and more complex models may both need to be considered (see the section on Future Directions in Exploring Fertility Relations and Chapter VIII on cross-population comparisons of marital fertility).

Use of Relations between the NX15 and MX15 EHR Time Parameters to Estimate Missing Data for the NX15 Sequence

EHR descriptions allow unusual years such as 1937 and 1949 to stand out from the trend. On the other hand, certain regularities (lasting 46 years) in the relations between the time parameters for the NX15 and MX15 sequences permit estimations of the trend in the NX15 sequence for 22 additional years for which fertility data by duration of marriage are not available.[12] For these estimations, some assumptions about α_i^*, $\beta_{i\cdot T}^*$, and T_i (the sum of age-specific rates) are necessary. The procedure is illustrated using the combination of assumptions in the accompanying list; the reader may wish to try other combinations.

1. For the period 1921–1923, T_i for the NX15 sequence is assumed to be approximately .52 births per woman lower than T_i for the MX15 sequence, in accord with the trend in that period. For the period 1895–1910, calculations are based on two assumed levels of T_i for the NX15 sequence: .45 and .50 below the level for the MX15 sequence (Fig. 7.10). For the period 1892–1894, the two assumed lev-

els are higher: only .35 and .40 below the level for the MX15 sequence. This is an estimated correction to bring the rates for the years 1892–1894 into line with those following the 1895 change to the practice of recording births by the mother's exact age as calculated from her date of birth (see Example 2 in the section on Level-compensated Change in Marital Fertility).

2. The nearly constant α_i^* parameter for the NX15 sequence is assumed to have values approximately .035 higher than α_i^* for the MX15 sequence in the periods 1921–1923 and 1892–1910 and to show no more fluctuation in the 1892–1910 period than does α_i^* for the MX15 and other sequences (Fig. 7.11).

3. The $\beta_{i\cdot T}^*$ parameter for the NX15 sequence, which has values variously slightly above or slightly below those for the MX15 sequence is assumed to have slightly lower values than those for the MX15 sequence from 1921 to 1923, in accord with the trend in that period, and to be approximately the same as $\beta_{i\cdot T}^*$ for the MX15 sequence from 1895 to 1910 (Fig. 7.11). For the years 1892–1894, the values of $\beta_{i\cdot T}^*$ for the NX15 sequence are assumed to be .1 higher than the unrevised values for the MX15 sequence, to be consistent with the correction applied to T_i for these three years.

4. The constant and regression coefficient from linear compensation of β_i^* for the NX15 sequence for total rate of fertility for the years 1911–1920 and 1924–1963 are assumed to apply also for the years 1892–1910 and 1921–1923.

Values of β_i^* for the NX15 sequence are estimated for the 1892–1910 and 1921–1923 periods from the following relation of EHR level-compen-

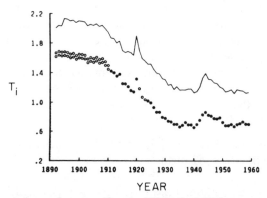

YEAR

Fig. 7.10   Reported sum of age-specific rates (T_i) for the MX15 sequence (——) from 1892 to 1959 and the NX15 sequence (● ● ●) from 1911 to 1920 and 1924 to 1959 and assumed sum of age-specific rates for the NX15 sequence (○ ○ ○) from 1892 to 1910 (on two levels) and 1921 to 1923.

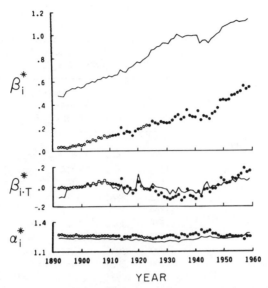

Fig. 7.11   EHR standard-form time parameters α_i^*, β_i^*, and $\beta_{i\cdot T}^*$ for the MX15 and NX15 sequences from 1892 to 1959: fitted values (——) for the MX15 sequence and fitted (● ● ●) and approximated (○ ○ ○) values for the NX15 sequence.

sated parameters and the level of fertility:

$$\hat{\beta}_i^* = k_1 + k_2 \hat{T}_i^{1/2} + \hat{\beta}_{i\cdot T}^*.$$

In the present case, $k_1 = 1.068$ and $k_2 = -.807$ (Table 7.4). The inverse relation between β_i^* and the total rate means that only a relatively narrow range for the total rate can be logically assumed for any given year. The values of $\hat{\beta}_i^*$ estimated for the lower level of fertility from 1892 to 1910 are included in Fig. 7.11.

Cumulative fertility distributions are calculated from the A_j^* and B_j^* age standards for the NX15 sequence and the estimated time parameters by

$$\hat{F}_{ij} = \hat{\alpha}_i^* A_j^* + \hat{\beta}_i^* B_j^*.$$

These distributions are then de-transformed from the folded square root scale to the raw fraction scale (see Chapter VIII for the procedure) to provide the distributions shown in Table 7.6.[13] The extent to which the higher of the two $\hat{\beta}_i^*$ values for a given year places a larger proportion of childbearing at the younger ages can be detected by comparing the two estimated distributions for the same year. These distributions, de-cumulated and multiplied by the corresponding values of T_i assumed for these years, provide the estimated age-specific rates shown in Tables 7.7 and 7.8 for confinements occurring 9 months or more after marriage. The

TABLE 7.6

Cumulated, Normalized Fertility Distributions (Raw Fraction Scale) Calculated from
EHR-derived Age Standards A_j^* and B_j^* for the NX15 Sequence and Estimated Time
Parameters $\hat{\alpha}_i^*$ and $\hat{\beta}_i^*$ for the Years 1892–1910 and 1921–1923

Year	Age cut					
	19/20	24/25	29/30	34/35	39/40	44/45
Based on lower T_i estimates[a]						
1892	.1736	.3867	.5763	.7580	.9067	.9899
1893	.1735	.3874	.5778	.7598	.9080	.9904
1894	.1750	.3877	.5767	.7577	.9058	.9893
1895	.1751	.3861	.5736	.7543	.9033	.9885
1896	.1764	.3886	.5771	.7574	.9050	.9887
1897	.1779	.3916	.5812	.7610	.9070	.9890
1898	.1747	.3900	.5813	.7628	.9097	.9906
1899	.1792	.3943	.5848	.7642	.9087	.9893
1900	.1790	.3928	.5823	.7615	.9068	.9887
1901	.1804	.3955	.5859	.7647	.9086	.9890
1902	.1834	.4025	.5959	.7739	.9139	.9901
1903	.1829	.4014	.5945	.7727	.9132	.9900
1904	.1843	.4060	.6015	.7794	.9175	.9911
1905	.1854	.4047	.5980	.7751	.9139	.9896
1906	.1892	.4121	.6079	.7838	.9185	.9903
1907	.1873	.4103	.6063	.7830	.9187	.9908
1908	.1905	.4164	.6146	.7902	.9225	.9913
1909	.1885	.4125	.6094	.7851	.9201	.9910
1910	.1910	.4157	.6127	.7878	.9207	.9906
Based on higher T_i estimates[b]						
1892	.1714	.3823	.5702	.7526	.9037	.9895
1893	.1713	.3830	.5718	.7545	.9051	.9900
1894	.1728	.3833	.5707	.7524	.9029	.9889
1895	.1729	.3816	.5676	.7489	.9004	.9880
1896	.1741	.3842	.5710	.7520	.9020	.9883
1897	.1756	.3872	.5751	.7556	.9040	.9886
1898	.1725	.3855	.5752	.7575	.9068	.9902
1899	.1770	.3898	.5787	.7588	.9057	.9888
1900	.1768	.3883	.5762	.7562	.9039	.9883
1901	.1781	.3910	.5798	.7594	.9057	.9885
1902	.1811	.3980	.5898	.7686	.9110	.9896
1903	.1805	.3969	.5883	.7673	.9103	.9895
1904	.1819	.4014	.5953	.7741	.9146	.9906
1905	.1831	.4001	.5918	.7697	.9110	.9891
1906	.1869	.4076	.6018	.7785	.9157	.9899
1907	.1850	.4057	.6002	.7776	.9159	.9904
1908	.1882	.4119	.6085	.7849	.9197	.9909
1909	.1861	.4079	.6032	.7803	.9173	.9906
1910	.1886	.4109	.6063	.7824	.9178	.9902

TABLE 7.6 (continued)

	Age cut					
Year	19/20	24/25	29/30	34/35	39/40	44/45
Based on T_i estimates[c]						
1921	.2017	.4347	.6370	.8080	.9306	.9917
1922	.2071	.4406	.6426	.8113	.9309	.9906
1923	.2083	.4438	.6471	.8153	.9332	.9912

[a] In the estimation of β_i^* from T_i and $\beta_{i\cdot T}^*$, T_i is assumed to be .40 births per woman lower than T_i for the MX15 sequence for the years 1892–1894 and .50 births per woman lower for the years 1895–1910.
[b] T_i is assumed to be .35 births per woman lower than T_i for the MX15 sequence for the years 1892–1894 and .45 births per woman lower for the years 1895–1910.
[c] T_i is assumed to be .52 births per woman lower than T_i for the MX15 sequence for the years 1921–1923.

reported age-specific rates of marital fertility for age groups 30–34 and higher for these years are shown in Table 7.7 for comparison.

We shall assume that the reported marital fertility rates for the four highest age groups for the years 1892–1910 and 1921–1923 are as negligibly influenced by confinements occurring less than 9 months after marriage as are the rates for the years 1911–1920 and 1924–1963. If the estimated NX15 rates for these age groups for the years 1892–1910 and 1921–1923 are very close to the reported MX15 rates, we then have some confirmation that our estimation procedures for supplying missing fertility data are based on sound assumptions. For the years 1921–1923, the estimated and reported rates for age groups 30–34 and higher are extremely close (Table 7.7). For the years 1892–1910, EHR estimates at the lower assumed levels of fertility are again extremely close and sometimes identical to the reported rates for age groups 35–39, 40–44, and 45–49 and are even quite close to the reported rates for age group 30–34 when the higher-level estimates are closer. We therefore adopt the set of lower-level rates as our estimated rates for confinements occurring 9 months or more after marriage in age groups 15–19, 20–24, and 25–29 in these years (Table 7.8).[14] Revision of the faulty MX15 rates for the years 1892–1894 using EHR parameters and MX15–MC15 intersequence relations will be outlined in the next section.

Cohort Marital Fertility and Its Relation to Cohort Overall Fertility

The MC15 cohort marital fertility sequence is the shortest of the Swedish sequences analyzed, covering only 42 cohorts. It includes, however, most

TABLE 7.7

	Age group					
	30–34			35–39		
Year	Low estimate	Reported	High estimate	Low estimate	Reported	High estimate
1892	.293	.300	.304	.240	.236	.252
1893	.297	.308	.308	.242	.244	.254
1894	.294	.305	.304	.241	.240	.252
1895	.294	.309	.305	.243	.244	.254
1896	.292	.305	.302	.239	.240	.251
1897	.288	.298	.298	.233	.233	.245
1898	.292	.301	.303	.236	.236	.248
1899	.283	.285	.294	.228	.229	.240
1900	.287	.296	.297	.232	.232	.244
1901	.285	.293	.295	.229	.230	.241
1902	.282	.289	.292	.222	.223	.233
1903	.274	.282	.284	.216	.214	.227
1904	.277	.285	.287	.215	.212	.226
1905	.273	.283	.283	.214	.211	.225
1906	.274	.279	.284	.210	.210	.221
1907	.270	.275	.280	.208	.207	.218
1908	.270	.273	.280	.204	.205	.214
1909	.264	.268	.275	.202	.204	.212
1910	.254	.255	.264	.193	.198	.203
	Estimate	Reported			Estimate	Reported
1921	.204	.200			.146	.149
1922	.181	.184			.129	.135
1923	.175	.177			.123	.129

of the cohorts that experienced the prominent changes in cohort overall fertility patterns examined in Chapter VI. The MC15 sequence therefore provides an opportunity to test the validity of our use of EHR overall fertility parameters to draw conclusions about underlying change in marital fertility patterns. In addition, the age 15–19 intersection of the MC15 and MX15 sequences provides a means for estimating corrections to faulty age-specific fertility rates for the years 1892–1894 using cohort and cross-sectional EHR marital fertility parameters.

Marital Fertility Rates for Age Groups 30–34 to 45–49 for the Years 1892–1910 and
1921–1923 Reported and Calculated from EHR Age Parameters, Estimated Time
Parameters, and Estimated Sums of Age-specific Rates for the NX15 Sequence

			Age group		
	40–44			45–49	
Low estimate	Reported	High estimate	Low estimate	Reported	High estimate
.135	.132	.143	.016	.019	.017
.135	.133	.143	.016	.019	.017
.136	.137	.144	.017	.020	.019
.139	.136	.147	.019	.018	.020
.136	.134	.144	.018	.018	.020
.131	.130	.140	.018	.018	.019
.130	.129	.139	.015	.016	.016
.127	.125	.135	.017	.017	.018
.131	.128	.139	.018	.017	.019
.128	.123	.136	.018	.017	.019
.121	.121	.129	.016	.015	.017
.118	.115	.126	.015	.016	.017
.114	.116	.122	.014	.015	.015
.117	.116	.124	.016	.016	.017
.112	.115	.119	.015	.015	.016
.110	.110	.118	.014	.014	.015
.106	.106	.113	.013	.014	.014
.106	.104	.114	.014	.014	.015
.101	.100	.109	.014	.013	.015
	Estimate	Reported		Estimate	Reported
	.073	.075		.010	.009
	.064	.069		.010	.009
	.060	.066		.009	.008

Relations between Marital and Overall
Fertility Change

The evidence in Chapter VI indicated that: one, change in the age
pattern of overall fertility for the cohorts aged 15 from 1893 to 1910 could
be largely accounted for by a decline in childbearing at ages 30 and higher;
and two, change for subsequent cohorts was largely dependent on change
in the age pattern of entry into marriage and dependent to only a small

TABLE 7.8

Rates of Childbearing Occurring 9 Months or
More After Marriage for Age Groups 15–19 to
25–29 for the Years 1892–1910 and 1921–1923
Estimated from EHR Parameter Relations
between the NX15 and MX15 Sequences

	Age group		
Year	15–19	20–24	25–29
1892	.2804	.3441	.3062
1893	.2836	.3499	.3113
1894	.2844	.3456	.3072
1895	.2854	.3439	.3057
1896	.2857	.3438	.3053
1897	.2846	.3420	.3033
1898	.2813	.3465	.3080
1899	.2832	.3398	.3010
1900	.2864	.3421	.3031
1901	.2877	.3431	.3037
1902	.2907	.3473	.3065
1903	.2807	.3355	.2963
1904	.2865	.3448	.3040
1905	.2855	.3377	.2976
1906	.2952	.3478	.3055
1907	.2866	.3411	.3000
1908	.2934	.3479	.3052
1909	.2828	.3361	.2953
1910	.2770	.3257	.2857
1921	.2401	.2772	.2408
1922	.2226	.2511	.2172
1923	.2167	.2448	.2115

degree on further change in marital fertility patterns. The MC15 time parameters and total rates confirm this interpretation in a comparison with time parameters and total rates for the corresponding portion of the C15 overall fertility sequence (Fig. 7.12).

Trends for 1892 to 1910 Cohorts   The cohorts aged 15–19 from 1892 to 1910 experienced only small differences in the age pattern of marriage (see Fig. 6.8). These are the cohorts with the youngest mean age of level-standardized overall fertility since the cohorts aged 15–19 from 1811 to 1826 (see Fig. 6.17). The steady rise in the value of β_i^* for the MC15 sequence (Fig. 7.12) is synchronous with the rise in the value of β_i^* for the C15 sequence and signals the increasing shift of the marital fertility distribution (like the overall fertility distribution) toward a younger age pattern of childbearing. The fact that a steady decline in total marital fertility rate as well as total overall fertility rate accompanies the shift confirms that the decline of marital fertility at higher ages is a factor in the observed change in the overall fertility pattern for these cohorts.

Linear compensation of β_i^* for the MC15 sequence for change in the level of completed marital fertility reveals in $\beta_{i\cdot T}^*$ the extent to which change in β_i^* is not inversely related to change in level across the sequence. Adapting to marital fertility parameters the interpretive scheme outlined in Chapter VI for overall fertility parameters, we consider both the sign of $\beta_{i\cdot T}^*$ and the direction of change in $\beta_{i\cdot T}^*$. For the cohorts aged 15–19 from 1895 to 1901, $\beta_{i\cdot T}^* \simeq 0$; for the cohorts aged 15–19 from 1902 to 1909, $\beta_{i\cdot T}^* > 0$ and $\Delta\beta_{i\cdot T}^* > 0$. We can therefore say that the shift toward younger ages according to the pattern determined by the B_j^* vector either equals or is increasingly greater than the change that would correspond, on the average, to the decline in the level of fertility for these cohorts.

Trends for 1914 to 1933 Cohorts   In contrast to the cohorts aged 15–19 from 1892 to 1910, cohorts which experienced little change in marriage

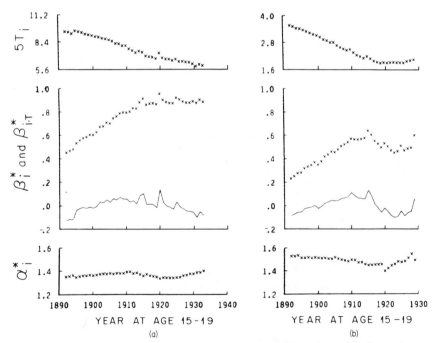

Fig. 7.12   EHR standard-form time parameters α_i^*, and β_i^* ($\times\times\times$), and $\beta_{i\cdot T}^*$ (——), and total rate of fertility $5T_i$: (a), MC15 sequence, cohorts aged 15–19 from 1892 to 1933; (b), C15 sequence, segment for cohorts aged 15–19 from 1892 to 1929.

pattern but progressive change in marital fertility, the cohorts aged 15–19 from 1914 to 1933 maintained a relatively steady age pattern of marital fertility as viewed through EHR time parameters. Aside from single-cohort departures, the value of β_i^* for the MC15 sequence shows only a very slight rise—confirmation that the change toward an older pattern of overall fertility described by the prominent decline in the value of β_i^* for the C15 sequence does not depend on marital fertility change toward an older pattern but on the pronounced change in the age pattern of entry into marriage.

Turning to the level-compensated time parameter $\beta_{i\cdot T}^*$ for the MC15 sequence, we find a gradual decline across the 20 cohorts from 1914 to 1933 that is punctuated by brief departures from trend. The increasingly negative value of $\beta_{i\cdot T}^*$ for the cohorts aged 15–19 after 1926 indicates a slightly lower proportion of total fertility at the youngest ages and a slightly higher proportion at older ages than would correspond, on the average, to the level of fertility.

Departures from Trend   The brief positive deviations in the value of β_i^* for the MC15 sequence represent period effects on cohort behavior that were either fully or partially brought into the fitted parameters. For example, the 1914, single-year increase in childbearing at ages 15–19 is reflected by a peak in the value of β_i^*, indicating a younger age pattern of fertility for the cohort aged 15–19 in 1914 than for adjacent cohorts. The postwar burst of fertility in 1920 is reflected in peaks for the cohort aged 15–19 in 1920 and the cohort aged 15–19 in 1915 (and therefore aged 20–24 in 1920). The corresponding prominent peaks in the value of $\beta_{i\cdot T}^*$ emphasize how much younger a childbearing pattern these cohorts had than would have been predicted from the level of fertility in the context of the MC15 sequence. The 1915, 1920, and 1925 cohort peaks in the value of β_i^* for the MC15 sequence are all reflected to some extent in the overall fertility pattern described by β_i^* for the C15 sequence and $\beta_{i\cdot T}^*$ derived for the "CC15" sequence.[15]

These examples of departure from trend illustrate two points:

1. the influence of change at *younger* ages on the marital fertility pattern;
2. the importance of bringing both change in pattern and change in level of fertility into the interpretation of change.[16]

The influence of period-specific events on cohort fertility and the relations of marital and overall fertility patterns can be further examined in the corresponding sets of residuals for cohort marital and overall fertility (Fig. 7.13). The residuals for marital fertility exhibit an almost identical lagged pattern to that already considered for overall fertility in Chapter IV (Figs. 4.7 and 4.8). The major negative departures, related to the beginning of World War I and the years after 1933, tend to be larger for overall fertility than for marital fertility. Much of this difference is removed, however, when the residuals are multiplied by the corresponding sums of age-specific rates T_i, which are only about one-third as high for overall fertility as for marital fertility.

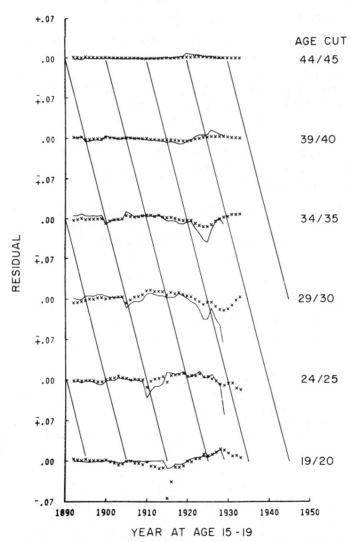

Fig. 7.13 Time-sequence plot of residuals by age cut (raw fraction scale) from double multiplicative EHR fits to the MC15 sequence ($\times\times\times$, cohorts aged 15–19 from 1892 to 1933) and the C15 sequence (——, segment for cohorts aged 15–19 from 1892 to 1929).

Use of EHR Parameters for Related Sequences to
Revise Faulty Data

Revision of the 1892–1894, age 15–19 rates to correct for the misreporting of the mother's age at the time of confinement, discussed earlier, depends on viewing the rates in both cohort and cross-sectional contexts. Revised estimates of α_i^*, β_i^*, and T_i values for both the MC15 and MX15 sequences are selected to meet the following requirements:

1. to predict essentially the same fertility rate at age 15–19 for a given year 1892–1894 whether the rate is calculated from the MC15 or the MX15 parameters;
2. to make only small changes in the MC15 rates for age groups 20–24 and higher because these rates would have been affected only slightly or not at all by the pre-1895 misreporting of the mother's age at the time of confinement;
3. to provide values of the level-compensated parameter $\beta_{i \cdot T}^*$ that are consistent with the post-1894 trends in the value of $\beta_{i \cdot T}^*$ for the MC15 and MX15 sequences.

One set of estimated parameters that satisfies these requirements quite well is shown in Table 7.9.[17] Substitution of these values of $\hat{\alpha}_i^*$ and $\hat{\beta}_i^*$ with the values for the corresponding set of age standards A_j^* and B_j^* for either the MC15 or MX15 sequence in the equation

$$\hat{F}_{ij} = \hat{\alpha}_i^* A_j^* + \hat{\beta}_i^* B_j^*$$

leads to the folded square root expression of cumulative, normalized age-specific fertility rates. De-transformation to the raw fraction scale (see Chapter VIII for the procedure), de-cumulation, and multiplication by $\hat{T}_i$

TABLE 7.9

Derived and Revised EHR Time Parameters α_i^* and β_i^*; Reported and Revised Sum of Age-specific Fertility Rates T_i for the MX15 and MC15 Sequences: Basis of Revised Marital Fertility Rates for the Years 1892–1894

Year	Sequence	α_i^*	$\hat{\alpha}_i^*$	β_i^*	$\hat{\beta}_i^*$	T_i	$\hat{T}_i$	$\hat{f}(15\text{--}19)$
1892	MC15	1.347	1.34	.451	.490	1.89	1.92	.550
	MX15	1.236	1.23	.481	.500	2.00	2.08	.555
1893	MC15	1.351	1.34	.467	.503	1.88	1.93	.563
	MX15	1.239	1.23	.475	.507	2.04	2.10	.565
1894	MC15	1.361	1.34	.481	.516	1.85	1.92	.570
	MX15	1.235	1.23	.473	.514	2.03	2.11	.573

TABLE 7.10

Reported and Revised Marital Fertility Rates for Age Groups 15–19 to 25–29 for the
Years 1892–1894

	Age group					
	15–19		*20–24*		*25–29*	
Year	*Reported*	*Revised*	*Reported*	*Revised*	*Reported*	*Revised*
1892	.515	.555	.444	.458	.358	.364
1893	.519	.565	.454	.463	.363	.367
1894	.512	.573	.461	.466	.358	.368

provides the age-specific rates in Tables 7.9 and 7.10. Note that the two
estimates of $f(15-19)$ for a given year are very close, as required, but the
rates for this age group are revised upward by .04 to .06.

Future Directions in Exploring Overall and Marital Fertility Relations

We have spent considerable time examining trends and departures from
trend in marital fertility, not only the evidence of change in childbearing at
older ages, but also the evidence of change in premarital pregnancy and in
the delay or limitation of births at younger ages. The latter two are variations in aggregate fertility patterns that more narrowly focused models
have not attempted to describe. Their description is possible here because
of the high proportion of the systematic variability in the data that is
brought into the fitted descriptions by the robust–resistant fitting procedures, the standard-form re-presentation adopted for the fitted parameters, and the additional level-compensation step that permits the examination of change in pattern of fertility apart from change in level. On these
bases, we can now propose further steps of exploration in seeking the
most concise and useful description possible of a population's reported
childbearing experience both within and outside of legal marriage.

First, we need to step back for a broader view of the situation that we
hope to model more fully using aggregate data in time sequence. Age-
specific marital fertility schedules form a problematical subset for the
description of childbearing experience. Actual populations depart to varying degrees from the idealized one in which all exposure to the possibility
of pregnancy occurs within marriage, and populations are not static in

their degree of departure. Social customs of the time and place determine first the size and age composition of the nonmarried group exposed to the possibility of pregnancy and then, for members of this group, strongly influence the outcome of pregnancy in terms of abortion, illegitimate birth, or conception legitimated by marriage before the birth. With a given proportion of unmarried women pregnant, quite different age patterns of marital fertility can result, depending on the separation by age into two groups—those marrying and those not marrying before giving birth to a nonmaritally conceived child—and the relation in magnitude and age distribution between premaritally conceived legitimate births and post-maritally conceived births.

The categorization of births may be complicated by the fact that ongoing unions not legalized by marriage account for nonnegligible fractions of total fertility in quite diverse populations, from high fertility populations to some of the lowest fertility ones. Both the level and the age pattern of fertility within consensual unions, however, may differ from those within legal marriage. Therefore, even when the number of women by age in each of these types of unions is known and when births are recorded not only by the age of mother but also by the type of union, these groups may need to be viewed as subpopulations of the whole. The distinction between legal and informal unions appears to be important in considering Swedish fertility levels for recent years (Gendell, 1980). Marital dissolution and remarriage also have new degrees of influence on the age distribution of fertility in many populations as the incidence of separation and divorce at lower ages increases.[18]

In the broader focus of the EHR time-sequence analyses, such variable departures of actual populations from model populations become the sources of transitions in aggregate experience that are described as closely as possible. The demographic importance of both the timing of the first birth and the length of the first interbirth interval are strong arguments for seeking more informative ways to include in the analysis those portions of aggregate data that cover the beginning of childbearing. When total fertility is low, the inclusion of *all* births becomes particularly necessary to the understanding of childbearing patterns. The next exploratory steps might therefore productively concentrate on the border between marital and nonmarital childbearing in the decades after 1890.

Making full use of the available data on women by age and marital status and births by mother's age, marital status, and duration of marriage, we should submit to exploration a variety of potentially useful subpopulation sequences that are related in specific ways to each other and to sequences already analyzed. These sequences would at least include the following:

1. a legitimate overall fertility sequence to pair with the age 15–49 marital fertility sequence extended to include the most recent data available;
2. two sequences for unmarried women—one for births not legitimated by marriage before birth of the child and one approximating births legitimated by marriage (that is, births occurring less than 8 months after marriage);
3. a sequence that approximates birth rates resulting from nonmarital conceptions, whether legitimated by marriage or not, to pair with a sequence for births occurring 8 months or more after marriage.

All of these sequences would be analyzed not only by calendar year but also by cohorts with completed childbearing experience. A cohort illegitimate fertility sequence has already been fit (Breckenridge, 1976).

In the effort to achieve useful descriptions of the systematic variability in these subpopulation sequences, we should again make full use of the data guiding and flexibility of the EDA approach. This means not only using the fitting conditions and the standard form of re-presentation adopted for the previously analyzed sequences but also testing modifications of these procedures. Choices to be given particular attention include:

1. the linearizing re-expression applied to the data before fitting;
2. the degree of resistance to outliers in the fitting procedures;
3. the number of components to fit;
4. the choice of the standard form—to simplify descriptions but at the same time permit useful cross-sequence comparisons of standard age patterns and time patterns of change both before and after linear compensation for the level of fertility.

Data re-expressions other than the folded square root re-expression may be more appropriate for some of these sequences. A three-component fit,

$$\hat{F}_{ij} = \alpha_i^* A_j^* + \beta_i^* B_j^* + \gamma_i^* C_j^*,$$

is likely to be useful on several counts.

1. Both the EHR fits to the traditional overall and marital fertility sequences for Sweden (Chapters VI and VII) and the preliminary cross-population comparisons (Chapter VIII) indicate that fitting the third component $\gamma_i^* C_j^*$ may be necessary to bring some of the most recent low-fertility variations of pattern into the fit.
2. Even when the type of variation expressed by the $\gamma_i^* C_j^*$ component makes only a small contribution to the description of a fertility time

sequence, bringing more of the systematic variation into the fit makes the nature of isolated deviations more evident in the residuals. This helps to identify responses to unusual circumstances or the existence of data errors.

3. Having three components to submit to the re-presentation procedures (Chapter V) permits standardization of the form of the second age parameter as well as the first. This can enhance cross-sequence comparisons even when the analyst decides to retain only the first two of the three re-presented components.

4. Having one more component than might be preferred for the final fit gives the analyst more information on which to base efforts to simplify the description or to seek an appropriate balance between parsimony and completeness of description.

These analyses should result in more information about the nature of societal changes over time, not only in nonmarital conceptions leading to the birth of a child, but also in the decision to marry or not marry before giving birth to a nonmaritally conceived child.

Summary

This chapter begins with marital fertility descriptions that have met the first goal of our fertility modeling: a closely fitting description in a small number of parameters for each cross-sectional and cohort sequence. Because we have adopted a broader focus on marital fertility than modeling the decline of fertility at higher ages—because we want to identify transitions, whatever their cause—we have set as the second goal of the modeling the achievement of stable, interpretable descriptions of marital fertility for the full 15–49 age range as well as the more frequently modeled 20–49 age range. This chapter demonstrates that the second goal has been met, not only for marital fertility across seven decades, but also for the subset that includes only births occurring 9 months or more after marriage.

As a baseline from which to view the additional contributions made by EHR modeling, the standard-form EHR parameters are compared at the outset with the parameters of the previously derived and more narrowly focused Coale model of marital fertility. Although both models describe similarly the progression of the major change in fertility—the development of a younger childbearing pattern accompanying the decline of fertility at higher ages—the EHR model captures this trend more fully in a single age standard and a single variable time parameter. This is the result of at least two factors: the closer EHR fits, which bring more of the systematic variability of the time-sequence data into the fitted parameters, and the choice of the standard form of the fitted parameters, which deliberately transfers to one component the type of systematic variation associated with the decline of fertility across the sequence. Other consequences important for a broader description of marital fertility time sequences follow directly from these characteristics of the EHR descriptions.

The smaller or more subtle variations in the trend toward a younger pattern and brief departures from trend can be identified in the EHR time parameters. Standardizing the descriptions for the inverse relation between the level of fertility and the shift of the distribution toward younger ages then provides an indicator of an additional type of transition: systematic change in the relative contributions of marital fertility reduction at younger and older ages that affects both the age pattern and the level of fertility, at least from 1908 onward.

The selected standard form and the retention of total rate as one dimension of the data also enhance the interpretability of the marital fertility descriptions in other ways. Although derived empirically, the nearly constant EHR standard pattern of the cumulation of births with age that underlies the 7-decade sequence of age 20–49 fertility and the comparable pattern that underlies the age 15–49 sequence for births occurring 9 months or more after marriage prove to closely approximate the age pattern of fertility in "natural" fertility schedules that have some of the highest levels of marital fertility on record. For each sequence, level standardization of the time parameter associated with the decline of fertility leads to identification of the high level of fertility that would correspond to the nearly constant, approximately "natural" pattern of the cumulation of births with age. For the age 20–49 sequence the predicted level is 11.2 births per woman.

Building on the results for overall fertility in Chapter VI, a series of intersequence comparisons relates change in marital fertility patterns, marriage patterns, and overall fertility patterns through cross-sectional and cohort standard-form parameters. The parallel evidence of period effects on cohort marital and overall fertility patterns is examined in the corresponding sets of residuals. The use of EHR parameters for related sequences to estimate missing data and estimate corrections for data errors is illustrated with the incomplete sequence for births occurring 9 months or more after marriage and with the faulty age-specific marital fertility rates for the years 1892–1894.

This chapter provides the methodological basis for a more detailed examination of the variable border between marital and nonmarital childbearing. Further exploratory analyses should thus reveal more information about the nature of societal changes over time, not only in the incidence of nonmarital conceptions leading to birth of a child, but also in the decision to marry or not marry before giving birth to a nonmaritally conceived child.

Notes for Chapter VII

1. For a description of the derivation of the A_j^* and α_i^* parameters, see Chapter V on the standard-form re-presentation of fits.

2. An analog of the Coale model that provides an alternate solution by duration of marriage incorporates a logarithmic departure from $n(a_j)$ at marriage durations greater than 2 years (Page, 1977).

3. Age 15–19 marital fertility has customarily been omitted from pattern considerations as too highly influenced by premarital pregnancy. In populations with a late marriage pattern, premarital pregnancy at ages 20–24 may also have a nonnegligible effect on fertility patterns.

4. Either least squares regression or a robust–resistant iteratively weighted regression procedure may be used. When results of the two regression procedures differ markedly, the analyst should explore the reasons for the difference. With the natural fertility schedules tested, the least squares and robust–resistant fits differed in only the fourth decimal place on the raw fraction scale at any age cut.

5. The similarity of these distributions does not imply a similarity of causal factors, but means only that the aggregate effects were the same. We know that the population for the NX15 sequence includes for the first time each year a number of women aged 15–19, 20–24, and 25–29 who are of proven fecundity (who had a premaritally conceived child in the preceding year) and that some of these women would be in a period of postpartum subfecundity in the year of first inclusion. Age 15–49 distributions closely fit as a weighted sum of the NX15 age standards may contain both some premarital pregnancy and some adolescent subfecundity.

6. Least squares regression of the β_i^* vectors for the MX15 and MX20 sequences independently on the $\bar{m}_i$ vector provides the following conversions of β_i^* to the scale of $\bar{m}_i$: MX15 sequence, $\beta_i' = (\beta_i^* - .0195)/(.5212)$; MX20 sequence, $\beta_i' = (\beta_i^* - .2579)/(.7401)$.

7. This problem with M_i may, in some instances, be of consequence in the use of the Coale–Trussell model fertility schedules, which incorporate the Coale model of marital fertility except for the omission of M_i:

$$f_i(a_j) = G_i(a_j)n(a_j) \exp[m_i \cdot v(a_j)],$$

where $f_i(a_j)$ is the age-specific overall fertility rate and $G_i(a_j)$ the age-specific proportion of women ever married. To the extent that variable aspects of the age pattern of marital fertility for an actual population would have been incorporated in M_i these aspects would be absorbed by $G_i(a_j)$, thus attributing to the age pattern of marriage some of the variation in the overall fertility distribution that is actually due to marital fertility.

8. The reader should refer to Chapter V for a detailed consideration of the roles of α_i^* and β_i^* in describing change in these sequences.

9. Comparisons between overall and marital fertility sequences in regard to the time pattern of change are appropriate for both the age 15–49 and age 20–49 sequences; however,

similarity in the magnitude of change in specific age groups is confined largely to age groups 30–34 and higher for the age 20–49 sequences (see Tables 5.5, 5.11, and 5.12).

10. Note that the scale for $\beta_{i\cdot T}^*$ is expanded over that for β_i^* in Fig. 7.4 to make the variations in $\beta_{i\cdot T}^*$ easier to examine.

11. Note certain similarities between the EHR standardization procedures and the level-standardization procedures adopted in the Coale (1967) indices of fertility and of proportion married—indices subsequently applied in a series of monographs on the decline of fertility in Europe (Coale, Anderson, and Harm, 1979; Knodel, 1974; Lesthaeghe, 1977; Livi-Bacci, 1971, 1977; Van de Walle, E., 1974). To look at the time pattern of change in nuptiality and fertility, the Coale indices are standardized to the Hutterite age-specific marital fertility schedule for 1921–1930 marriages—a schedule that represents one of the highest levels of natural fertility on record.

The overall fertility Σf_i and the marital fertility Σg_i for a study population are related to the fertility ΣF_i for the standard population by two indices: an index of overall fertility I_f and an index of marital fertility I_g, which use as weights the number of all women w_i and of married women m_i in each 5-year age group i in the study population. These relations are expressed by the equations

$$I_f = \sum w_i f_i \Big/ \sum w_i F_i \quad \text{and} \quad I_g = \sum m_i g_i \Big/ \sum m_i F_i.$$

When illegitimate fertility is negligible, the index of proportion married I_m equals I_f/I_g.

For the purpose of expressing change in fertility over time in terms that *retain the age structure of fertility in the summary measures*, the EHR procedures derive *internal* standards for the age patterns of marital and overall fertility and standardize in the time dimension for the relation between these patterns and fertility decline across the time sequence. We have seen that the tight cluster of level-standardized marital fertility distributions expressed by M'_{ij} are very close to the pattern of the Hutterite schedule that was used as the external standard in the Coale indices and that the level of marital fertility $5T_m = 11.22$ associated with the standard age pattern underlying the M'_{ij} distributions is approximately that of the Hutterite schedule.

12. The NX15 sequence for confinements occurring 9 months or more after marriage is one of a number of similarly constructed sequences that could have been selected to illustrate the use of exploratory analysis results in this section. This sequence has some intrinsic interest because its first fitted component $\alpha_i^* A_j^*$ describes an age pattern of fertility that is very close to those identified with the term "natural fertility". In addition, the NX15 set of A_j^* and B_j^* age standards proves in Chapter VIII to describe quite well the type of marital fertility pattern found in a number of other countries.

13. The near identity of some of these generated distributions and some "natural fertility" distributions is considered earlier in the chapter.

14. If we recall the method of constructing the NX15 sequence (Chapter III), we see that we can use the estimated NX15 rates for the years 1892–1910 and 1921–1923 to estimate the number of confinements at ages 15–19, 20–24, and 25–29 that occur 9 months or more after marriage as well as the number that occur less than 9 months after marriage in these years. To make these calculations, we solve for $e_i(a_j)$ in the equation

$$f_i(a_j) = \frac{c_i(a_j) - e_i(a_j)}{w_i(a_j) - e_i(a_j)},$$

where $f_i(a_j)$ is the modified rate of confinements for year i and age group $j = 1$ to n, $c_i(a_j)$ the number of confinements for legitimate births for year i and age group $j = 1$ to n, $e_i(a_j)$ the number of confinements for year i and age group $j = 1$ to n that result in a legitimate birth less than 9 months after marriage, and $w_i(a_j)$ the number of married women in year i and age group $j = 1$ to n.

15. We use "CC15" to designate the 1892–1929 cohort portion of the C15 sequence. The $\beta^*_{i \cdot T}$ values for the CC15 sequence are derived by regressing the 1892–1929 cohort portion of the β^*_i vector for the C15 sequence on the corresponding vector of $T_i^{1/2}$ to confine the level-compensation to these 38 cohorts apart from the rest of the 155-cohort sequence. The resulting $\beta^*_{i \cdot T}$ values for the CC15 sequence therefore differ slightly from those for the C15 sequence shown in Fig. 6.17 for the same cohorts.

16. Without consideration of change in level, the increases in β^*_i for the 1914, 1915, 1920, and 1925 cohorts would have been traditionally interpreted as due to increased control of marital fertility at higher ages.

17. $\hat{\beta}^*_{i \cdot T}$ is calculated from the linear compensation equation

$$\hat{\beta}^*_i = k_1 + k_2 \hat{T}_i^{1/2} + \hat{\beta}^*_{i \cdot T},$$

where k_1 and k_2 are the regression constant and coefficient, respectively, for the MC15 or the MX15 sequence (Table 7.4).

18. An increase in the divorce rate during the prime ages of childbearing can have significant effects not only on overall fertility patterns but also on marital fertility patterns if those women divorcing differ in marriage and fertility history from those remaining married—for example, if teenage marriage, premarital pregnancy, or childlessness is highly associated with divorce. High incidence of remarriage with renewed childbearing would further affect aggregate fertility patterns.

VIII

Preliminary Cross-population Comparisons of Fertility Patterns: Evidence for the Generality of EHR Age Standards

Introduction

EHR analysis has produced extraordinarily close-fitting descriptions of all the Swedish age-specific overall and marital fertility time sequences tested, including fertility in both cross-sectional and cohort perspectives, for ages 15–49 and 20–49, by 5-year age groups, and by single year of age. Age standards derived from national data have proved appropriate for comparisons of fertility change in the individual counties of Sweden over the period of a century. Now we ask, are the standard-form age parameters derived from the Swedish data particular to Sweden or are they of general use in comparing age-specific fertility schedules across populations? Can these parameters serve as the basis for a complete EHR analysis of changing age distributions of fertility across time and place?

Support for the generality and usefulness of the derived standard age patterns comes from four lines of evidence that are based on the least squares regression of diverse fertility schedules on the standard-form age vectors:

1. fits to a group of "natural fertility" schedules, as reported in Chapter VII;
2. fits to a 58-year time sequence of U.S. overall fertility distributions;
3. fits to a series of Coale–Trussell (1974) model schedules considered to cover a wide range of pace of entry into marriage and parity-dependent control of marital fertility;
4. fits to overall and marital fertility schedules for 48 countries in the 1960s and 1970s, representing a variety of levels of fertility and including short time sequences for 15 countries.

Examination of the fitted parameters and the residuals leads to three groups of conclusions. First, changes in U.S. overall fertility distributions across time can be as closely and coherently described on the basis of the EHR standard age parameters as can changes in Swedish fertility. A variety of Coale–Trussell model schedules with pace of entry into marriage ranging from about one-half to four times their model standard pace and "parity-dependent control" up to two times the highest found for Sweden by the Coale method can also be closely fit as a weighted sum of the EHR age standards. Overall fertility schedules as diverse as those for Tunisia in 1966, with a total fertility rate of 6.8 births per woman, and the German Democratic Republic in 1973, with a total fertility rate of 1.6 births per woman, can also be closely described by the EHR parameters. Therefore, useful few-parameter comparisons of fertility patterns across populations can be made on the basis of the EHR standards even before a complete cross-population analysis of age-specific fertility patterns is carried out.

Second, some regularity remains in the generally small residuals for fits to the cross-population overall fertility series and the age 20–49 marital fertility series. One would expect to bring this regularity into fitted descriptions in a complete EHR analysis. The pronounced regularity remaining in the residuals for a group of age 15–49 marital fertility schedules suggests an analytic approach to the influence of premarital pregnancy on aggregate marital fertility distributions.

Third, in a complete dissection of age-specific fertility, a single set of age standards for overall fertility and a single set for marital fertility would not necessarily be the outcome and should not necessarily be the goal. Sets with a common A_j^* vector, perhaps a common B_j^* vector, and a family of C_j^* vectors might be more expected—and more useful in relating fertility change to other demographic and social change.

We shall now summarize the procedure for expressing schedules in terms of the standard age parameters so far derived; in a later section we shall discuss the evidence for their general applicability and usefulness.

Procedure for Expressing Age-specific Fertility Schedules in Terms of EHR-derived Age Standards

To express a schedule of age-specific fertility rates $f_i(a_j)$ as a weighted sum of EHR standard-form age vectors, six steps are followed:

1. Cumulate the schedule $f_i(a_j)$ to obtain the fertility rates for women a given age and younger, with age cuts at 19/20, 24/25, . . . , 49/50 for schedules by 5-year age groups covering the full age 15–49 range or with age cuts starting at 24/25 when fertility rates for ages 20–49 only are used.

2. Normalize the cumulated schedule—that is, divide by $T_i = \Sigma_{j=1}^{n} f_i(a_j)$, the rate at age cut 49/50, to give f_{ij}, the proportion of all births achieved by a given age.

3. Linearize this cumulative distribution by expressing it as its folded square root:

$$F_{ij} = (f_{ij})^{1/2} - (1 - f_{ij})^{1/2}$$

4. Select an appropriate set of EHR age standards such as one from the following tabulation.

Age standard	Age cut					
	19/20	24/25	29/30	34/35	39/40	44/45
X202 Sequence						
A_j^*	−.5822	−.3432	−.1070	.1328	.3807	.6077
B_j^*	.2788	.4913	.5648	.4905	.3264	.1217
C_j^*	−.4560	−.6849	−.0239	.3781	.2036	−.3716
X15 Sequence						
A_j^*	−.6016	−.3915	−.1375	.1170	.3600	.5680
B_j^*	.2870	.5074	.5525	.4754	.3291	.1438
MX20 Sequence						
A_j^*	—	−.3428	−.0547	.2102	.4908	.7711
B_j^*	—	.4521	.5622	.5451	.4008	.1474
MX15 Sequence						
A_j^*	−.4816	−.2238	−.0058	.2093	.4468	.6888
B_j^*	.5056	.5140	.4788	.4042	.2757	.1075
NX15 Sequence						
A_j^*	−.3940	−.1374	.0712	.2844	.4990	.7007
B_j^*	.2479	.4068	.5479	.5410	.3980	.1476

5. By least squares regression of F_{ij} on the selected set of age vectors, determine the schedule-specific regression coefficients α_i^*, β_i^*, and γ_i^* (if fitted) and the residuals z_{ij}.

6. Obtain the fitted schedule and the residuals on the original raw fraction scale by de-transformation as follows.

    a. The fitted cumulative distribution on the folded square root scale is equal to $F_{ij} - z_{ij} = \hat{F}_{ij}$.

    b. The fitted cumulative distribution on the raw fraction scale is equal to

$$\tfrac{1}{2}(1 + \hat{F}_{ij}\sqrt{2 - \hat{F}_{ij}^2}) = \hat{f}_{ij}.$$

    c. The residuals for the cumulative distribution on the raw fraction scale are equal to $f_{ij} - \hat{f}_{ij}$.

    d. The fitted, cumulated rates are equal to $T_i \hat{f}_{ij}$.

Whichever set of EHR age standards is selected for the regression, the implications of a small difference in each schedule-specific regression coefficient may be reviewed in Chapter V.

Cross-Population Comparisons of Fertility Patterns

A Time Sequence of U.S. Overall Fertility Distributions

The 1917–1968 portion of the U.S. age-specific overall fertility sequence tested here for fit to EHR age standards was one of the data sets used by McNeil and Tukey (1975) in the initial development of EHR analysis. There, the concerns were methodological rather than demographic. Such matters as examination of the residuals in time sequence for their relation to specific years or periods and re-presentation of fitted parameters in a demographically useful standard form for interpretation of changes across time did not come under consideration.

The 52-year sequence is extended here to include data for the years 1969–1974 (United Nations, 1976), and regressions are carried out with two sets of EHR-derived age standards: A_j^* and B_j^* for the X15 sequence and A_j^*, B_j^*, and C_j^* for the X202 sequence. Two major questions need to be answered: Do close fits result from this process? If the fits are close, what do the fitted time parameters reveal about U.S. fertility patterns across six decades? Examination of the residuals answers the first question with an unequivocal yes—close fits result with either set of age standards.[1]

The fitted time parameters provide a coherent picture of fertility change that can be compared to the results for Sweden. These parameters for either two- or three-component fits reveal a persistently younger age pat-

tern of childbearing in the United States than in Sweden and a similarity in
the rates of change in pattern for the two countries over almost half of the
sequence. For the description of U.S. fertility change, the chief advantages of the three-component fits are the additional standardization of the
descriptions and the detection of the recent onset of a variation in fertility
patterns that has been evident for Sweden since the mid-1950s and appears in the EHR descriptions of fertility for a number of other countries.
The bases for these statements become apparent on the detailed examination of the time parameters α_i^*, β_i^*, and γ_i^*.

For the United States, the description by two time parameters gives
essentially the same picture as the description by three time parameters
(Fig. 8.1): α_i^* is approximately .01 higher and β_i^* approximately .1 higher
in every year with the use of X15 than with the use of $X202$ standards; γ_i^*
with $X202$ standards is zero for all practical purposes except for the years
1924–1931, when it has a small negative value (between $-.01$ and $-.016$),
the years 1945–1946, when it has a small positive value (.013 and .020),
and from the late 1960s through the end of the sequence in 1974, when a
steady rise appears (from .01 to .04). We found in Table 5.8 that absolute
values of γ_i^* less than about .02 make only a negligible difference in the
fitted schedule. We can therefore, at least for the years 1917–1968, approximate the observed very close fits of three components with a two-
component model in which the first age standard A_j^* is constrained to be

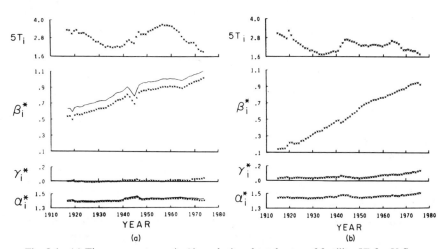

Fig. 8.1 (a) Time parameters α_i^*, β_i^*, and γ_i^* and total rates of fertility $5T_i$ for U.S. age-
specific overall fertility distributions (1917–1974) expressed as weighted sums of the A_j^* and
B_j^* age standards for the Swedish X15 sequence (———) and the A_j^*, B_j^*, and C_j^* age standards
for the Swedish $X202$ sequence ($\times\times\times$); (b) time parameters α_i^*, β_i^*, and γ_i^* and total rates of
fertility $5T_i$ for the Swedish $X202$ sequence (1915–1976 segment).

as linear as possible and the second age standard B_j^* is constrained to be as quadratic as possible. This is an example of the advantage that can sometimes be gained by fitting one extra component, re-presenting all components in a standard form, and then simplifying by using the $n - 1$ components that now all approximate known forms.

Referring again to Table 5.8 on the effects of small changes or differences in α_i^*, β_i^*, and γ_i^* on the age distribution of fertility, we confirm that childbearing has had a younger age pattern in the United States than in Sweden over the entire 1917–1974 time period included in Fig. 8.1. For the United States, the lower α_i^*, higher β_i^*, and lower γ_i^* values (in this case γ_i^* is negligible up to 1969) throughout the period are a reinforcing combination. The values of all these parameters place more births in age groups 15–19 and 20–24 and fewer births in age group 30–34 than do the corresponding values for Sweden. At the same time, the total rate of fertility is higher in the United States than in Sweden in every year until 1973 except for 1944 and 1945.

From 1920 to 1941, similarities in the *rates of change* for the two countries are apparent in the shift toward a younger childbearing pattern expressed by positive change in β_i^* and in the 1922–1935 parallel declines of total fertility rate. This suggests that fertility decline at higher ages is similarly important for change in fertility patterns in the United States and Sweden during this period. As seen through EHR parameters, both World War I and World War II effects on fertility differed, however, and changes in the age pattern of childbearing for the two countries diverge noticeably after 1941. Resumption of nearly parallel change does not occur until 1966.

The relatively brief U.S. involvement in World War I is reflected in the singular decline in β_i^* in 1919, followed by the 1920–1921 rise in β_i^* to a level slightly above its 1917–1918 levels. This means that the depressed total fertility rate for 1919 and the catch-up increase for 1920 to 1921 involve age group 20–24 in particular and age groups 25–29 and 15–19 to a lesser extent. In Sweden, the effects of the war appear as extensions of pre-1914 trends. (See Fig. 6.12 to place the 1917–1974 Swedish fertility experience in the context of a longer time sequence.) The 1915–1918 plateau that occurs in the value of β_i^* (Fig. 8.1) while the total rate continues to decline indicates a steady proportional contribution to the decline across all age groups. The 1920–1921 postwar burst in total rate for Sweden is a more prominent catch-up response than occurred in the United States, but the comparable increases in β_i^* indicate that the age group responses in Sweden are proportional to the age group responses in the United States.

In both countries, the trend toward a younger childbearing pattern continues through the nadir in total rate that occurs in the 1930s. For the United States, this trend accelerates after 1933 while the total rate remains low but terminates in the major disruption of childbearing patterns during World War II. The influence of the war is seen in both time parameters: the 1941–1947 increase in α_i^*, similar to that for Sweden, and the 1943–1946 decrease in β_i^*. Together these changes describe a period in which childbearing at ages 30–39 has relatively more importance and childbearing at ages 15–24 has relatively less importance for the age distribution of fertility than in the immediately preceding or following years. The total rate, however, declines only for the period 1944–1945.

In contrast to the tendency in Sweden, any tendency in the United States for an increasingly younger age pattern of childbearing is strongly damped from 1947 to 1965. In this period, which includes the postwar "baby boom", the near plateaus in β_i^* for the years 1951–1954 and 1957–1964 reflect the extent to which the prominent rise in total rate and its subsequent decline were shared across all age groups proportionately (according to the age pattern determined by the second EHR age standard B_j^*). Not until 1966 does the trend toward a younger childbearing pattern resume.

For Sweden, a slight recovery in total rate of fertility begins in 1936, sooner than in the United States, but slows briefly from 1940 to 1941. The small increase in α_i^* from 1941 to 1946, the very small increase in γ_i^* from 1942 to 1944, and the brief decrease in β_i^* from 1942 to 1944 appear as small aberrations in the trend toward a younger childbearing pattern. All of these changes indicate that from 1942 to 1944 women aged 25 and older contributed relatively more to the burst in total fertility than did those younger than 25 but that age group 20–24 in particular and also age groups 25–29 and 15–19 assume greater importance for the age pattern of fertility after 1944 for a period of about 10 years. New childbearing patterns then emerge that are reflected in the simultaneous increases in α_i^*, β_i^*, and γ_i^*. These increases reinforce each other by placing a higher proportion of births in age group 25–29 than occurred previously even as the total rate of fertility rises again and then falls to a new low.

Nearly parallel changes in the age pattern of childbearing in the United States and Sweden resume about 1966 as the United States partially adopts the new pattern that began to appear in Sweden in the mid-1950s. The rates of positive change in β_i^* and also in γ_i^* once more become very similar; the difference in change of pattern lies in the almost negligible change in α_i^* for the United States but continued steady rise in α_i^* to the end of the sequence for Sweden. Judging by the higher β_i^*, lower γ_i^*, and lower and relatively unchanged α_i^* values—with the α_i^* parameter reflecting the continued importance of teenage childbearing for the age pattern of fertility in the United States—this country maintains a younger pattern than does Sweden even as the total rate of fertility in the two countries reaches the same low level after 1971.

The successful use of the same EHR age standards to describe time-sequence change in fertility patterns for both the United States and Sweden points to further steps of analysis. Subpopulation trends in fertility patterns, such as the 1945–1969 U.S. trends examined by Rindfuss and Sweet (1977), should now be summarized in EHR terms for both countries. Differentials by place of residence (already examined for geographic areas of Sweden in Chapter VI), education, income level, and ethnicity (also important in Sweden for recent years because of high in-migration) would all be of interest. Because each EHR time parameter is associated with a standard age pattern, the EHR expressions provide more information about the nature of difference or change than do the usual summary measures, such as total fertility rate, when used alone. At the same time, the EHR expressions capture the age-group detail in a small number of parameters that can be compared graphically. With these characteristics, EHR summaries of subpopulation fertility trends should contribute an additional perspective to the study of factors that underlie national trends.

Coale–Trussell Model Schedules of the Age Distribution of Fertility

The example of the U.S. fertility time sequence demonstrates that the standard-form EHR age parameters derived from Swedish data are appropriate for description of a younger childbearing pattern than that for Sweden. Evidence of their capacity to accommodate a wide variety of fertility patterns in which childbearing begins at an early age will now be presented.

For this test, 30 schedules were selected from the 700 Coale–Trussell (1974) model fertility schedules, which are concerned only with the age pattern of fertility and are considered by their authors to cover the full range of possible age distributions of childbearing for any population. This set of model schedules for an idealized population without illegitimacy, premarital pregnancy, divorce, or widowhood were constructed on the basis of two previously derived models: the Coale model of marital fertility (Coale, 1971), which is described in detail in Chapter VII; and the Coale–McNeil model of the age pattern of entry into first marriage (Coale, 1971; Coale and McNeil, 1972).[2] To describe variations in the age pattern of marital fertility, the model schedules use only the parameter m, termed the "degree of parity-dependent control". The Coale–Trussell schedules are not intended to describe other types of fertility control, such as the delay of a first birth within marriage or the spacing of subsequent births, and they omit the original marital fertility model's second variable parameter M. (Trussell (1979) points out that the M parameter does appear to contain part of the description of "degree of control" in schedules for actual populations.) The model schedules do incorporate both of the marriage-model parameters: a_0, the earliest age of a significant number of marriages, and k, a measure of the pace of entry into marriage in relation to the standard pattern of entry. The smaller the value of k below 1, the more rapid the pace of entry in relation to the standard pattern; the higher the value of k above 1, the slower the pace of entry in relation to the standard pattern.

The 30 schedules used to test a set of EHR parameters were selected with a_0 values of 14.85 to 15.40 years, the earliest marriage ages appropriate for fertility standards that start with age 15. In addition, the schedules were selected to cover the full range of k and m that the model schedules allow with such values of a_0. The pace of entry parameter k then has a range of .25 to 1.80—that is, four times faster to 80 percent slower than the pace of entry of the standard pattern. The parity-dependent control parameter m has a range of .10 to 3.89—that is, from approximately "natural" fertility to about two and a half times the highest degree of control found for Swedish schedules by the Coale method. The schedules were cumulated to seven 5-year age cuts—19/20, 24/25, . . . , 49/50—for regression on the A_j^*, B_j^*, and C_j^* age standards for the $X202$ sequence, the most general set of EHR overall fertility standards so far derived.

Table 8.1 shows the Coale–Trussell parameters and the EHR parameters for all 30 schedules grouped generally by the value of k and listed within groups by decreasing values of m as one logical way of viewing such diversity.[3] The six schedules of least good fit (that is, those having a residual with an absolute value greater than .019 at any age cut) are indicated by square brackets. Examples of fits to the other 24 schedules are shown in Table 8.2. Selected for variety in the combinations of Coale–Trussell model parameters and not as "best fits", they illustrate the closeness of the fitted descriptions obtained for the large majority of the schedules tested.

It is apparent that a weighted sum of $X202$ standard-form age parameters can describe well a wide variety of schedules with ranges of 1 to 22 percent of total fertility achieved below age 20, 13 to 65 percent achieved below age 25, and 39 to 88 percent achieved below age 30. For all of the schedules less closely fit, the departures have the same pattern: negative

TABLE 8.1

Parameters of Coale–Trussell (1974) Model Fertility Schedules and EHR Parameters α_i^*, β_i^*, and γ_i^* that Express the Model Schedules as Weighted Sums of EHR Standard-form Age Parameters A_j^*, B_j^*, and C_j^* for the *X202* Sequence: Selected Schedules with Earliest Marriage Age a_0 Near Age 15 Grouped by Pace of Entry into Marriage k, and Listed within the Groups by Decreasing Parity-dependent Control of Marital Fertility m

Schedule	Coale–Trussell parameters					EHR parameters[a]		
	a_0	k	m	μ	σ	α_i^*	β_i^*	γ_i^*
1	15.23	.350	3.024	24	4.5	[1.376	1.333	−.001]
2	15.13	.250	2.469	24	5.0	1.334	1.283	−.039
3	15.40	.250	1.885	25	5.5	1.360	1.118	−.020
4	15.06	.300	1.393	26	6.0	1.372	.951	−.012
5	15.44	.250	.910	27	6.5	1.370	.782	−.018
6	15.10	.250	.468	28	7.0	1.352	.614	−.034
7	15.39	.300	.282	29	7.0	1.378	.475	−.013
8	14.94	.550	3.888	24	4.0	[1.413	1.388	.042]
9	15.18	.400	2.373	25	5.0	[1.406	1.163	.025]
10	14.95	.450	1.810	26	5.5	1.419	.991	.035
11	14.91	.450	1.285	27	6.0	1.420	.819	.031
12	15.07	.400	.779	28	6.5	1.407	.646	.016
13	15.18	.500	.629	29	6.5	1.435	.502	.041
14	15.17	.400	.096	30	7.0	1.393	.331	.001
15	15.05	.600	3.089	25	4.5	[1.450	1.213	.076]
16	14.96	.650	2.421	26	5.0	[1.467	1.035	.090]
17	14.95	.650	1.804	27	5.5	1.471	.856	.087
18	15.03	.600	1.210	28	6.0	1.460	.677	.071
19	14.97	.800	1.159	29	6.0	1.488	.529	.097
20	14.99	.650	.493	30	6.5	1.450	.352	.056
21	15.06	.750	.309	31	6.5	1.455	.196	.059
22	14.96	1.050	3.456	26	4.5	[1.511	1.083	.152]
23	15.02	1.000	2.622	27	5.0	1.518	.895	.148
24	15.06	.900	1.854	28	5.5	1.511	.710	.129
25	14.97	1.050	1.133	30	6.0	1.505	.372	.111
26	14.97	1.550	2.223	29	5.5	1.538	.556	.155
27	15.05	1.450	2.145	29	5.5	1.538	.556	.155
28	14.96	1.400	1.145	31	6.0	1.510	.210	.109
29	15.04	1,350	1.110	31	6.0	1.510	.211	.110
30	15.17	1.800	1.130	32	6.0	1.504	.044	.094

[a] The square brackets indicate schedules of least good fit (those having a residual with an absolute value > .019 at any age cut).

TABLE 8.2

Examples of Coale–Trussell (1974) Model Fertility Schedules and Their EHR Fits as Weighted Sums of the A_j^*, B_j^*, and C_j^* Age Standards for the $X202$ Sequence

Example[a]	Age cut					
	19/20	24/25	29/30	34/35	39/40	44/45
Schedule 3						
Model	.1768	.5757	.8241	.9387	.9857	.9988
EHR fit	.1858	.5678	.8228	.9387	.9868	.9991
Residual	−.0090	.0079	.0013	.0000	−.0011	−.0003
Schedule 7						
Model	.0859	.3409	.5816	.7786	.9226	.9906
EHR fit	.0855	.3393	.5855	.7783	.9204	.9909
Residual	.0004	.0016	−.0039	.0003	.0022	−.0003
Schedule 11						
Model	.0980	.4360	.7185	.8837	.9682	.9970
EHR fit	.1096	.4251	.7137	.8851	.9707	.9977
Residual	−.0116	.0109	.0048	−.0014	−.0025	−.0007
Schedule 28						
Model	.0182	.1709	.4625	.7369	.9196	.9917
EHR fit	.0149	.1751	.4678	.7365	.9153	.9913
Residual	.0033	−.0042	−.0053	.0004	.0043	.0004

[a] Examples are selected from the schedules described in Table 8.1.

residuals at age cut 19/20, positive residuals at age cuts 24/25 and 29/30. This means the EHR standards would predict that a higher proportion of total births would occur at ages 15–19 and a smaller proportion at ages 20–24. When the residual has a higher positive value at age cut 29/30 than at age cut 24/25, the EHR standards would predict that a slightly smaller proportion of total births would occur at ages 25–29 also.

For all of the schedules that are least well fit, the typical pattern of departure from fit is most often associated with a particular combination of schedule characteristics: a mean age of childbearing that is well in the lower half of the possible range and with low standard deviation, a pace of entry into marriage that is usually rapid, and a very high degree of parity-dependent control of marital fertility. In other words, these schedules express a high degree of concentration of fertility in a fairly narrow, low age range. The departures from fit are in the opposite direction than would be expected, however, if the EHR parameters could not accommodate early childbearing well—that is, the EHR fits predict a *higher* proportion of births at ages 15–19 than the model schedules allow. This circumstance leads to an examination of both the EHR standards and the Coale–Trussell model standards.

Page's (1977) evidence of a marriage duration effect on the distribution of marital fertility has led Trussell (1979) to express concern about the need for inclusion of the marriage duration parameters a_0 and k in the marital fertility component of the model used to generate the Coale–Trussell model schedules. Such a revision would lead to slightly different model schedules when childbearing is spread out by a high incidence of delay in marriage coupled with parity-dependent control. Also, and equally important, such a revision would lead to slightly different schedules when childbearing is concentrated by a combination of high incidence of early marriage and a very high degree of parity-dependent control. In turn, a complete EHR analysis of the full range of age distributions of fertility across populations may lead to age standards that better accommodate the latter type of extreme fertility distribution than do the age standards derived from Swedish data. We should expect a variation of the C_j^* standard to draw into the fitted description the pattern of departure we have observed with some model schedules—negative residuals at age cut 19/20, positive residuals at age cuts 24/25 and 29/30.

The variety of tested model schedules that are well fit as a weighted sum of EHR parameters provides a temptation to attach causal meaning to the EHR parameters. Such an effort would at the least be premature until a fuller EHR analysis across populations has been carried out and until contemplated revisions have been incorporated in the Coale–Trussell schedules so that complete sets of refined parameters are available for comparison. Consider, however, the following two groups of observations.

First, even with refined parameters any causal meaning assigned to the Coale–Trussell parameters must refer to cohort experience under the model population assumptions of no illegitimacy or premarital pregnancy, no marital dissolution in the childbearing years, a "natural" pattern of marital fertility up to age 20, and parity-dependent control as the form of fertility control beyond age 20. Coale and Trussell (1974, p. 192) report that when these criteria are not met a close fit to an actual schedule can usually still be achieved, but this often requires a model schedule whose parameters a_0, k, and m imply a marriage pattern and degree of control of marital fertility very different from those existing in the population. As an example, they cite a distribution for Japan (1964) fit with a model schedule "embodying an implied mean age of first marriage (32.4 years) that bears no relation to the actual mean age at marriage in Japan (about 24 years)". Another example of the loss of demographic meaning in model parameters under real-world circumstances is found in the failure of the a_0, k, and m parameters of fitted model schedules to describe accurately the nuptiality and marital fertility conditions in Sweden and the United States or to provide coherent time-sequence descriptions of overall fertility change in these two countries (Trussell, 1974; see also the discussion in Chapter I and in Chapter VII). An additional assumption of the model schedules is that the proportion of women remaining celibate does not influence the age pattern of fertility but only the level of fertility, a factor that is not incorporated in the schedules (Coale and Trussell, 1974, p. 187). For actual schedules in time sequence, however, *change* in the proportion of women ever married does contribute to *change* in fertility pattern. This circumstance may further reduce the applicability of the parameter labels. In short, the Coale–Trussell expressions of caution about transferring the demographic meaning of parameters from model schedules to schedules that do not meet model assumptions should be heeded.

Second, the closely fitting, coherent EHR descriptions of time-sequence change in fertility for Sweden (see Chapters VI and VII) and for the United States (see the first section of this chapter) provide evidence that the EHR parameters are likely to be more useful to us *without labels assigning causal meaning and with total fertility rates retained as one dimension of the description.* As used with actual schedules, the standard form adopted for the parameters incorporates the advantages of a demographically guided representation of fertility patterns without introducing the problems of having a single causal meaning attached to any parameter. Interpretation proceeds from understanding what effect a given change in a time parameter has on the age pattern of fertility, considering change in pattern in relation to change in total rate, and routinely examining the residuals from fit for any additional valuable information they may hold.

Different purposes prompted the construction of the Coale–Trussell model fertility schedules and the development of the EHR descriptions of changing fertility patterns. Although the two are complementary for many purposes, each makes its own distinctive contribution to the study of the age distribution of fertility (see Appendix A).

Overall and Marital Fertility for Diverse Populations in Recent Years

We shall turn now from EHR descriptions of model schedules to preliminary EHR descriptions of reported schedules for a variety of populations. Because this is an exploratory step to guide a complete EHR analysis, the several hundred schedules tested were selected for the diversity of pattern, fertility level, and geographic location and for the high quality of data (Cho, 1973; Freedman, Fan, Wei, and Weinberger, 1977; United

Nations, 1966, 1976). Schedules for at least two years were included for most countries.[4]

Beginning with the cumulated, normalized schedules of age 15–49 overall fertility by 5-year age groups, then age 20–49 marital fertility, and finally age 15–49 marital fertility, we shall examine some of the results of expressing these distributions as weighted sums of the EHR age standards derived from Swedish time-sequence data: for overall fertility, A_j^* and B_j^* for the X15 sequence and A_j^*, B_j^*, and C_j^* for the X202 sequence; for marital fertility, A_j^* and B_j^* for the MX20, MX15, and NX15 sequences. For each set of schedules, the discussion will give first attention to the fitted parameters and how they distinguish between schedules or serve to group similar schedules. Then typical patterns of departure from fit will be pointed out as another means of grouping schedules and a means of identifying the type of adjustment of fit to be sought in a complete EHR analysis across populations.

Overall Fertility Time Sequences　Short time sequences of overall fertility for 15 countries are described in EHR terms in Fig. 8.2. Total fertility rate $5T_i$ ranges from 6.8 births per woman for Tunisia (1966) to 1.6 births per woman for Japan (1966). All of the countries except Ireland and Japan experience some decline in total rate over the years shown. The most prominent changes in fertility pattern are described in the β_i^* parameter, the measure of the extent to which the age distribution of childbearing is shifted from age 30 and higher to ages below 30. The sequence for Taiwan, described in the center of Fig. 8.2, provides a notable example of change—in the span of 13 years, the fertility pattern becomes less like the patterns for the countries to the left and more like those for the countries to the right. The generally inverse relation of β_i^* to the total rate $5T_i$ has some exceptions, however: Ireland achieves a younger pattern without decline in total rate and the four highest fertility countries—Tunisia, Ecuador, Honduras, and Venezuela—achieve some decline in total rate without increase in β_i^*. The sequence for Romania merits particular notice for the sudden 1966–1967 change in β_i^* that accompanies the recision of legal abortion (Teitelbaum, 1972), followed by the almost complete recovery of the former pattern but not the former level of fertility.

The α_i^* and γ_i^* parameters exhibit little change for most of these sequences. Their levels, however, are an important aspect of the differences between sequences. The slightly rising values of γ_i^* for some countries appear to announce the onset of new fertility patterns or the magnification of earlier tendencies. Recall that the α_i^* and γ_i^* parameters are measures of specific types of concentration in the fertility distribution and that they emphasize different age groups. Higher α_i^* values indicate a greater concentration of births in the central ages of the childbearing age range, drawing the distribution in fairly equally from both ends. Higher γ_i^* values indicate an uneven contraction of the distribution toward age group 25–29, primarily at the expense of age group 20–24, but also at the expense of age groups 15–19, 35–39, and 40–44 (see Table 5.8). The type of concentration expressed by γ_i^* would be logically associated with a high prevalence of those customs and activities that serve to confine childbearing more sharply to intermediate ages—for example, delay of marriage, age-related abortion, contraceptive delay of first and subsequent births, and marital dissolution (either separation or divorce) during the childbearing years.

The distributions for Ecuador, Honduras, and Venezuela, represented by the lowest α_i^* values and either negligible or slightly negative γ_i^* values, have the least age concentration of fertility described in Fig. 8.2. In contrast, for Japan the unusually high α_i^* and γ_i^* values, coupled with high β_i^* values, signal an extreme degree of age concentration of childbearing in maintaining a steady, low level of fertility.

More subtle differences in distributions can also be detected through the EHR parameters. The sequences for France, the United Kingdom, Canada, and the United States provide an example. These countries have almost the same level of fertility in 1966 and by 1973 the last three have experienced similar declines in level. Each of the four has a younger pattern of childbearing (higher β_i^* value) in 1973 than in 1966. Throughout the 1966–1973 period, however, the United States maintains the youngest pattern of the four (highest β_i^*, lowest γ_i^*, and lowest α_i^* values), Canada exhibits an older pattern (lower β_i^*, rising γ_i^* values) than either the United States or the United Kingdom, and France exhibits the oldest pattern of the four (lesser rise in the value of β_i^* after 1966, highest γ_i^* and highest α_i^* values) as well as the least decline in total rate. Taiwan provides a second example of the subtle differences detected. The sets of time parameters for 1961 through 1974a are for births tabulated by date of registration; the set shown as 1974b is for births tabulated by date of occurrence and includes births for that year that were registered by March of the following year (Freedman *et al.*, 1977).

Overall Fertility: Fits to Diverse Schedules The closeness of fit achieved with the current EHR age standards can be examined in Tables 8.3–8.6 for a variety of overall fertility distributions. The distributions for higher fertility countries (Table 8.3) are quite well fit by two time parameters and more closely fit by three time parameters, evidence that the third component has picked up additional systematic variation left in the generally small residuals. These distributions range from the relatively younger pattern for El Salvador (higher β_i^*, lower α_i^*, and negative γ_i^* values) to the relatively older pattern for Tunisia (lower β_i^*, higher α_i^*, and consider-

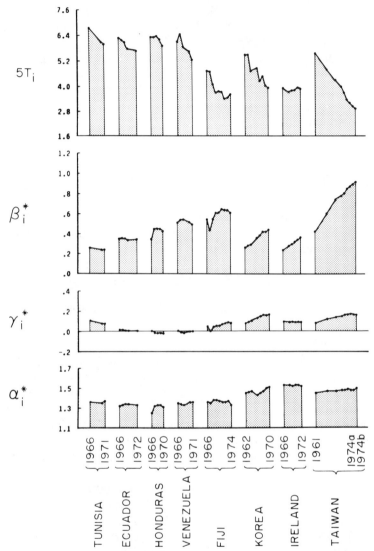

Fig. 8.2   (*Above and right*) EHR time parameters α_i^*, β_i^*, and γ_i^* and total rates of fertility $5T_i$ for selected countries from 1961 to 1974: time sequences of age-specific overall fertility distributions expressed as weighted sums of the A_j^*, B_j^*, and C_j^* age standards for the *X202* sequence.

ably higher γ_i^* values). The greater degree of concentration expressed by higher values of α_i^* and γ_i^* is apparent in a comparison of the distributions for Ecuador and Reunion with their similar β_i^* levels. For both distributions, 54 percent of total fertility is achieved by age 30, but for Reunion

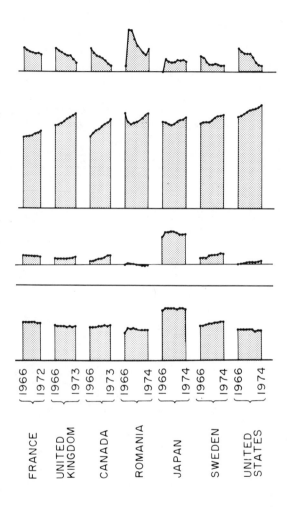

the lower proportions at each age cut below 29/30 and the higher proportions at each age cut above 29/30 confirm the greater contributions made to the similar total rates by women aged 25–34.

The distributions for low-fertility countries with quite varied age pat-

TABLE 8.3

Cumulative Distributions of Overall Fertility and Their EHR Fits as Weighted Sums of the A_j^* and B_j^* Standards for the X15 Sequence or the A_j^*, B_j^*, and C_j^* Standards for the X202 Sequence: Selected High Fertility Countries, 1966–1972

Schedule	Source of age standards	α_i^*	β_i^*	γ_i^*	Age cut						$5T_i$
					19/20	24/25	29/30	34/35	39/40	44/45	
El Salvador 1971											
Reported					.1212	.3655	.5936	.7829	.9235	.9819	6.16
Fitted	X202	1.302	.513	−.012	.1111	.3692	.6059	.7836	.9130	.9823	
Residual					.0101	−.0037	−.0123	−.0007	.0105	−.0004	
Reported					.1212	.3655	.5936	.7829	.9235	.9819	6.16
Fitted	X15	1.309	.605	—	.1089	.3562	.6085	.7962	.9174	.9754	
Residual					.0123	.0093	−.0149	−.0133	.0061	.0065	
Ecuador 1972											
Reported					.0748	.3025	.5404	.7326	.8991	.9781	5.70
Fitted	X202	1.330	.347	.007	.0780	.2988	.5377	.7394	.8944	.9799	
Residual					−.0032	.0037	.0027	−.0068	.0047	−.0018	
Reunion 1967											
Reported					.0516	.2824	.5401	.7564	.9151	.9910	6.03
Fitted	X202	1.426	.368	.020	.0552	.2279	.5386	.7574	.9160	.9916	
Residual					−.0036	.0045	.0015	−.0010	−.0009	−.0006	
Reported					.0516	.2824	.5401	.7564	.9151	.9910	6.03
Fitted	X15	1.448	.461	—	.0545	.2713	.5393	.7643	.9187	.9889	
Residual					−.0029	.0111	.0008	−.0079	−.0036	.0021	
Tunisia 1966											
Reported					.0413	.2249	.5001	.7341	.8986	.9701	6.77
Fitted	X202	1.359	.259	.107	.0440	.2210	.4987	.7385	.8958	.9718	
Residual					−.0027	.0039	.0014	−.0044	.0028	−.0017	
Reported					.0413	.2249	.5001	.7341	.8986	.9701	6.77
Fitted	X15	1.416	.329	—	.0476	.2364	.4907	.7217	.8931	.9808	
Residual					−.0063	−.0115	.0094	.0124	.0055	−.0107	

TABLE 8.4

Cumulative Distributions of Overall Fertility and Their EHR Fits as Weighted Sums of the A_i^* and B_j^* Standards for the X15 Sequence or the A_j^*, B_j^*, and C_j^* Standards for the X202 Sequence: Selected Low Fertility Countries, 1966–1973

Schedule	Source of age standards	α_i^*	β_i^*	γ_i^*	19/20	24/25	29/30	34/35	39/40	44/45	$5T_i$
							Age cut				
Romania 1966											
Reported	X202	1.385	.947	.002	.1343	.5029	.7644	.9082	.9747	.9976	1.88
Fitted					.1455	.4921	.7630	.9078	.9769	.9981	
Residual					−.0112	.0108	.0014	.0004	−.0022	−.0005	
Reported	X15	1.397	1.040	—	.1343	.5029	.7644	.9082	.9747	.9976	1.88
Fitted					.1461	.4866	.7607	.9120	.9793	.9970	
Residual					−.0118	.0163	.0037	−.0038	−.0046	.0006	
Romania 1967											
Reported	X202	1.429	.861	.019	.1095	.4536	.7245	.8941	.9757	.9984	3.66
Fitted					.1157	.4437	.7289	.8937	.9749	.9989	
Residual					−.0062	.0099	−.0044	.0004	.0008	−.0005	
Reported	X15	1.449	.995	—	.1095	.4536	.7245	.8941	.9757	.9984	3.66
Fitted					.1170	.4416	.7258	.8957	.9768	.9985	
Residual					−.0075	.0120	−.0013	−.0016	−.0011	−.0001	
Denmark 1973											
Reported	X202	1.508	.947	.133	.0677	.4088	.7641	.9344	.9894	.9995	1.93
Fitted					.0805	.3988	.7526	.9363	.9926	.9997	
Residual					−.0128	.0100	.0115	−.0019	−.0032	−.0002	
German Democratic Republic 1973											
Reported	X202	1.344	1.253	−.059	.2135	.6483	.8644	.9566	.9927	.9997	1.56
Fitted					.2247	.6364	.8664	.9570	.9924	.9999	
Residual					−.0112	.0119	−.0020	−.0004	.0003	−.0002	

TABLE 8.5

Cumulative Distributions of Overall Fertility for the United Kingdom, 1967 and 1973, and Their EHR Fits as Weighted Sums of the A_j^* and B_j^* Standards for the X15 Sequence and the A_j^*, B_j^*, and C_j^* Standards for the X202 Sequence: An Example of an Emerging Variation in the Age Pattern of Overall Fertility that Is Brought into the Fitted Description by the C_j^* Age Standard

Schedule	Source of age standards	α_i^*	β_i^*	γ_i^*	Age cut						$5T_i$
					19/20	24/25	29/30	34/35	39/40	44/45	
United Kingdom 1967											
Reported					.0922	.4065	.7199	.8947	.9772	.9985	2.63
Fitted	X202	1.455	.833	.064	.0945	.4057	.7158	.8968	.9775	.9986	
Residual					−.0023	.0008	.0041	−.0021	−.0003	−.0001	
Reported					.0922	.4065	.7199	.8947	.9772	.9985	2.63
Fitted	X15	1.494	.918	—	.0986	.4160	.7084	.8897	.9778	.9996	
Residual					−.0064	−.0095	.0115	.0050	−.0006	−.0011	
United Kingdom 1973											
Reported					.1084	.4318	.7662	.9232	.9840	.9990	2.03
Fitted	X202	1.445	.945	.083	.1081	.4378	.7571	.9246	.9862	.9987	
Residual					.0003	−.0060	.0091	−.0014	−.0022	.0003	
Reported					.1084	.4318	.7662	.9232	.9840	.9990	2.03
Fitted	X15	1.492	1.026	—	.1143	.4550	.7471	.9137	.9860	1.0000	
Residual					−.0059	−.0232	.0191	.0095	−.0020	−.0010	

TABLE 8.6

Cumulative Distributions of Overall Fertility and Their EHR Fits as Weighted Sums of the A_j^*, B_j^*, and C_j^* Standards for the $X202$ Sequence: Examples of a Degree of Age Concentration of Childbearing that Is Incompletely Described by Current EHR Age Standards

Schedule	Source of age standards	α_i^*	β_i^*	γ_i^*	Age cut						$5T_i$
					19/20	24/25	29/30	34/35	39/40	44/45	
Taiwan 1970											
Reported					.0500	.3475	.7138	.8975	.9713	.9963	4.00
Fitted	X202	1.481	.776	.150	.0641	.3399	.6918	.9008	.9798	.9965	
Residual					-.0141	.0076	.0220	-.0033	-.0085	-.0002	
Korea 1970											
Reported					.0164	.2277	.5774	.8061	.9421	.9912	3.98
Fitted	X202	1.506	.442	.168	.0247	.2196	.5596	.8106	.9503	.9920	
Residual					-.0083	.0081	.0178	-.0045	-.0082	-.0008	
Netherlands 1974											
Reported					.0426	.3383	.7396	.9197	.9824	.9989	1.79
Fitted	X202	1.529	.842	.182	.0546	.3357	.7122	.9237	.9898	.9988	
Residual					-.0120	.0026	.0274	-.0040	-.0074	.0001	
Japan 1970											
Reported					.0106	.2410	.7406	.9456	.9930	.9995	2.07
Fitted	X202	1.626	.840	.329	.0166	.2470	.7023	.9504	.9985	.9990	
Residual					-.0060	-.0060	.0383	-.0048	-.0055	.0005	

257

terns of childbearing, including the very young pattern for the German Democratic Republic, are also well fit by three time parameters and sometimes by two time parameters (Table 8.4). The distributions for Romania (1966) and Denmark (1973) with identical β_i^* values and 76 percent of fertility achieved by age cut 29/30 provide a second example of the greater degree of concentration expressed by higher α_i^* and γ_i^* values. The nature of the sudden 1966–1967 change in the distribution for Romania is well captured by two time parameters and still better by three time parameters. The small increase in the values of α_i^* and γ_i^* accompanied by a greater decrease in the value of β_i^* indicates that the burden of doubled total rate fell on all age groups, but disproportionately on those women aged 30–39.

The point in a time sequence at which fitting the third component becomes more than a refinement will depend on our purposes—whether we are interested in broad comparisons or more subtle distinctions. The increasing importance of the type of variation captured in the $\gamma_i^* C_j^*$ component is apparent, for example, in a comparison of residuals from two-component and three-component fits for the United Kingdom (1967 and 1973, Table 8.5). With a two component fit, the distribution of the residuals by sign is the same for the two years, but by 1973 the size of the residuals has increased appreciably at the four central age cuts. Fitting the third component improves the fit for both years, as expected.

More extreme examples of the concentration of childbearing in a narrow age range can be examined in Table 8.6. Here, the $\gamma_i^* C_j^*$ component is not a refinement but a requirement for adequate description. At very different total rates, a similarity in the distributions and their EHR descriptions for the Netherlands and Taiwan is clear. Comparison of the distributions for Taiwan and Korea, which have the same total rate and similar degrees of concentration expressed by α_i^* and γ_i^*, reveals vividly the younger age distribution of fertility associated with higher values of β_i^*. The distributions for the Netherlands and Japan, which have a common level of β_i^*, provide a third example of the effects of higher values of α_i^* and γ_i^*, but at much higher degrees of concentration of fertility than we saw in the distributions for El Salvador and Reunion or Romania and Denmark.

With the highly concentrated distributions shown in Table 8.6, a further pattern of departure from fit emerges in the prominent positive residual at age cut 29/30 accompanied by negative residuals at age cuts 19/20 and 34/35. These departures represent the "worst fits" to any of the overall fertility schedules tested. Although the largest of these residuals multiplied by the sum of age-specific rates T_i yields a difference of no more than

.016 births per woman between the reported and fitted rate at any age cut (or for de-cumulated schedules, a difference of no more than .020 between the reported and fitted rate for any age group), improvement of fit would be expected in a complete EHR analysis.

The preliminary cross-population comparisons of overall fertility in EHR terms provide several conclusions.

1. The close fits to a variety of schedules from 48 countries indicate that broadly applicable choices have been made in deriving EHR age standards from Swedish fertility time sequences.

2. The importance of the third component $\gamma_i^* C_j^*$ in completing descriptions of fertility patterns for a number of low- and moderately low-fertility countries suggests the need for the inclusion of one or more versions of the C_j^* vector in a refined set of age standards.

3. The tendency for both α_i^* and γ_i^*, the two different degree-of-concentration parameters, to have a higher level in some time sequences and individual schedules than in others (that is, to not vary independently across populations) points to the first steps of the refinement of cross-population descriptions:

   a. a direct three-component fitting of a set of high quality schedules (preferably by single year of age) composed of short time sequences for countries with a range of age distributions of fertility;

   b. re-presentation of the fitted A_j and α_i values as in Chapter V to assure as complete a separation of α_i^* from γ_i^* and from the total rate as possible before proceeding to refine the B_j^* age standard and identify one or more C_j^* age standards.

High-fertility countries with early ages of entry into childbearing will admittedly be underrepresented in the set of schedules used in direct three-component fitting. Judging from the experience with the age standards derived from Swedish data, however, such distributions should still be well described by the more general EHR parameters in re-presented standard form.

Marital Fertility: Fits to Age 20–49 Schedules   Turning to marital fertility and to the age 20–49 distributions that have traditionally been used to study the decline of marital fertility with age, we find that a wide variety of patterns can be closely fit as a weighted sum of the A_j^* and B_j^* standards for the MX20 sequence (Table 8.7). The first time parameter α_i^* varies over the narrow range 1.02–1.16—very similar to the 1.08–1.14 range observed for the MX20 sequence. We know from Chapter VII that the $\alpha_i^* A_j^*$ component for the MX20 sequence closely approximates a "natural" fertility pattern. We can therefore relate the descriptions of the

TABLE 8.7

Cumulative Distributions of Age 20–49 Marital Fertility and Their EHR Fits as Weighted Sums of the A_j^* and B_j^* Standards for the MX20 Sequence: Selected Countries, 1960–1974

Schedule	α_i^*	β_i^*	Age cut					$5T_i$
			24/25	29/30	34/35	39/40	44/45	
Reunion 1961	1.126	.236						8.47
Reported			.3017	.5499	.7512	.9102	.9899	
Fitted			.3064	.5501	.7494	.9068	.9914	
Residual			-.0047	-.0002	.0018	.0034	-.0015	
El Salvador 1971	1.066	.269						5.85
Reported			.3229	.5590	.7586	.9086	.9781	
Fitted			.3301	.5654	.7529	.8993	.9831	
Residual			-.0072	-.0064	.0057	.0093	-.0050	
Ireland 1961	1.164	.368						7.27
Reported			.3287	.5985	.8038	.9430	.9960	
Fitted			.3376	.6006	.7987	.9377	.9978	
Residual			-.0089	-.0021	.0051	.0053	-.0018	
Chile 1960	1.091	.371						6.46
Reported			.3443	.6029	.7978	.9287	.9865	
Fitted			.3557	.6046	.7905	.9233	.9902	
Residual			-.0114	-.0017	.0073	.0054	-.0037	
Spain 1970	1.112	.605						4.62
Reported			.4105	.7019	.8679	.9635	.9961	
Fitted			.4243	.6937	.8655	.9627	.9973	
Residual			-.0138	.0082	.0024	.0008	-.0012	
France 1972	1.104	.744						3.17
Reported			.4606	.7522	.9047	.9765	.9983	
Fitted			.4705	.7450	.9025	.9778	.9985	
Residual			-.0099	.0072	.0022	-.0013	-.0002	
Hungary 1963	1.074	.877						2.04
Reported			.5227	.7999	.9278	.9833	.9993	
Fitted			.5200	.7921	.9316	.9868	.9982	
Residual			.0027	.0078	-.0038	-.0035	.0011	
German Democratic Republic 1974	1.024	1.075						1.54
Reported			.6149	.8605	.9596	.9928	.9997	
Fitted			.5949	.8574	.9669	.9959	.9975	
Residual			.0200	.0031	-.0073	-.0031	.0022	

diverse schedules in Table 8.7 to departure from such a pattern. We can consider that the values of β_i^*, which span the broad range of .24 for the distribution for Reunion to 1.08 for the distribution for the German Democratic Republic, express the degree of that departure according to the age pattern determined by B_j^*.

The information to be gained from such fitted descriptions is not limited to the measure of the extent to which childbearing is shifted toward lower ages according to the pattern determined by B_j^*. Examination of the residuals reveals that one of the variations of pattern detected in overall fertility is also apparent in marital fertility. Emergence of this specific type of departure from fit—lower than the predicted proportion of total fertility at age cut 24/25, higher than the predicted proportion at age cut 29/30—is illustrated in Table 8.8 by pairs of distributions, separated by 10 years, for the countries Australia, Denmark, and Japan. In each case this pattern of departure, already apparent (or prominent in the case of Japan) in the 1960s, is magnified by the 1970s. It is a type of systematic variation that was shown with overall fertility to be well fit by a third component $\gamma_i^* C_j^*$ that expresses the degree of concentration of fertility in age group 25–29. Such a C_j^* age standard would accommodate in the fitted parameters significant incidence of delay of a first birth and spacing of births within marriage.

Marital Fertility: Fits to Age 15–49 Schedules For the full age 15–49 marital fertility distributions, introduction of a third component $\gamma_i^* C_j^*$ appears to be essential for useful cross-population descriptions—at least to establish a standard form for a more generalized second age parameter B_j^*. Evidence for this comes from preliminary tests of fit by both of the sets of age 15–49 marital fertility age standards so far derived—one incorporating approximately known levels of premarital pregnancy, the other presumed to include a small degree of subfecundity at the lower ages.

Most of the schedules tested fall into one of three groups. At one extreme is the group of schedules quite well fit by the A_j^* and B_j^* standards for the MX15 sequence (see Table 8.9 for examples); at the other extreme is the group of schedules quite well described in terms of the A_j^* and B_j^* standards for the NX15 sequence (see Table 8.10 for examples). Some schedules do fall at, or beyond, the lower fringe of the latter group in having even a smaller proportion of births occur at ages 15–19 than the NX15 age standards can accommodate. The schedule for Japan (1960) is included in Table 8.10 to illustrate this point; it is also shown in decumulated form in Table 8.11, with the schedule for Japan (1970), as an example of increasing departure in this direction. (See Table 8.6 for some

TABLE 8.8

Cumulative Distributions of Age 20–49 Marital Fertility and Their EHR Fits as Weighted Sums of the A_i^* and B_j^* Standards for the MX20 Sequence: Examples of an Emerging Variation in the Age Pattern of Marital Fertility that Is Incompletely Described by Current EHR Age Standards

Schedule	α_i^*	β_i^*	Age cut					$5T_i$
			24/25	29/30	34/35	39/40	44/45	
Australia 1961								
Reported	1.126	.676	.4282	.7247	.8931	.9734	.9981	4.16
Fitted			.4434	.7195	.8868	.9734	.9990	
Residual			−.0152	.0052	.0063	.0000	−.0009	
Australia 1971								
Reported	1.154	.707	.4102	.7438	.9104	.9807	.9988	3.20
Fitted			.4464	.7297	.8978	.9803	1.0000	
Residual			−.0362	.0141	.0126	.0004	−.0012	
Denmark 1963								
Reported	1.109	.779	.4696	.7632	.9147	.9811	.9988	3.25
Fitted			.4802	.7571	.9117	.9819	.9991	
Residual			−.0106	.0061	.0030	−.0008	−.0003	
Denmark 1973								
Reported	1.138	.858	.4656	.7951	.9443	.9908	.9996	2.38
Fitted			.4985	.7838	.9331	.9914	1.0000	
Residual			−.0329	.0113	.0112	−.0006	−.0004	
Japan 1960								
Reported	1.113	.911	.4843	.8211	.9520	.9906	.9993	3.49
Fitted			.5215	.8025	.9424	.9928	1.0000	
Residual			−.0372	.0186	.0096	−.0022	−.0007	
Japan 1970								
Reported	1.139	.952	.4771	.8353	.9659	.9957	.9997	3.58
Fitted			.5284	.8152	.9526	.9967	.9997	
Residual			−.0513	.0201	.0133	−.0010	.0000	

TABLE 8.9

Cumulative Distributions of Age 15–49 Marital Fertility and Their EHR Fits as Weighted Sums of the A_j^* and B_j^* Standards for the MX15 Sequence: Selected Countries, 1960–1974

Schedule	α_i^*	β_i^*	Age cut						$5T_i$
			19/20	24/25	29/30	34/35	39/40	44/45	
Ireland 1961									
Reported	1.301		.2964	.5277	.7175	.8620	.9599	.9972	10.34
Fitted		.667	.3000	.5367	.7152	.8540	.9550	.9990	
Residual			−.0036	−.0090	.0023	.0080	.0049	−.0018	
Chile 1960									
Reported	1.232		.3258	.5579	.7323	.8637	.9520	.9909	9.58
Fitted		.707	.3358	.5620	.7278	.8548	.9479	.9947	
Residual			−.0100	−.0041	.0045	.0089	.0041	−.0038	
Faeroe Islands 1966									
Reported	1.209		.4541	.6721	.8179	.9104	.9685	.9981	9.14
Fitted		1.009	.4491	.6726	.8169	.9131	.9719	.9967	
Residual			.0051	−.0005	.0010	−.0027	−.0034	.0014	
Papua 1961									
Reported	1.311		.4115	.6601	.8185	.9237	.9863	1.0000	7.43
Fitted		1.014	.4164	.6589	.8180	.9233	.9839	.9999	
Residual			−.0049	.0012	.0005	.0004	.0024	.0001	
German Democratic Republic 1974									
Reported	1.156		.6844	.8785	.9560	.9872	.9977	.9999	4.86
Fitted		1.621	.6826	.8712	.9565	.9904	.9987	.9992	
Residual			.0018	.0073	−.0005	−.0032	−.0010	.0007	

263

TABLE 8.10

Cumulative Distributions of Age 15–49 Marital Fertility and Their EHR Fits as Weighted Sums of the A_j^* and B_j^* Standards for the NX15 Sequence: Selected Countries, 1960–1961

Schedule	α_i^*	β_i^*	Age cut						$5T_i$
			19/20	24/25	29/30	34/35	39/40	44/45	
Reunion 1961									
Reported	1.224		.2189	.4546	.6485	.8057	.9299	.9921	10.84
Fitted		.229	.2129	.4469	.6485	.8145	.9309	.9894	
Residual			.0060	.0077	.0000	-.0088	-.0010	.0027	
Martinique 1961									
Reported	1.217		.2227	.4653	.6648	.8179	.9326	.9919	9.88
Fitted		.266	.2202	.4582	.6620	.8250	.9355	.9895	
Residual			.0025	.0071	.0028	-.0071	-.0029	.0024	
Spain 1960									
Reported	1.195		.2778	.5604	.7695	.9005	.9705	.9968	6.79
Fitted		.570	.2733	.5478	.7697	.9075	.9735	.9945	
Residual			.0045	.0126	-.0002	-.0070	-.0030	.0023	
Japan 1960									
Reported	1.201		.3026	.6403	.8752	.9665	.9934	.9995	5.01
Fitted		.861	.3194	.6299	.8623	.9689	.9969	.9991	
Residual			-.0168	.0104	.0129	-.0024	-.0035	.0004	

TABLE 8.11

Noncumulated Distributions of Age 15–49 Marital Fertility for Japan, 1960 and 1970, and Their EHR Fits as Weighted Sums of the A_j^* and B_j^* Standards for the NX15 Sequence: An Example of an Increasing Degree of Age Concentration of Marital Fertility that is Incompletely Described by Current EHR Age Standards

Schedule	α_i^*	β_i^*	Age group							$5T_i$
			15–19	20–24	25–29	30–34	35–39	40–44	45–49	
Japan 1960										
Reported			.3026	.3377	.2349	.0913	.0269	.0061	.0005	5.01
Fitted	1.201	.861	.3194	.3105	.2324	.1066	.0280	.0022	.0008	
Residual			−.0168	.0272	.0025	−.0153	−.0011	.0039	−.0003	
Japan 1970										
Reported			.2435	.3610	.2709	.0988	.0225	.0031	.0002	4.73
Fitted	1.286	.814	.2894	.3192	.2431	.1168	.0305	.0006	.0004	
Residual			−.0459	.0418	.0278	−.0180	−.0080	.0025	−.0002	

265

reflection of Japan's 1970 marital fertility pattern in the overall fertility distribution at age cuts 29/30 and 34/35.)

A third group of schedules lies between the two sets of age standards, well fit by neither set, but departing from fit with each set in a typical pattern: using the A_j^* and B_j^* standards for the NX15 sequence, there is a higher proportion of total fertility at ages 15–19 and a lesser concentration of fertility at ages 20–29 than the standards would predict; using the A_j^* and B_j^* standards for the MX15 sequence, there is a lower proportion of total fertility at ages 15–19 and a greater concentration of fertility at ages 20–29 than the standards would predict. That this group of schedules includes the 1974 schedule for Sweden is evidence for prominent changes in Swedish marital fertility patterns in the 15 years following the end of the MX15 sequence for which the A_j^* and B_j^* standards provide very close fits (see Fig. 4.10). The increase in family formation outside of legal marriage and any change in the use of contraceptives to delay or space births should be contributing factors.

How these patterns of variation can be brought into useful fitted descriptions would be determined in a complete cross-population EHR analysis of the age distribution of fertility, both within legal marriage and within stable unions of other types. We would expect many of the similarities detected at this preliminary stage to persist and be sharpened with refined cross-population age standards, whereas others, more apparent than real, would be dissipated in new, more clearly defined groupings. We should also expect some new similarities to emerge that had been obscured by the use of age standards not fully appropriate to the range of systematic variation encountered.

The analysis, taking advantage of existing time sequences of single-year-of-age fertility schedules as well as 5-year-age-group sequences, would reasonably investigate other re-expressions of the data before three-component EHR fitting and would also give fresh consideration to the choice of constraints in the re-presentation of the fitted parameters in a standard form. The sufficiency of a single C_j^* age standard, the need for more than one, or the need for none at all with some schedules would emerge in such an analysis. Giving the fitting procedure a guided start with a refined A_j^* age standard similar to that for the NX15 sequence is a possibility to consider in efforts to transfer the effects of premarital pregnancy to the C_j^* standard or at least one version of C_j^*. If the age distribution of fertility within legal marriage and within stable unions of other types continues to hold interest for demographers, these analyses should make vigorous use of the data guiding and flexibility of the EDA approach in developing demographically useful descriptions of the full diversity of fertility distributions in changing social milieux.

Summary

This chapter accomplishes three purposes:

1. It establishes that the EHR age standards derived from Swedish fertility time sequences are not peculiar to Sweden but are broadly applicable.
2. It demonstrates how time parameters and residuals can be used to group diverse schedules.
3. It identifies types of systematic variation in fertility patterns that are not accommodated by the age standards so far derived and that a thorough cross-population EHR analysis would be expected to bring into the fitted parameters.

A simple regression procedure is described for the expression of any age-specific fertility schedule as a weighted sum of an appropriate set of EHR age standards. This procedure is then applied to overall and marital fertility schedules for 48 countries and Coale–Trussell model fertility schedules that have a wide range of patterns.

The applicability of the EHR standard-form parameters is prominently established by the finding that changes in twentieth-century U.S. overall fertility patterns are as closely and coherently described on this basis as are changes in Swedish patterns. Similarities and differences in the child-bearing experience of the two countries over six decades are clearly revealed in the time parameters. Short overall fertility time sequences for 15 countries further illustrate the cross-population comparisons that can be based on EHR age standards.

The capacity of sets of EHR standard-form parameters to represent quite well both actual and hypothetical fertility distributions that did not contribute to their derivation is further demonstrated by fits and residuals for a variety of isolated distributions. For overall fertility, the well-fitted schedules are as diverse as those in the 1960s and 1970s for Tunisia, El Salvador, Korea, the German Democratic Republic, and Romania (both before and after the recision of legal abortion). Close fits to hypothetical distributions are illustrated with Coale–Trussell model fertility schedules that incorporate a pace of entry into marriage ranging from one-half to four times the model's standard pace and a "degree of parity-dependent control" ranging from "natural" fertility to about twice the highest degree found for Sweden by the Coale method.

For marital fertility, the age 20–49 distributions that are closely fit as a weighted sum of EHR age standards have total rates ranging from 8.5 to 1.5 births per woman. An important finding is that an essentially constant component underlies these diverse schedules, as it did for the Swedish schedules—a pattern of cumulation of births with age that closely approximates the natural fertility patterns examined in Chapter VII. The differences between the distributions are expressed in a single variable time parameter that measures the extent to which childbearing is shifted toward younger ages according to the pattern determined by the second EHR age standard.

The EHR age standards distinguish three groups of marital fertility distributions for the full 15–49 age range: schedules well described by the set of standards that incorporates an approximately known, high level of premarital pregnancy at ages 15–19; schedules well described by the set of standards that is presumed to include little premarital pregnancy but a small degree of subfecundity at the lower ages; and schedules whose underlying patterns are shown in the residuals to lie between the two sets of age standards, departing from each in a systematic way.

The first contribution of this chapter, then, is the evidence that useful few-parameter comparisons of fertility patterns across populations can be made on the basis of EHR age standards so far derived even before a complete cross-population analysis of age-specific overall and marital fertility patterns is carried out. The second, but equally important, contribution is the guidance provided by these fits—both in the fitted parameters and the residuals—for improving the description of fertility patterns in a thorough cross-population exploratory analysis. The residuals reveal that the major systematic variation in both overall and marital patterns that needs to be more fully accommodated by refined age standards is the increasing concentration of childbearing in a narrow age range centered on ages 25–29 observed for a number of countries in the 1960s and 1970s. A full exploration would continue to place first emphasis on obtaining close fits in few parameters and using residual patterns to group similar schedules in seeking improvements to the fit. Data re-expressions in addition to the folded square root should be considered. Alternative constraints in the re-presentation of the second age parameter and second time parameter in a three-component fit should also be considered. Finally, total fertility rate should enter the analysis as a separate dimension of the data in the expectation that the refined schedule-specific parameters, like the time parameters in Chapters VI and VII, will be better understood through the additional step of level compensation.

Notes for Chapter VIII

1. With the X15 standards, residuals at 307 of the 348 age cuts do not exceed the third decimal place on the raw fraction scale. The remaining 41 residuals range in size from .010 to

.022. Only three of these residuals have an absolute value greater than .015, and they appear as fewer births than predicted at age cut 24/25 from 1972 to 1974. With the *X202* standards, the only residuals with an absolute value greater than .009 are two in 1945 (more births than predicted at age cut 19/20, fewer than predicted at age cut 29/30) and six from 1972 to 1974 (more births than predicted at age cut 19/20, fewer than predicted at age cut 24/25).

2. These two models are incorporated in one overall fertility model by means of the equation

$$f(a) = G(a)n(a) \exp[m \cdot v(a)],$$

where $f(a)$ is the age-specific overall fertility rate, $G(a)$ the age-specific proportion of women ever married, and $n(a) \exp[m \cdot v(a)]$ the age pattern of marital fertility; $f(a)$ is then normalized so that $\Sigma f'(a) = 1$. To generate the marital fertility component, the two age standards $n(a)$ for ages 20 and higher by 5-year age groups and $v(a)$ for ages 25 and higher by 5-year age groups are retained from the original marital fertility model but are interpolated to give values by single year of age that sum to the original values by 5-year age groups. Because $n(a)$, the average natural fertility schedule used in the original model, lacks values below age 20, single-year estimations are added for ages 12–19 to form a smooth curve. To provide a smooth curve for $v(a)$, the logarithmic pattern of departure from natural fertility by age, $v(a)$ is assumed to have its nonzero values begin at age 20 instead of age 25. The standard pattern in the marriage model, derived from Swedish marriage entry data for the years 1865–1869, is described by the convolution of a normal curve and a double exponential curve and is expressed in two variable parameters, a_0 and k.

3. In considering the EHR parameters that describe Coale–Trussell model schedules, recall the difference between β_i^* for overall fertility used here and β_i^* for marital fertility. The counterpart of the Coale–Trussell model parameter m is β_i^* for *marital fertility* (see Chapter VII), a measure of the extent to which the marital fertility distribution is shifted toward younger ages according to the pattern determined by the marital fertility age standard B_j^*. The β_i^* parameter for *overall fertility* describes the net effect of the several factors (including the marital fertility pattern) that influence the extent to which the overall fertility distribution is shifted from ages 30 and higher to ages below 30 according to the pattern determined by the overall fertility age standard B_j^* (see Chapter V). In the EHR descriptions of the model schedules of overall fertility, β_i^* is therefore determined by the two factors specified by the Coale–Trussell model: the age pattern of entry into first marriage and the decline of marital fertility with age. We see in Table 8.1 that as delay in marriage, expressed by a higher value of k, becomes a more prominent factor in the age pattern of overall fertility, the degree of decline of marital fertility with age m becomes a less important factor in the degree of shift of overall fertility toward younger ages, which is measured by β_i^* for overall fertility.

4. Preliminary work with World Fertility Survey data for 17 Asian, Central American, and South American countries (not reported here) indicates that the EHR standard age patterns are appropriate for description of these data also.

IX

Conclusion

The success of the exploratory analyses reported in this book can be judged from several points of view:

1. as a response to the need for a time-sequence model of the age pattern of fertility;
2. as a demonstration of the value of exploratory data analysis in demography;
3. as a source of additional questions and guidance on ways to approach further exploratory analyses.

The analyses of two centuries of Swedish overall fertility and seven decades of marital fertility have accomplished their original purposes: the development of close-fitting, stable, and interpretable descriptions of change in the age pattern of fertility in both cross-sectional and cohort perspectives. Trends and transitions have been clearly identified. Transitions in the aggregate pace or timing of childbearing as well as transitions associated with the decline of fertility at higher ages have been well described in the variable time parameters. The nature of departures from trend that are related to unusual circumstances or inaccuracies in the data has been made apparent by the close fits to the time sequences of single-year schedules and the re-presentation of fitted parameters in a standard form. The possibility of including recent low-fertility variations on fertility patterns in the model has been illustrated.

Several innovations in demographic modeling have contributed to the interpretability of the parameters. The separation of modeling into two stages—fitting and standard-form re-presentation of fits—applies the concept that the form in which the closest fits are achieved need not be the form in which the fits are examined and interpreted. The choice of a standard form has been guided by knowledge of the demographic processes that underlie fertility patterns. The retention of total fertility rate as a separate dimension of the data to be used in further steps of parameter dissection has permitted the interpretation of some changes in the age pattern of fertility that are missed or misconstrued in models based on pattern alone.

Several advantages have followed directly from parallel analyses of related fertility time sequences: in cross-sectional and cohort perspectives, by 5-year age groups and by single year of age, for the full 15–49 age range and truncated for childbearing at ages 20–49 only, for overall and marital fertility, and for births occurring 9 months or more after marriage. Interpretation of the evidence of change has been further enhanced by this adoption of multiple points of view. Clues have been elicited that fertility limitation by means other than late and nonuniversal marriage existed at an earlier time in the nineteenth century and that the delay and spacing of births at younger ages had importance for fertility levels earlier in the twentieth century than is commonly supposed. The period around 1910 has been repeatedly identified, from every viewpoint, as one of major transition in the age pattern of fertility that involved childbearing at younger as well as older ages and marital as well as overall fertility. Intersequence relations of standard-form parameters have led to estimates for missing data and to estimated corrections for obvious data errors. Valuable information has been extracted from flawed eighteenth- and early nineteenth-century data that had been subjected to little previous analysis.

The value of the modeling has extended beyond the specific sequences analyzed. The standard age patterns developed for the country as a whole have proved to be a useful basis for characterizing subpopulation differences from the whole. The age standards have proved to be widely applicable for preliminary cross-population comparisons of fertility patterns. This work has been cited (Stoto, 1982) as an example of a relational model approach to fertility modeling that should lead to more effective population projections.

These results demonstrate clearly that exploratory data analysis (EDA) is an analytic style that has much to offer demographers who deal with large amounts of data that are often incomplete or flawed. The contributions come both from the philosophy of this approach and from its tools. The effective description depends on considering the data from a number of different viewpoints to see which will be useful. Stepwise dissection of the data and attention to the residuals is central to the detection of patterns that underlie the long time sequences. The examination of residuals for remaining structure takes precedence over summarizing their size. The absence of assumptions about the distribution of data and residuals leads to pattern detection without interference from the unusual observations or data misclassifications common in demographic data. An emphasis on simplifying the descriptions—expressing the systematic variability of the data in as few parameters as possible—leads to the use of linearizing re-expression of the data before seeking underlying patterns and also to the re-presentation of the fitted descriptions in a standard form selected to reduce the number of parameters when appropriate. Graphic displays are used to force attention to the unexpected.

The effectiveness of the EDA approach to demographic data is apparent not only in the coherent descriptions so far derived for age patterns of fertility across time—a result not achieved by other approaches to aggregate fertility data—but also in the additional questions that the explorations raise, including questions that appear to be newly amenable to study in aggregate data. Three examples will serve to illustrate.

For flawed historical data covering an extended period of time, can the exploratory analysis identification of patterns and departures from pattern direct the estimation of data corrections that meet the tests of demographic consistency? Sundbärg's previous adjustments of census and registration data in a reconstitution of Swedish population statistics by age and sex for the period 1750–1860 led to estimated fertility rates by 5-year periods that have been used for both official and research purposes since the early twentieth century. The rationale underlying some of his adjustments has now been questioned by some Swedish demographers. The dual cohort–cross-sectional exploratory analysis of the extended fertility time sequence, which appends later-nineteenth-century and twentieth-century data to the single-year historical data on which Sundbärg based his revisions, brings out the strong patterns that underlie the early data and tie them to the later data. Both the fitted parameters and the residuals indicate the nature of possible errors. Some first steps in the exploration of possible adjustments have been outlined; later steps would be guided by the intermediate results. If demographically consistent adjustments resulted, their value for historical studies might lie partly in the confirmation or revision of Sundbärg's fertility rate estimates for 5-year periods, but their chief value would be in returning to active status a large body of single-year data and enhancing its usefulness.

What have been the systematic variations across time in the age pattern of nonmarital conception leading to birth of a child? What have been the systematic variations in the tendency to marry or not marry before giving birth to a nonmaritally conceived child? How well can such variations be detected in available fertility data? Exploratory analysis has described well the trends and transitions in the age pattern of marital fertility that is highly influenced by premarital pregnancy and the changes in the age pattern of births occurring 9 months or more after marriage. Systematic change should be equally detectable in other sets of related time sequences constructed from the available data on women by age and marital status and on births by mother's age, marital status, and marriage duration. Continuing the exploratory philosophy of considering a body of data from a number of viewpoints, the proposed analyses would focus on the variable border between marital and nonmarital childbearing from the point of view of the mothers' marital status at the time of conception as well as the mothers' marital status at the time of delivery. This would bring under consideration an aspect of fertility change over time that has generally been avoided in aggregate fertility modeling. One of the values of successful identification of the structure that underlies this portion of childbearing experience would be clarifying the relation between the traditional overall and marital fertility time sequences when the possibility of pregnancy is not confined to married women.

How well can recently evolved variations on the age pattern of fertility in many low-fertility countries be brought into a few-parameter model? Preliminary cross-population comparisons based on the age standards derived from the Swedish sequences have identified a specific variation in both overall and marital fertility patterns that needs to be more fully accommodated by refined age standards: an increasing concentration of childbearing in a narrow age range centered on ages 25–29. Some early steps for seeking such an accommodation have been outlined. Making vigorous use of the data guiding and flexibility of the EDA approach, the first emphasis would continue to be on obtaining close fits and using residual patterns to group similar schedules in seeking improvements to the fit. The choice of the standard form in which to examine the fits would continue to have considerable importance in efforts to describe still greater diversity in a small number of demographically interpretable parameters. The success of such an effort would have particular value in population projections, comparisons of subpopulation fertility experience, and models relating recent demographic change to economic and social change.

The value of the fertility modeling reported in this book is not that it provides a "finished" model of time-sequence change in fertility patterns, but that it has taken informative and provocative steps in the ongoing search for useful and more refined ways of considering demographic change in changing social milieux. Its approach is in the spirit of the "demographic view of society" that Winsborough (1978) sees as having an increasingly important role in the social sciences "as a way of dealing with the problem of aggregating the effects of individual behaviors into change at the societal level".

APPENDIX A

The Relationship of Empirical Analysis to More Narrowly Modeled Analysis*

by JOHN W. TUKEY

Princeton University, Princeton, New Jersey
and Bell Laboratories, Murray Hill, New Jersey

Kinds of Models

The word "model" is one of those words that mean quite different things to different people or to the same person at different times. At one extreme a model may be both almost completely normative and very precise, as in the mathematical expressions that describe the motion of two (or three) bodies under Newtonian gravitation. With such a model the discovery of "unexplained" (meaning "beyond the narrow model") deviations can be of great importance, as occurred when knowledge of the advance of the perihelion of Mercury was vital in the assessment of Einstein's theory of relativity. The existence of such precise normative models almost always depends on a long series of interactions between experiment or experience on the one hand and concepts and theory on the other.

At another extreme lie models that are highly adaptable because they involve so many more constants that can be adjusted to give a good fit and that, because of the diverse kinds of behavior to which they are adapted,

* Prepared in part in connection with research at Princeton University sponsored by the Army Research Office (Durham). This appendix originally appeared with the technical report by Breckenridge (1978).

are thought of almost entirely as providing empirical descriptions. In this case the emphasis is on the ability to describe very diverse phenomena in a single way, and the discovery of more or less systematic deviations is often a call to increased flexibility—to the use of still more general models to absorb these deviations.

In general, a model tends to contain two elements: the collection of things (the "stock") from which one is to be selected to describe a particular instance, and explicit or implied guidance for interpreting whichever element of the stock is selected. However, especially in the two extremes just discussed, the "guidance" element is often very weak or even nonexistent.

In the context of multiple regression, Mosteller and I (1977, p. 302ff) introduce the word "stock" (the word "posse" has also been used) for the collection of possibilities to be fit—from which one is to be selected as a useful description. In the extremely flexible case just described we are concerned with "broad stocks". By contrast, a stock involving only a few (and one hopes well-selected) constants would be a "narrow stock".

The second extreme, in which flexibility is emphasized but guidance has yet to be included, is reasonably referred to by the term "broad empirical models". The fact that guidance is initially avoided does not mean that it cannot be added as Breckenridge (1978) illustrates. It may be very desirable to start with an emphasis on adaptability and consequent good fit and then move to an emphasis on guidance in the interpretation of specific fits.

Still another extreme is given by relatively narrow (few-parameter) models where the way in which the constants enter into the algebraic or other expressions is such that we can make useful interpretations of changes in any particular constant. A good example is compartment models in biology, in which the passage of a traceable substance through the body—perhaps in and out of the blood stream—is modeled in terms of very simple differential equations (differential equations in which only the rate constants are to be fitted to the observed data.) In this case a change in one constant may be rightly given a different interpretation than change in another constant. However, no close similarity between what actually occurs and what can be modeled is essential (or even very likely). Deviations, if not too large, are often recognized as something to be anticipated and overlooked. Such models might be termed "separating models" because their main purpose is to separate information into pieces that relate to separate aspects of what is being studied. Guidance is an important part of the model.

A very important class of models (unfortunately frequent, some would say, and sometimes hard to separate from the previous class) are those described as "narrow empirical models". These models describe most of the detail of some behavior in terms of a few constants. This offers two great advantages: one, situations can often be compared more effectively and more intuitively if they are described in terms of only a few numbers; two, precision can usually be gained by estimating only a few constants from the data and leaving the bulk of the impact of irregularities, deviations, and sampling fluctuations in the residuals. Compared with broad empirical models, these models would involve fewer constants, perhaps many fewer. For narrow empirical models, in contrast to separating models, guidance is prominent by its absence and fit may be less than, or even far from, perfect. Imperfection of fit is accepted in return for the two advantages of such a model.

The last class of models we shall choose to mention is a system of "transferring models" with which we hope to effectively transfer into common terms what can be learned from observations of very different sorts. Economists hope that some of their models are of this kind, as when they compare the results of cross-sectional studies with the results of time-series studies. In these models, guidance is likely to be much more important than stock. Bridgman's (1927) discussion of operational constructs in physics in which, for example, masses measured in different ways represent different concepts illustrates the delicacy of such transfers.

In considering the model types just sketched—normative models, broad empirical models, separating models, narrow empirical models, and transferring models (or model systems)—we must remember that these types have been isolated as characteristic extremes and that many real situations are likely to be mixtures of at least two of them.

Finally, a mathematician might hope for the very frequent occurrence of "interpolative models" with which careful measurements in a few well-selected situations tell us what will happen in many other intermediate situations. Such models are at least very close to being precise normative models. The models used in studying the strength of materials and the rates of chemical reactions often come close to doing just this. Outside of the physical sciences, however, such models occur infrequently.

The General Character of Combinational Broad Stocks

It is important to recognize that the expressions fitted in empirical higher rank (EHR) analysis are selected from broad stocks and belong to some class of very flexible stocks. These classes make very little, if any, use of an understanding of the mechanism that underlies the data. They strive to mobilize their intrinsic flexibility and be guided by the data in the way that they dispose this flexibility to provide relatively close description. As Breckenridge (1978) has emphasized, they are usually well adapted to relatively automatic generalization—something that can be more difficult for narrower models.

The classes of flexible models so far of greatest importance are defined in terms of the simplest arithmetic operations, beginning with one or two additions. Additive fits with two crossed categories take the form

$$\hat{y}_{ij} = a + b_i + c_j$$

and are often most usefully written

$$y_{ij} = q(\text{data}_{ij}),$$

where q is a well-chosen monotone function [$q(z) = \log z$ is one frequent choice]. This approach not only underlies the widespread ramifications of the analysis of variance (perhaps the most widely used of the nonelementary statistical procedures) but also plays a key role in axiomatized fundamental measurement (Luce and Tukey, 1964).

Multiplicative fits are almost a twin to additive fits, as the formula

$$Y_{ij} = AB_iC_j$$

and the transfer rule

$$\text{lower case letter} = \log \text{ of capital letter}$$

shows for multiplicative fits involving only positive values of A, B_i, and C_j. Their importance lies not in this twin relation but in their facility for generalization. Not only

$$A + B_iC_j \quad \text{but} \quad B_iC_j + D_iE_j \quad \text{and} \quad A + B_iC_j + D_iE_j$$

offer generalizations of simple multiplicative models conveniently described as higher-rank models. Using this general term for a special-appearing class is reasonable because its twin,

$$a(b_i + c_j)(d_i + e_j),$$

has not yet often proved to be a stage of description that is helpful on our way to understanding. We can go easily to still higher complexities, to stocks in which more terms of the form (function of row) × (function of column) are summed.

Comments on EHR Analysis

A number of comments about the use of EHR analysis and the corresponding stocks deserve attention. The most important concern re-expression and re-presentation. Re-expression can greatly influence the satisfactoriness with which a well-selected example from a given kind of stock describes the data. We are familiar with this in circumstances where we understand in detail what is happening. We tend to forget that it is almost equally likely to be so when we face less understood (perhaps impenetrable) situations in a very empirical manner.

If we were given the volumes, cross-sectional areas, and lengths for a collection of cylinders, we would disagree with anyone who proposed to fit volumes with

(a function of cross section) PLUS (a function of length)

because we would recognize the need for TIMES instead of PLUS. Even in this case, we might not stop to think that, if we worked with the logarithm of volume instead of volume, a very simple re-expression, we could use the additive broad stock very effectively.

If we had data on blood pressures, I fear we would be much less likely to shun the PLUS analysis of raw blood pressures and much less likely to pounce on the advantages of a PLUS analysis of the *logarithm* of blood pressure, although such an opportunity would exist. As we move toward even less well-understood data, we are even more likely to miss an opportunity when re-expression could help. There is no intrinsic reason for this; we have only failed to take advantage of our opportunities.

The issue of re-presentation is of a very different kind (Breckenridge, 1978). Where re-expression sought for us a way to find better, and therefore more useful fits, we are now trying to do a more useful job of looking at the exact same fit. As a simple example, consider a fit $2A_iB_j + 2C_iD_j$, which can also be written as $(A_i + C_i)(B_j + D_j) + (A_i - C_i)(B_j - D_j)$. These two forms are algebraically identical, as can easily be seen by multiplying out the second form. Here there is no question of changing the fit, only of rewriting the fit.

If we are to compare the results of such a fit applied to two or more sets of data, we need to seek out a distinguished re-presentation of each fit so that the results will at least be conveniently comparable. If one fit looks like

$$2A_iB_j + 2C_iD_j$$

when the other looks like

$$(A_i + C_i)(B_j + D_j) + (A_i - C_i)(B_j - D_j),$$

we may miss an instance of a striking resemblance, something we should take only the least possible chance of doing.

Another way in which re-presentation can be important arises when we can find a re-presentation such as

$$E_iF_j + G_iH_j$$

in which one factor (say F_j) is very nearly constant. This offers us the opportunity to try a less general stock such as

$$E_i^* + G_iH_j,$$

where E_i^* is approximately given by E_i times the nearly common value of F_j.

Empirical fits with broad stocks need not and often should not be thought of as ends in themselves. They often play important roles in leading us to simpler fits that may or may not gain a more or less normative character.

The Structure of the Coale–Trussell Model

We shall now consider the internal structure of what might be thought of, by some at least, as almost the antithesis of the higher-rank broad stocks. The Coale–Trussell model schedules are traditionally considered to involve one constant, m, and one variable function of age, $G(a)$, in the form

$$f(a) = G(a)n(a) \exp[m \cdot v(a)],$$

where $n(a)$ and $v(a)$ are fixed functions of the age a.

If we want to study a single population at several dates (or in several cohorts) or compare several populations, we need to subscript m and $G(a)$. We shall also subscript a because we will be using discrete age ranges. This gives us the equation

$$f_i(a_j) = G_i(a_j)n(a_j) \exp[m_i \cdot v(a_j)]$$

and, once we take the natural logarithm, the equation

$$\ln f_i(a_j) = \ln n(a_j) + \ln G_i(a_j) + m_i \cdot v(a_j),$$

which is of the form

$$y_{ij} = K_j + C_iD_j + E_iL_j,$$

where K_j and L_j are fixed. This is now obviously a special case of

$$B_j + C_iD_j + E_iF_j,$$

an often useful but special case of the rank-three stock

$$A_i B_j + C_i D_j + E_i F_j.$$

There is therefore no necessary antithesis between the Coale–Trussell and the EHR models, although there may be differences in purpose and style. If we thought of EHR analysis as an end in itself, there might indeed be a vast gap between the two approaches. But if we think of such analyses as a first step in which the regular behavior of the data is to be encompassed as thoroughly as possible (going to still higher rank when necessary), so that we are ready to seek out as great a simplification of the EHR fit as we believe the data and our purposes will sustain, there will be no antithesis and the gap between approaches may be very small. It may not be possible to find effective fewer-constant fits or to convert them into higher-rank form, if they exist, by re-expressing the response. When this happens, we must work with the facts as they are, but we should not accept that it has happened without careful inquiry.

Comparison of the Breckenridge EHR and Coale–Trussell Models

The first major difference between the two models is in the chosen response: for the Coale–Trussell model, fertility at an age (for an age interval); and for the Breckenridge EHR model, fertility cumulated to an age-cut, as a fraction of total fertility. The fact that one takes the logarithm of the former response but the folded square root of the latter response is also important, but perhaps not as important. The question of how complicated or simple a stock one uses (how broad or narrow) is mainly a matter of detailed purposes. I argue strongly that the most practical way to begin is to fit the broad stock and then proceed to whatever degree of reduction is appropriate to the combination of data behavior and the purposes of the analyst.

What are the main issues of choice in this situation? I believe that the purposes toward which the Coale–Trussell schedules are directed combine, to various degrees, those typical of descriptive models, separating models, and transferring models, in order of decreasing emphasis. (Ansley Coale chose to emphasize the first two of these in an independent assessment.)

For the purpose of description, we want to make our fit to the diversity of the real world as good as possible, subject to holding the number of parameters to a minimum. For this purpose, it should not be important whether we work with fertility in age ranges or with accumulated fertility. Equally, it should not matter what re-expression proves to be useful.

The analysis suggested by Breckenridge (1978), in which EHR analysis would be applied to data from a wide variety of countries and time periods, is a natural first step in the search for the most useful descriptions. To be fully effective, such an analysis should explore the advantages not only of data by age range versus data cumulated to age cuts but also of varied re-expressions of each form. The absence of effective, tested techniques for guiding the exploration of re-expression in such situations is to be regretted, but we must start to learn somewhere.

Once we clearly understand how we can do very well with both broad-stock and narrow-stock fits, it will be time to ask how well the results serve our needs as separating and transferring models. We can then sensibly consider what changes in the structure of the empirically best-fitting models are wise or reasonable to make to do better in separating and transferring. We ought, in "Student's" words (1938, p. 365), plan to use "all the principles of allowed witchcraft".

References

Breckenridge, M. B.
  1978 "An Empirical Higher-Rank Analysis Model of the Age Distribution of Fertility." Department of Statistics, Princeton University, Princeton, New Jersey, Technical report no. 143, series 2.
Bridgman, P. W.
  1927 "The Logic of Modern Physics." New York: MacMillan.
Luce, R. D., and Tukey, J. W.
  1964 Simultaneous conjoint measurement. *Journal of Mathematical Psychology* 1:1–27.
Mosteller, F., and Tukey, J. W.
  1977 "Data Analysis and Regression." Reading, Massachusetts: Addison-Wesley.
"Student"
  1938 Comparison between balanced and random arrangements of field plots. *Biometrika* 29:363–379.

APPENDIX B

Robust–Resistant Fitting
Procedures and a
Robust–Resistant Measure
of Fit

Iteratively Weighted Fitting of Two or Three Multiplicative Components to an $m \times n$ Matrix

The iteratively weighted fitting procedures used to fit the multiplicative components $\alpha_i A_j$, $\beta_i B_j$, and $\gamma_i C_j$ to a fertility matrix F_{ij}, where $i = 1, 2, \ldots, m$ and $j = 1, 2, \ldots, n$, can be summarized as follows (see Mosteller and Tukey, 1977, pp. 353–364, and McNeil and Tukey, 1975, for further detail). Cellwise weights for the residuals z_{ij} are based on the biweight function

$$w(u) = (1 - u^2)^2 \quad \text{with} \quad u = (F_{ij} - \hat{F}_{ij})/cS = z_{ij}/cS,$$

where $\hat{F}_{ij}$ is the cellwise incomplete fit developed up to that point, S the median $|F_{ij} - \hat{F}_{ij}|$, which equals the median $|z_{ij}|$, and c a constant of assigned value. Thus at each iteration we assign to the residuals an updated set of weights

$$w_{ij} = \begin{cases} \left[1 - \left(\dfrac{F_{ij} - \hat{F}_{ij}}{cS}\right)^2\right]^2 & \text{when} \quad \left(\dfrac{F_{ij} - \hat{F}_{ij}}{cS}\right)^2 < 1, \\ 0 & \text{otherwise.} \end{cases}$$

This means that residuals of size greater than c times the median absolute deviation from the incomplete fit are given zero weight in seeking improvements to the fit and residuals less than about $c/2$ times the median absolute deviation are weighted about equally at the next iteration. Values of c between 6 and 9 are usually appropriate in starting an exploratory analysis. Optimal values of c vary with the data and with the analyst's purposes (see the discussion in Chapter III).

Because $\hat{F}_{ij}$ depends on w_{ij} and w_{ij} depends on $\hat{F}_{ij}$, a start to the iterative fitting procedure is needed. One frequently useful start is the assumption of temporary identical values for all of the members of one vector: for example, $\alpha_i^1 = 1$ for a row vector, if we want to emphasize pattern detection in the column dimension. We begin with weights

$$w_{ij}^1 = [1 - (F_{ij}/cS_1)^2]^2,$$

where S_1 is the median $|F_{ij}|$. A first approximation for A_j is

$$A_j^1 = \sum_{i=1}^{m} F_{ij}w_{ij}^1 \Big/ \sum_{i=1}^{m} w_{ij}^1.$$

The residuals after any iteration p are designated

$$z_{ij}^p = F_{ij} - \alpha_i^p A_j^p$$

and the new weights for use in iteration $p + 1$ are designated

$$w_{ij}^p = [1 - (z_{ij}^p/cS_p)^2]^2,$$

where S_p is the median $|z_{ij}^p|$. At iteration $p + 1$, the estimators of α_i are improved on the basis of A_j^p according to the equation

$$\alpha_i^{p+1} = \alpha_i^p + \sum_{j=1}^{n} z_{ij}^p w_{ij}^p A_j^p \Big/ \sum_{j=1}^{n} w_{ij}^p (A_j^p)^2,$$

and the estimators of A_j are improved according to

$$A_j^{p+1} = A_j^p + \sum_{i=1}^{m} z_{ij}^p w_{ij}^p \alpha_i^{p+1} \Big/ \sum_{i=1}^{m} w_{ij}^p (\alpha_i^{p+1})^2$$

and normalized so that $\Sigma A_j^2 = 1$. After adjustment of α_i^{p+1} to take into account the normalization of A_j^{p+1}, the residuals z_{ij}^{p+1} can be calculated. Iterative improvements in α_i and A_j are continued until a selected convergence criterion is met, typically when

$$1 - \sum (cS_{p+1})^2 \Big/ \sum (cS_p)^2 < \varepsilon$$

for a specified small value of $\varepsilon > 0$. The residuals

$$z_{ij}^{p+1} = F_{ij} - \alpha_i^{p+1} A_j^{p+1}$$

from this first stage of the fitting procedure are then examined in the same way for additional pattern in the column dimension. We begin the second stage of fitting with

$$\beta_i^1 = 1,$$

$$w_{ij}^1 = \begin{cases} [1 - (z_{ij}^{p+1}/cS_{p+1})^2]^2 & \text{for } z_{ij}^{p+1}/cS_{p+1} < 1, \\ 0 & \text{otherwise,} \end{cases}$$

$$B_j^1 = \sum_{i=1}^{m} z_{ij}^{p+1} w_{ij}^1 \Big/ \sum_{i=1}^{m} w_{ij}^1.$$

The residuals after any iteration r are designated

$$z_{ij}^r = z_{ij}^{p+1} - \beta_i^r B_j^r$$

and the new weights for use in iteration $r + 1$ are designated

$$w_{ij}^r = [1 - (z_{ij}^r/cS_r)^2]^2,$$

where S_r is the median $|z_{ij}^r|$. The iterative improvements in β_i and B_j are continued until the convergence criterion is met at some iteration $r + 1$.

For a fit in two multiplicative components, $\alpha_i A_j + \beta_i B_j$, the two-stage procedure is repeated for the residuals

$$z_{ij}^{r+1} = F_{ij} - \alpha_i^{p+1} A_j^{p+1} - \beta_i^{r+1} B_j^{r+1}$$

obtained up to this point and for subsequent sets of residuals—alternately seeking further adjustments to the $\alpha_i A_j$ and $\beta_i B_j$ components—until convergence of the fit in the final estimates of A_j, α_i, B_j, and β_i. For a fit in three components, $\alpha_i A_j + \beta_i B_j + \gamma_i C_j$, the residuals z_{ij}^{r+1} after the second stage are instead examined for additional pattern C_j in the column dimension and corresponding estimates of γ_i. Then the three-stage procedure is repeated, refining, in turn, α_i and A_j, β_i and B_j, and γ_i and C_j until convergence in the final estimates of all these parameters.

With some data sets, a guided start to the fitting and alternative convergence criteria for the intermediate stages of fitting may need to be tested. Orav (1977) has suggested the possibility of basing convergence on the robust measure of variance of the residuals.

A Robust–Resistant Measure of Fit

One summary measure of fit that is highly resistant to outliers is a robust measure of the variance of the biweighted residuals (s_{bi}^2). This is a refinement of a measure of scale derived by Lax (1975) from the asymptotic variance of the biweight location estimator (the estimator that is the basis of the iteratively weighted fitting procedures). The form of s_{bi}^2 adopted by Orav (1977) and used in Chapter IV, a slight modification of the form described by Mosteller and Tukey (1977, pp. 207–208), is given by

$$ns_{bi}^2 = \frac{n \sum' (z_i - \overset{\shortmid}{z_i})^2 (1 - u_i^2)^4}{\left[\sum' (1 - u_i^2)(1 - 5u_i^2)\right]\left[-e + \sum' (1 - u_i^2)(1 - 5u_i^2)\right]},$$

where $\overset{\shortmid}{z_i}$ is the median value of z_i,

$$e = n \Big/ \sum' (1 - u_i^2)(1 - 5u_i^2),$$

$$u_i = (z_i - \overset{\shortmid}{z_i})/cS,$$

c is a constant of assigned value, S is the median $|z_i - \overset{\shortmid}{z_i}|$, the second factor of the denominator of ns_{bi}^2 is never taken to be less than 1, and $\sum'$ indicates summation for $u_i^2 \le 1$ only. When the values of u_i are small, this expression of ns_{bi}^2 approaches

$$\sum (z_i - \overset{\shortmid}{z_i})^2/(n - 1),$$

an expression very similar to the customary measure of sample variance

$$s^2 = \sum (y_i - \bar{y}_i)^2/(n - 1).$$

The degree of resistance of s_{bi}^2 to outliers is determined by the value assigned to the constant c. Setting c equal to 9 is a commonly appropriate choice.

APPENDIX C

Re-presentation of EHR Fits in a Standard Form

A Selected Standard-form Re-presentation of a Rank-two Fit

We shall re-present the $m \times n$ matrix

$$\hat{F}_{ij} = \alpha_i A_j + \beta_i B_j \tag{1}$$

in the algebraically equivalent form

$$\hat{F}_{ij} = k_1 \alpha_i^{**} A_j^{**} + k_2 \beta_i^{**} B_j^{**} = \alpha_i^* A_j^* + \beta_i^* B_j^* \tag{2}$$

for all i and j so that the following conditions are met:

1. α_i^{**} for $i = 1, 2, \ldots, m$ is as constant as possible;
2. A_j^{**} for $j = 1, 2, \ldots, n$ is as linear as possible;
3. $\Sigma A_j^{*2} = \Sigma B_j^{*2} = 1$ for standardization.

Step 1 We first apply the linear transformation

$$\alpha_i^{**} = p\alpha_i + q\beta_i \tag{3}$$

and constrain α_i^{**} to be as constant as possible by least squares multiple regression (with zero intercept) of a vector of identical constants (for example, $K_i = 1$ for $i = 1, 2, \ldots, m$) on vectors α_i ($i = 1, 2, \ldots, m$) and β_i ($i = 1, 2, \ldots, m$). The regression coefficients equal p and q in Eq. (3) and indicate the proportions of α_i and β_i, respectively, that would bring the members of the new vector α_i^{**} as close as possible to a constant value. The values of p and q for all the fertility sequences fitted by two components are shown in Table C.1.

TABLE C.1

Derived Coefficients for Standard-form Re-presentation of EHR Fitted Parameters: Selected
Fertility Time Sequences, 1775–1976

| | Coefficient | | | | | | Eigenvalue for first |
| | | | | | | | canonical variate |
Sequence	p	q	r	s	t	u	
By least squares regression				*By canonical correlation*			
C15	.9505	−.0249		.9934	−.0886		.9989
C20	1.075	−.2428		.9415	−.2808		.9997
X15	.6867	.0062		.9875	−.0899		.9989
X20	.8403	−.2862		.8948	−.2724		.9996
XX15	.6880	−.0997		.9532	−.2536		.9997
XX20	.8061	−.2560		.9321	−.3562		.9999
MX15	.6951	−.4293		.8070	−.5936		.9994
MX20	.7808	−.5033		.9463	−.3288		.9999
By least squares regression				*By minimization of summed second differences*			
SYAC13	.2319	−.0343		1.00	−.1651		
X202	.6898	.0117	−.2913	1.00	−.0799	−.0290	
MC15	.6619	−.3230		1.00	−.5920		
NX15	.7090	−.4533		1.00	−.2284		

Step 2   We next apply the linear transformation

$$A_j^{**} = sA_j + tB_j \qquad (4)$$

and constrain A_j^{**} to be as linear as possible by either of the following
methods that lead to the same values for the re-presented and standardized parameters A_j^* and B_j^*.

METHOD 1   A canonical correlation analysis uses two sets of variables
as the input: the vectors A_j and B_j form one set; two linearly independent
straight lines form the other set. The analysis identifies, in the eigenvector
for the first canonical variate, the linear combination of A_j and B_j that is
maximally correlated with a linear combination of the two straight lines;
that is, it identifies s and t, the proportions of A_j and B_j that bring the
members of the new vector A_j^{**} as close as possible to linearity. The
squared canonical correlation coefficient for the first canonical variate
(that is, the eigenvalue of the first canonical variate) expresses the proportion of the variance in A_j^{**} that is accounted for by a single straight line.
For a detailed discussion of canonical correlation analysis see, for example, Van de Geer (1971). The values of s and t and the proportion of the
variance explained are shown in Table C.1 for all the fertility time sequences for which this procedure was used.

METHOD 2   We shall minimize the sum of the $n - 2$ squared second differences[1] between the n members of the new vector A_j^{**} by minimizing

$$\sum [\Delta^2(sA_j + tB_j)]^2.$$

If A_j^{**} were exactly linear, all the second differences in A_j^{**} would be zero. Therefore, the smaller the sum of the squared second differences, the closer A_j^{**} is to linearity.

To identify a value for t, we set $s = 1$ and multiply[2]:

$$\sum [\Delta^2(A_j + tB_j)]^2 = \sum \Delta^2 A_j \, \Delta^2 A_j + t \sum \Delta^2 A_j \, \Delta^2 B_j + t^2 \sum \Delta^2 B_j \, \Delta^2 B_j. \quad (5)$$

Taking the derivative of Eq. (5) with respect to t,

$$\partial/\partial t = \sum \Delta^2 A_j \, \Delta^2 B_j + 2t \sum \Delta^2 B_j \, \Delta^2 B_j = 0, \quad (6)$$

and solving for t, we obtain the equation

$$t = -\sum \Delta^2 A_j \, \Delta^2 B_j \Big/ \sum \Delta^2 B_j \, \Delta^2 B_j. \quad (7)$$

The values of t when $s = 1$ are shown in Table C.1 for all the fertility time sequences for which this procedure was used.

Example. The accompanying tabulation uses the A_j and B_j age vectors for the NX15 sequence (see Table 5.1) to illustrate first and second differences for the vector members. The second differences result in the following value of t:

$$t = -\sum \Delta^2 A_j \, \Delta^2 B_j \Big/ \sum \Delta^2 B_j \, \Delta^2 B_j = -.01269/.05556 = -.22842.$$

A_j	ΔA_j	$\Delta^2 A_j$	B_j	ΔB_j	$\Delta^2 B_j$
−.29339			.48264		
	.26709			.01834	
−.02630		−.04717	.50098		.00897
	.21992			.02731	
.19362		−.03100	.52829		−.15621
	.18892			−.12890	
.38254		−.03100	.39939		−.14233
	.15792			−.27123	
.54046		−.03709	.12816		−.10400
	.12083			−.37523	
.66129			−.24707		

Step 3   We next calculate the β_i^{**} and B_j^{**} vectors that correspond to the α_i^{**} and A_j^{**} vectors such that

$$\hat{F}_{ij} = k_1 \alpha_i^{**} A_j^{**} + k_2 \beta_i^{**} B_j^{**}.$$

From Eqs. (3) and (4) we obtain the following expressions for α_i and A_j:

$$\alpha_i = (\alpha_i^{**} - q\beta_i)/p \qquad (8)$$

$$A_j = (A_j^{**} - tB_j)/s. \qquad (9)$$

Substituting Eqs. (8) and (9) for α_i and A_j in Eq. (1), we obtain

$$\hat{F}_{ij} = [(\alpha_i^{**} - q\beta_i)/p][(A_j^{**} - tB_j)/s] + \beta_i B_j. \qquad (10)$$

Multiplying, we obtain

$$\hat{F}_{ij} = (1/ps)(\alpha_i^{**}A_j^{**}) + (1/ps)(-q\beta_i A_j^{**}) \\ + (1/ps)(-t\alpha_i^{**}B_j) + (1 + qt/ps)\beta_i B_j, \qquad (11)$$

which can also be expressed as

$$\hat{F}_{ij} = \frac{\alpha_i^{**}A_j^{**}}{ps} + \left(\frac{ps + qt}{ps}\right)\left[\beta_i B_j + \left(\frac{-q\beta_i A_j^{**}}{ps + qt}\right) + \left(\frac{-t\alpha_i^{**}B_j}{ps + qt}\right)\right]. \qquad (12)$$

To cast Eq. (12) in the form of Eq. (2), we add to the second component and subtract from the first component of Eq. (12) the quantity $xy\alpha_i^{**}A_j^{**}[(ps + qt)/ps]$, where $x = -t/(ps + qt)$ and $y = -q/(ps + qt)$, the coefficients of $\alpha_i^{**}B_j$ and $\beta_i A_j^{**}$ in Eq. (12). The second component then becomes

$$[(ps + qt)/ps](\beta_i + x\alpha_i^{**})(B_j + yA_j^{**})$$

and the first component becomes

$$(1/ps)\alpha_i^{**}A_j^{**} - xy\alpha_i^{**}A_j^{**}[(ps + qt)/ps].$$

With x and y expressed in terms of p, s, q, and t, we combine terms to obtain

$$\hat{F}_{ij} = \left(\frac{1}{ps + qt}\right)\alpha_i^{**}A_j^{**} + \left(\frac{ps + qt}{ps}\right)\left(\beta_i - \frac{t\alpha_i^{**}}{ps + qt}\right)\left(B_j - \frac{qA_j^{**}}{ps + qt}\right) \qquad (13)$$

$$= \left(\frac{1}{ps + qt}\right)\alpha_i^{**}A_j^{**} + \left(\frac{ps + qt}{ps}\right)\beta_i^{**}B_j^{**}, \qquad (14)$$

where $\beta_i - t\alpha_i^{**}/(ps + qt) = \beta_i^{**}$, $B_j - qA_j^{**}/(ps + qt) = B_j^{**}$, $1/(ps + qt) = k_1$, and $(ps + qt)/ps = k_2$ in Eq. (2).

Step 4 We next calculate A_j^*, B_j^*, α_i^*, and β_i^* from Eq. (14). We standardize A_j^{**} and B_j^{**} according to

$$A_j^* = A_j^{**}/\sqrt{\Sigma A_j^{**2}} \qquad \text{and} \qquad B_j^* = B_j^{**}/\sqrt{\Sigma B_j^{**2}}$$

so that $\Sigma A_j^{*2} = \Sigma B_j^{*2} = 1$. Equation (14) then becomes

$$\hat{F}_{ij} = [\sqrt{\Sigma A_j^{**2}}/(ps + qt)]\alpha_i^{**}A_j^* + [(ps + qt)\sqrt{\Sigma B_j^{**2}}/ps]\beta_i^{**}B_j^*. \qquad (15)$$

Incorporating the coefficients of $\alpha_i^{**}A_j^*$ and $\beta_i^{**}B_j^*$ in the time parameters, we obtain the algebraically equivalent form of Eq. (1) that was the goal of the re-presentation:

$$\hat{F}_{ij} = \alpha_i A_j + \beta_i B_j = \alpha_i^* A_j^* + \beta_i^* B_j^*.$$

A Selected Standard-form Re-presentation of a Rank-three Fit

We shall re-present the $m \times n$ matrix

$$\hat{F}_{ij} = \alpha_i A_j + \beta_i B_j + \gamma_i C_j \tag{16}$$

in the algebraically equivalent form

$$\hat{F}_{ij} = k_1\alpha_i^{**}A_j^{**} + k_2\beta_i^{**}B_j^{**} + k_3\gamma_i^{**}C_j^{**} = \alpha_i^* A_j^* + \beta_i^* B_j^* + \gamma_i^* C_j^* \tag{17}$$

for all i and j so that the following conditions are met:

1. α_i^{**} for $i = 1, 2, \ldots , m$ is as constant as possible;
2. A_j^{**} for $j = 1, 2, \ldots , n$ is as linear as possible;
3. B_j^{**} for $j = 1, 2, \ldots , n$ is as quadratic as possible;
4. slow change in β_i^{**} is maximized so that β_i^{**} expresses the major long-term trend of systematic change in the data sequence;
5. $\Sigma A_j^{*2} = \Sigma B_j^{*2} = \Sigma C_j^{*2} = 1$ for standardization.

We shall choose a two-stage re-presentation that meets conditions 1 and 2 in the first stage and conditions 3, 4, and 5 in the second stage, which is carried out on the remainder of the fit:

$$\hat{F}_{ij} - \alpha_i^* A_j^* = \beta_i'' B_j'' + \gamma_i'' C_j''.$$

First Stage of Re-presentation

Step 1   We first apply the linear transformation

$$\alpha_i^{**} = p\alpha_i + q\beta_i + r\gamma_i \tag{18}$$

and constrain α_i^{**} to be as constant as possible by least squares multiple regression (with zero intercept) of a vector of identical constants (for example, $K_i = 1$ for $i = 1, 2, \ldots , m$) on the vectors α_i ($i = 1, 2, \ldots , m$), β_i ($i = 1, 2, \ldots , m$) and γ_i ($i = 1, 2, \ldots , m$). The regression coefficients equal $p, q,$ and r in Eq. (18) and indicate the proportions of $\alpha_i, \beta_i,$ and γ_i, respectively, needed to bring the members of the new vector α_i^{**} as close as possible to a constant value. Values of $p, q,$ and r

for the *X202* fertility sequence, which is fitted by three components, are shown in Table C.1.

Step 2   We next apply the linear transformation

$$A_j^{**} = sA_j + tB_j + uC_j \tag{19}$$

and constrain A_j^{**} to be as linear as possible by either of the following methods that lead to the same values for the re-presented and standardized parameter A_j^*.

METHOD 1   We carry out a canonical correlation analysis as in the re-presentation of a rank-two fit. The vectors A_j, B_j, and C_j form one variable set and two linearly independent straight lines form the other variable set. The analysis identifies in the eigenvector of the first canonical variate the linear combination of A_j, B_j, and C_j that is maximally correlated with a linear combination of the straight lines; that is, it identifies s, t, and u, the proportions of A_j, B_j, and C_j, respectively, that bring the members of the new vector A_j^{**} as close as possible to linearity.

METHOD 2   We shall minimize the sum of the $n - 2$ squared second differences between the n members of the new vector A_j^{**} by minimizing

$$\sum [\Delta^2(sA_j + tB_j + uC_j)]^2.$$

To identify values for t and u in this expression, we set $s = 1$ and multiply[3]:

$$\sum [\Delta^2(A_j + tB_j + uC_j)]^2 = \sum \Delta^2 A_j \Delta^2 A_j + 2t \sum \Delta^2 A_j \Delta^2 B_j$$
$$+ 2u \sum \Delta^2 A_j \Delta^2 C_j + t^2 \sum \Delta^2 B_j \Delta^2 B_j$$
$$+ 2tu \sum \Delta^2 B_j \Delta^2 C_j + u^2 \sum \Delta^2 C_j \Delta^2 C_j. \tag{20}$$

When we take the derivative of Eq. (20) with respect to t and with respect to u, we obtain

$$\partial/\partial t = \sum \Delta^2 A_j \Delta^2 B_j + t \sum \Delta^2 B_j \Delta^2 B_j + u \sum \Delta^2 B_j \Delta^2 C_j = 0, \tag{21}$$
$$\partial/\partial u = \sum \Delta^2 A_j \Delta^2 C_j + t \sum \Delta^2 B_j \Delta^2 C_j + u \sum \Delta^2 C_j \Delta^2 C_j = 0. \tag{22}$$

Solving Eqs. (21) and (22) for t and u, we obtain

$$t = \frac{(\sum \Delta^2 A_j \Delta^2 C_j)(\sum \Delta^2 B_j \Delta^2 C_j) - (\sum \Delta^2 A_j \Delta^2 B_j)(\sum \Delta^2 C_j \Delta^2 C_j)}{(\sum \Delta^2 B_j \Delta^2 B_j)(\sum \Delta^2 C_j \Delta^2 C_j) - (\sum \Delta^2 B_j \Delta^2 C_j)(\sum \Delta^2 B_j \Delta^2 C_j)}, \tag{23}$$

$$u = \left(-t \sum \Delta^2 B_j \Delta^2 C_j - \sum \Delta^2 A_j \Delta^2 C_j\right) \Big/ \sum \Delta^2 C_j \Delta^2 C_j. \tag{24}$$

Values of t and u calculated by method 2 for the *X202* fertility sequence are shown in Table C.1.

Step 3   We next determine the constant k_1 that satisfies the equation

$$\hat{F}_{ij} - k_1 \alpha_i^{**} A_j^{**} = \beta_i'' B_j'' + \gamma_i'' C_j'', \tag{25}$$

where k_1 is expressed in terms of the constants p, q, r, s, t, and u from steps 1 and 2,

$$\hat{F}_{ij} = \alpha_i A_j + \beta_i B_j + \gamma_i C_j \tag{26}$$

expresses the three-component fit before re-presentation,

$$\begin{aligned}
k_1 \alpha_i^{**} A_j^{**} &= k_1(p\alpha_i + q\beta_i + r\gamma_i)(sA_j + tB_j + uC_j) \\
&= k_1(ps\alpha_i A_j + pt\alpha_i B_j + pu\alpha_i C_j) \\
&+ k_1(qs\beta_i A_j + qt\beta_i B_j + qu\beta_i C_j) \\
&+ k_1(rs\gamma_i A_j + rt\gamma_i B_j + ru\gamma_i C_j) \tag{27}
\end{aligned}$$

expresses the portion of $\hat{F}_{ij}$ that has been re-presented in a standard form in steps 1 and 2, and

$$\beta_i'' B_j'' + \gamma_i'' C_j'' = f(\alpha_i, A_j, \beta_i, B_j, \gamma_i, C_j, p, q, r, s, t, u)$$

expresses the portion of $\hat{F}_{ij}$ that remains to be re-presented in a standard form.

METHOD   We begin with the equation

$$\begin{aligned}
\hat{F}_{ij} - k_1 \alpha_i^{**} A_j^{**} &= a_{11}\alpha_i A_j + a_{12}\alpha_i B_j + a_{13}\alpha_i C_j \\
&+ a_{21}\beta_i A_j + a_{22}\beta_i B_j + a_{23}\beta_i C_j \\
&+ a_{31}\gamma_i A_j + a_{32}\gamma_i B_j + a_{33}\gamma_i C_j, \tag{28}
\end{aligned}$$

where the coefficients a_{gh} are the differences between the set of coefficients in Eq. (26) and the set of coefficients in Eq. (27) for all combinations of α_i, β_i, and γ_i with A_j, B_j, and C_j. If the determinant of the array a_{gh} is zero, then the right-hand side of Eq. (28) can be expressed in two components as in Eq. (25)[4]:

$$\hat{F}_{ij} - k_1 \alpha_i^{**} A_j^{**} = \beta_i'' B_j'' + \gamma_i'' C_j''.$$

From Eqs. (26) and (27) we obtain the determinant

$$\det[a_{gh}] = \begin{vmatrix} 1 - k_1 ps & -k_1 pt & -k_1 pu \\ -k_1 qs & 1 - k_1 qt & -k_1 qu \\ -k_1 rs & -k_1 rt & 1 - k_1 ru \end{vmatrix} = 0. \tag{29}$$

Expanding the determinant and solving for k_1, we find that

$$k_1 = 1/(ps + qt + ru), \tag{30}$$

so Eq. (25) becomes

$$\hat{F}_{ij} - \alpha_i^{**} A_j^{**}/(ps + qt + ru) = \beta_i'' B_j'' + \gamma_i'' C_j''. \tag{31}$$

Step 4 We next calculate A_j^* and α_i^* from A_j^{**}, α_i^{**}, and k_1. If

$$A_j^* = A_j^{**}/\sqrt{\Sigma\, A_j^{**2}}$$

so that $A_j^{*2} = 1$ for standardization, then

$$\alpha_i^* = [\sqrt{\Sigma\, A_j^{**2}}/(ps + qt + ru)]\alpha_i^{**}.$$

We can therefore express Eq. (31) as

$$\hat{F}_{ij} - \alpha_i^* A_j^* = \beta_i'' B_j'' + \gamma_i'' C_j''. \tag{32}$$

Step 5 We next identify a solution for the parameters β_i'', B_j'', γ_i'', and C_j'' in Eq. (32). Note that any conveniently achieved solution is satisfactory at this point in the re-presentation. A standard form that incorporates demographically guided constraints on $\beta_i'' B_j'' + \gamma_i'' C_j''$ is then achieved in the second stage of re-presentation.

METHOD The $m \times n$ matrix $\hat{F}_{ij} - \alpha_i^* A_j^*$ can be viewed as the product of three matrices:

$$\mathbf{X}_{m \times n} = \mathbf{V}_{m \times 3} \mathbf{Y}_{3 \times 3} \mathbf{W}_{3 \times n}, \tag{33}$$

where $\mathbf{Y} = a_{gh}$ is the matrix of coefficients obtained in the solution of Eq. (29), $\mathbf{v}_1 = \alpha_i$, $\mathbf{v}_2 = \beta_i$ and $\mathbf{v}_3 = \gamma_i$ for $i = 1, 2, \ldots, m$, and $\mathbf{w}_1 = A_j$, $\mathbf{w}_2 = B_j$, and $\mathbf{w}_3 = C_j$ for $j = 1, 2, \ldots, n$. One procedure for solving Eq. (32) is to find a matrix $\mathbf{U}$ that transforms the asymmetric matrix $\mathbf{Y}$ in Eq. (33) into a diagonal matrix $\mathbf{D} = \mathbf{U}^{-1}\mathbf{Y}\mathbf{U}$. That is, we express $\mathbf{Y}$ as

$$\mathbf{Y} = \mathbf{U}\mathbf{D}\mathbf{U}^{-1}, \qquad \text{where} \quad \mathbf{D} = \begin{bmatrix} \lambda_1 & 0 & 0 \\ 0 & \lambda_2 & 0 \\ 0 & 0 & \lambda_3 \end{bmatrix}, \tag{34}$$

the eigenvalues of $\mathbf{Y}$ are ordered from large to small as the diagonal entries λ_1, and the columns of $\mathbf{U}$ consist of the associated eigenvectors of $\mathbf{Y}$.[5]

Because the product of the eigenvalues of $\mathbf{Y}$ equals the determinant of $\mathbf{Y}$, which we know is zero from step 4, we know that λ_3 equals zero. By substitution of Eq. (34) for $\mathbf{Y}$ in Eq. (33), we obtain

$$\mathbf{X} = \mathbf{V}\mathbf{U}\mathbf{D}\mathbf{U}^{-1}\mathbf{W}. \tag{35}$$

Then, if we let

$$\mathbf{V}^* = \mathbf{V}\mathbf{U}\mathbf{D} \qquad \text{and} \qquad \mathbf{W}^* = \mathbf{U}^{-1}\mathbf{W},$$

we obtain the following solution of Eq. (32):

$$\mathbf{v}_1^* = \gamma_i^\dagger, \qquad \mathbf{v}_2^* = \beta_i^\dagger, \qquad \mathbf{v}_3^* = 0, \qquad \mathbf{w}_1^* = C_j^\dagger, \qquad \text{and} \qquad \mathbf{w}_2^* = B_j^\dagger$$

so that

$$\hat{F}_{ij} - \alpha_i^* A_j^* = \beta_i^\dagger B_j^\dagger + \gamma_i^\dagger C_j^\dagger. \tag{36}$$

An alternative procedure by which we can decompose any matrix $\mathbf{Y}$ into a triple product

$$\mathbf{Y} = \mathbf{P\Delta Q'} \tag{37}$$

depends on finding the eigenstructure of the 3×3 symmetric matrix $\mathbf{Y'Y}$ (Green, 1976, pp. 232–237). In this solution, $\mathbf{\Delta}$ is a diagonal matrix with diagonal elements that are the square roots of the eigenvalues of matrix $\mathbf{Y'Y}$ ordered from large to small, $\mathbf{Q}$ is a matrix with columns that are the associated eigenvectors of $\mathbf{Y'Y}$, matrices $\mathbf{P}$ and $\mathbf{Q}$ are orthonormal by columns, and $\mathbf{P} = \mathbf{YQ\Delta}^{-1}$. Again, λ_3 equals zero. By substitution of Eq. (37) for $\mathbf{Y}$ in Eq. (33), we obtain

$$\mathbf{X} = \mathbf{VP\Delta Q'W}. \tag{38}$$

Then, if we let

$$\mathbf{V^*} = \mathbf{VP\Delta} \quad \text{and} \quad \mathbf{W^*} = \mathbf{Q'W},$$

we find that we have again obtained a solution of Eq. (32) that can be expressed as

$$\mathbf{v}_1^* = \gamma_i^\dagger, \quad \mathbf{v}_2^* = \beta_i^\dagger, \quad \mathbf{v}_3^* = 0, \quad \mathbf{w}_1^* = C_j^\dagger, \quad \text{and} \quad \mathbf{w}_2^* = B_j^\dagger,$$

although this solution represents a different linear combination of α_i, β_i, γ_i, A_j, B_j, C_j, and the coefficients of matrix $\mathbf{Y}$ than would be obtained through diagonalizing $\mathbf{Y}$ by means of $\mathbf{Y} = \mathbf{UDU}^{-1}$.

Whatever method we use to diagonalize $\mathbf{Y}$, the resulting $B_j^\dagger$ and $C_j^\dagger$ vectors are standardized according to

$$B_j'' = B_j^\dagger / \sqrt{\Sigma\, B_j^{\dagger 2}} \quad \text{and} \quad C_j'' = C_j^\dagger / \sqrt{\Sigma\, C_j^{\dagger 2}}$$

so that $\Sigma\, B_j''^2 = \Sigma\, C_j''^2 = 1$. Then,

$$\beta_i'' = \beta_i^\dagger (\sqrt{\Sigma\, B_j^{\dagger 2}}) \quad \text{and} \quad \gamma_i'' = \gamma_i^\dagger (\sqrt{\Sigma\, C_j^{\dagger 2}})$$

and we carry forward to the second stage of re-presentation the equation

$$\hat{F}_{ij} - \alpha_i^* A_j^* = \beta_i'' B_j'' + \gamma_i'' C_j''$$

to re-present $\beta_i'' B_j'' + \gamma_i'' C_j''$ in a demographically guided standard form.

Second Stage of Re-presentation

Step 1   Starting with

$$\hat{F}_{ij} - \alpha_i^* A_j^* = \beta_i'' B_j'' + \gamma_i'' C_j'', \tag{39}$$

we shall apply the linear transformation

$$B_j^{**} = B_j'' + gC_j'',$$ (40)

where g is selected to constrain B_j^{**} to be as quadratic as possible.

METHOD   We shall minimize the sum of the $n - 3$ squared third differences between the n members of the new vector B_j^{**} by minimizing $\Sigma [\Delta^3(B_j'' + gC_j'')]^2$. If B_j^{**} were exactly quadratic, all the third differences in B_j^{**} would be zero. Therefore, the smaller the sum of the squared third differences, the closer B_j^{**} is to being quadratic. To identify a value for g, we multiply to obtain

$$\sum [\Delta^3(B_j'' + gC_j'')]^2 = \sum \Delta^3 B_j'' \, \Delta^3 B_j''$$
$$+ 2g \sum \Delta^3 B_j'' \, \Delta^3 C_j'' + g^2 \sum \Delta^3 C_j'' \, \Delta^3 C_j''.$$ (41)

Taking the derivative of Eq. (41) with respect to g, we then obtain

$$\partial/\partial g = 2 \sum \Delta^3 B_j'' \, \Delta^3 C_j'' + 2g \sum \Delta^3 C_j'' \, \Delta^3 C_j'' = 0.$$ (42)

Solving Eq. (42) for g, we obtain

$$g = -\sum \Delta^3 B_j'' \, \Delta^3 C_j'' \Big/ \sum \Delta^3 C_j'' \, \Delta^3 C_j''.$$ (43)

Step 2   We next apply the linear transformation

$$\beta_i^{**} = \beta_i'' - f\gamma_i'',$$ (44)

where f is selected to maximize slow change in β_i^{**} so that it expresses the major long-term trend of systematic change in the data sequence.

METHOD   We shall minimize

$$\sum [\Delta(\beta_i'' - f\gamma_i'')]^2 \Big/ \sum [\beta_i'' - f\gamma_i'']^2$$

by solving for f in the following function of this expression:

$$\frac{\partial/\partial f \sum [\Delta(\beta_i'' - f\gamma_i'')]^2}{\sum [\Delta(\beta_i'' - f\gamma_i'')]^2} = \frac{\partial/\partial f \sum [\beta_i'' - f\gamma_i'']^2}{\sum [\beta_i'' - f\gamma_i'']^2}.$$

Squaring and taking the derivatives, we obtain

$$\frac{-2 \sum \Delta\beta_i'' \, \Delta\gamma_i'' + 2f \sum \Delta\gamma_i'' \, \Delta\gamma_i''}{\sum \Delta\beta_i'' \, \Delta\beta_i'' - 2f \sum \Delta\beta_i'' \, \Delta\gamma_i'' + f^2 \sum \Delta\gamma_i'' \, \Delta\gamma_i''}$$
$$= \frac{-2 \sum \beta_i''\gamma_i'' + 2f \sum \gamma_i''\gamma_i''}{\sum \beta_i''\beta_i'' - 2f \sum \beta_i''\gamma_i'' + f^2 \sum \gamma_i''\gamma_i''},$$ (45)

which reduces to

$$f^2\left[\left(\sum \beta_i''\gamma_i''\right)\left(\sum \Delta\gamma_i'' \, \Delta\gamma_i''\right) - \left(\sum \gamma_i''\gamma_i''\right)\left(\sum \Delta\beta_i'' \, \Delta\gamma_i''\right)\right]$$
$$+ f\left[\left(\sum \gamma_i''\gamma_i''\right)\left(\sum \Delta\beta_i'' \, \Delta\beta_i''\right) - \left(\sum \beta_i''\beta_i''\right)\left(\sum \Delta\gamma_i'' \, \Delta\gamma_i''\right)\right]$$
$$+ \left(\sum \beta_i''\beta_i''\right)\left(\sum \Delta\beta_i'' \, \Delta\gamma_i''\right) - \left(\sum \beta_i''\gamma_i''\right)\left(\sum \Delta\beta_i'' \, \Delta\beta_i''\right) = 0.$$ (46)

Because Eq. (46) is a quadratic of the form $af^2 + bf + c = 0$, it can readily be solved for the two values of f by substitution of the coefficients of f in the quadratic formula

$$f = (-b \pm \sqrt{b^2 - 4ac})/2a.$$

The values of f lead to alternative solutions for Eq. (44) that are carried forward to step 3 for calculation of the γ_i^{**} and C_j^{**} vectors corresponding to each solution. Although each set of β_i^{**}, γ_i^{**}, and C_j^{**} vectors, with their common B_j^{**} vector, provides an algebraically accurate description of the data in the form of Eq. (47), often only one set proves to be a demographically useful description of a time sequence.[6]

Step 3 We shall determine the C_j^{**} and γ_i^{**} vectors that correspond to the B_j^{**} vector from step 1 and to each of the two vector solutions for β_i^{**} from step 2 so that

$$\beta_i'' B_j'' + \gamma_i'' C_j'' = k_2 \beta_i^{**} B_j^{**} + k_3 \gamma_i^{**} C_j^{**} = \beta_i^* B_j^* + \gamma_i^* C_j^*. \qquad (47)$$

METHOD From Eqs. (40) and (44) we obtain the following expressions for β_i'' and B_j'':

$$\beta_i'' = \beta_i^{**} + f\gamma_i'', \qquad (48)$$

$$B_j'' = B_j^{**} - gC_j''. \qquad (49)$$

Substituting Eqs. (48) and (49) for β_i'' and B_j'' in the left-hand side of Eq. (47), we obtain

$$\beta_i'' B_j'' + \gamma_i'' C_j'' = (\beta_i^{**} + f\gamma_i'')(B_j^{**} - gC_j'') + \gamma_i'' C_j''. \qquad (50)$$

By multiplying we obtain

$$\beta_i'' B_j'' + \gamma_i'' C_j'' = \beta_i^{**} B_j^{**} + f\gamma_i'' B_j^{**} - g\beta_i^{**} C_j'' + (1 - fg)\gamma_i'' C_j'', \qquad (51)$$

which can also be expressed as

$$\beta_i'' B_j'' + \gamma_i'' C_j''$$

$$= \beta_i^{**} B_j^{**} + (1 - fg)\left[\gamma_i'' C_j'' + \left(\frac{f}{1 - fg}\right) \gamma_i'' B_j^{**} + \left(\frac{-g}{1 - fg}\right) \beta_i^{**} C_j''\right]. \qquad (52)$$

To cast Eq. (52) in the form of Eq. (47), we add to the second component and subtract from the first component of Eq. (52) the quantity $xy\beta_i^{**}B_j^{**}(1 - fg)$, where $x = -g/(1 - fg)$ and $y = f/(1 - fg)$, the coefficients of $\beta_i^{**}C_j''$ and $\gamma_i''B_j^{**}$ in Eq. (52). The second component then becomes

$$(1 - fg)(\gamma_i'' + x\beta_i^{**})(C_j'' + yB_j^{**})$$

and the first component becomes

$$\beta_i^{**} B_j^{**} - (xy\beta_i^{**}B_j^{**})(1 - fg).$$

With x and y expressed in terms of f and g, we combine terms to obtain

$$\beta_i'' B_j'' + \gamma_i'' C_j'' = \left(\frac{1}{1 - fg}\right) \beta_i^{**} B_j^{**}$$

$$+ (1 - fg)\left(\gamma_i'' - \frac{g\beta_i^{**}}{1 - fg}\right)\left(C_j'' + \frac{fB_j^{**}}{1 - fg}\right) \tag{53}$$

$$= [1/(1 - fg)]\beta_i^{**} B_j^{**} + (1 - fg)\gamma_i^{**} C_j^{**}, \tag{54}$$

where $\gamma_i'' - g\beta_i^{**}/(1 - fg) = \gamma_i^{**}$, $C_j'' + fB_j^{**}/(1 - fg) = C_j^{**}$, $1/(1 - fg) = k_2$, and $1 - fg = k_3$ in Eq. (47).

Step 4 We next calculate B_j^*, C_j^*, β_i^*, and γ_i^* from Eq. (54). We first standardize B_j^{**} and C_j^{**} according to

$$B_j^* = B_j^{**}/\sqrt{\Sigma B_j^{**2}} \qquad \text{and} \qquad C_j^* = C_j^{**}/\sqrt{\Sigma C_j^{**2}}$$

so that $\Sigma B_j^{*2} = \Sigma C_j^{*2} = 1$. Equation (54) then becomes

$$\beta_i'' B_j'' + \gamma_i'' C_j'' = [\sqrt{\Sigma B_j^{**2}}/(1 - fg)]\beta_i^{**} B_j^*$$

$$+ (1 - fg)\sqrt{\Sigma C_j^{**2}} \, \gamma_i^{**} C_j^{**}. \tag{55}$$

Incorporating the coefficients of $\beta_i^{**} B_j^*$ and $\gamma_i^{**} C_j^*$ in the time parameters, we obtain the algebraically equivalent form of Eqs. (39) and (47) that was the goal of the second stage of the re-presentation:

$$\hat{F}_{ij} - \alpha_i^* A_j^* = \beta_i'' B_j'' + \gamma_i'' C_j'' = \beta_i^* B_j^* + \gamma_i^* C_j^*.$$

Transposing $\alpha_i^* A_j^*$, we see that we have achieved the overall goal of re-presentation of the rank-three fit by expressing Eq. (17),

$$\hat{F}_{ij} = \alpha_i A_j + \beta_i B_j + \gamma_i C_j,$$

in the algebraically equivalent form of Eq. (18),

$$\hat{F}_{ij} = \alpha_i^* A_j^* + \beta_i^* B_j^* + \gamma_i^* C_j^*,$$

that incorporates all of the selected constraints to provide a demographically interpretable standard form for the parameters.

Notes for Appendix C

1. The following designations for differences between vector members are used throughout this appendix:

Δ the $n - 1$ first differences between the n members of a vector: for example,

$$\Delta x_j = x_{j+1} - x_j,$$

where $j = 1$ to $n - 1$

Δ^2,   the second differences between the n members of a vector, that is, the $n - 2$ differences between first differences: for example,

$$\Delta^2 x_j = \Delta x_{j+1} - \Delta x_j$$

$$= (x_{j+2} - x_{j+1}) - (x_{j+1} - x_j),$$

where $j = 1$ to $n - 2$

Δ^3 the third differences between the n members of a vector, that is, the $n - 3$ differences between second differences: for example,

$$\Delta^3 x_j = \Delta^2 x_{j+1} - \Delta^2 x_j$$

$$= (\Delta x_{j+2} - \Delta x_{j+1}) - (\Delta x_{j+1} - \Delta x_j),$$

where $j = 1$ to $n - 3$

2. Any convenient value can be assigned to s because t scales proportionately with s and A_j^{**} and B_j^{**} are subsequently standardized as A_j^* and B_j^* such that $\Sigma A_j^{*2} = \Sigma B_j^{*2} = 1$.

3. As for the two-component re-presentation, any convenient value can be assigned to s because the values of t and u are scaled proportionately with s and each of the re-presented vectors is subsequently standardized so that $\Sigma x_j^2 = 1$.

4. This result can be deduced from the discussion on matrix rank presented by Green (1976, pp. 167–174).

5. This transformation is only possible if the eigenvectors are linearly independent so that $\mathbf{U}$ is a nonsingular matrix and therefore has an inverse matrix $\mathbf{U}^{-1}$ (see Green, 1976, pp. 219–220).

6. For the $X202$ sequence, the values $g = -.3750$ and $f = .2432$ carried forward to step 3 are those that apply when β_i'', B_j'', γ_i'', and C_j'' are obtained for the sequence from Eq. (38). If matrix $\mathbf{Y}$ were diagonalized by other procedures that resulted in different solutions for $\beta_i'' B_j'' + \gamma_i'' C_j''$, different values of g and f would, of course, be required to bring these parameters to the selected standard form.

References

Anderson, B. A.
1975 Male age and fertility results from Ireland prior to 1911. *Population Index* **41**:561–566.
1982 Migration and modernization. Manuscript, Department of Sociology, Brown University, Providence, Rhode Island.
Anderson, B. A., and McCabe, J. L.
1977 Nutrition and the fertility of younger women in Kinshasa, Zaire. *Journal of Development Economics* **4**:343–363.
Anscombe, F. J.
1967 Topics in the investigation of linear relations fitted by the method of least squares. *Journal of the Royal Statistical Society Series B* **29**:11–52.
Bernhardt, E. M.
1971 "Trends and Variations in Swedish Fertility—A Cohort Study." Stockholm: National Central Bureau of Statistics.
Brass, W.
1974 Perspectives in population prediction: illustrated by the statistics of England and Wales. *Journal of the Royal Statistical Society Series A* **137**:532–583.
1975 "Methods for Estimating Fertility and Mortality from Limited and Defective Data." Chapel Hill: University of North Carolina, International Program of Laboratories for Population Statistics.
Breckenridge, M. B.
1976 Time series model of age-specific fertility: an application of exploratory data analysis. Ph.D. Dissertation, Department of Sociology, Princeton University, Princeton, New Jersey. Available from University Microfilms.
1978 "An Empirical Higher-Rank Analysis Model of the Age Distribution of Fertility." Department of Statistics, Princeton University, Princeton, New Jersey, Technical report no. 143, series 2.
Campbell, A. A.
1974 Beyond the demographic transition. *Demography* **11**:549–561.
Charbonneau, H.
1979 Les régimes de fécondité naturelle en Amérique du Nord: bilan et analyse des observations. *In* "Natural Fertility" (H. Leridon and J. Menken, eds.), pp. 441–491. Liège: Ordina Editions.

Cho, L.-J.
1973 The own-children approach to fertility estimation: an elaboration. *In* "International Population Conference, Liège 1973," vol. 2, pp. 263–279. Liège: International Union for the Scientific Study of Population.

Coale, A. J.
1967 Factors associated with the development of low fertility: an historic summary. *In* "Proceedings of the World Population Conference, Belgrade 1965," vol. 2, pp. 205–209. New York: United Nations, Department of Economic and Social Affairs.
1971 Age patterns of marriage. *Population Studies* **25**:193–214.

Coale, A. J., and Demeny, P.
1966 "Regional Modal Life Tables and Stable Populations." Princeton, New Jersey: Princeton Univ. Press.

Coale, A. J., and McNeil, D. R.
1972 The distribution by age of the frequency of first marriage in a female cohort. *Journal of the American Statistical Association* **67**:743–749.

Coale, A. J., and Trussell, T. J.
1974 Model fertility schedules: variations in the age structure of childbearing in human populations. *Population Index* **40**:185–258.
1978 Technical note: finding the two parameters that specify a model schedule of marital fertility. *Population Index* **44**:203–213.

Coale, A. J., Anderson, B. A., and Harm, E.
1979 "Human Fertility in Russia Since the Nineteenth Century." Princeton, New Jersey: Princeton Univ. Press.

Davis, K.
1963 The theory of change and response in modern demographic history. *Population Index* **29**:345–366.

D'Souza, S.
1974 "Closed Birth Intervals." New Delhi: Sterling.

Dupâquier, J.
1979 Etude comparative des données sur la fécondité dans 25 monographies concernant le bassin Parisien a la fin du XVIIe siècle et au debut du XVIIIe. *In* "Natural Fertility" (H. Leridon and J. Menken, eds.), pp. 409–439. Liège: Ordina Editions.

Eriksson, I., and Rogers, J.
1978 "Rural Labor and Population Change: Social and Demographic Developments in East-Central Sweden During the Nineteenth Century," Studia Historica Upsaliensia, no. 100. Stockholm: Almqvist and Wiksell International for Uppsala Universitet.

Ewbank, D. C.
1974 An examination of several applications of the standard pattern of age at first marriage. Ph.D. Dissertation, Department of Economics, Princeton University, Princeton, New Jersey.

Ewbank, D. C., Gomez de Leon, J. C., and Stoto, M. A.
1983 A reducible four-parameter system of model life tables. *Population Studies* **37**.

Freedman, R., Fan, G., Wei, S., and Weinberger, M. B.
1977 Trends in fertility and in the effects of education on fertility in Taiwan, 1961–1974. *Studies in Family Planning* **8**:11–18.

Friedlander, D.
1969 Demographic responses and population change. *Demography* **6**:359–381.

Gendell, M.
1980 Sweden faces zero population growth. *Population Bulletin* **35**(2). A publication of the Population Reference Bureau, Inc., Washington, D. C.

Glass, D. V.
1967 "Population Policies and Movements in Europe." London: Cass.
Green, P. E.
1976 "Mathematical Tools for Applied Multivariate Analysis." New York: Academic Press.
Hansen, H. O.
1979 From natural to controlled fertility: studies in fertility as a factor in the process of economic and social development in Greenland c. 1851–1975. *In* "Natural Fertility" (H. Leridon and J. Menken, eds.), pp. 493–547. Liège: Ordina Editions.
Henry, L.
1961 Some data on natural fertility. *Eugenics Quarterly* **8**:81–91.
1979 Concepts actuels et résultats empiriques sur la fécondité naturelle. *In* "Natural Fertility" (H. Leridon and J. Menken, eds.), pp. 15–28. Liège: Ordina Editions.
Hofsten, E.
1971 Birth variations in populations which practice family planning. *Population Studies* **24**:315–326.
Hofsten, E., and Lundstrom, H.
1976 "Swedish Population History: Main Trends from 1750 to 1970." Stockholm: National Central Bureau of Statistics.
Hyrenius, H.
1946 The relation between birth rates and economic activity in Sweden 1920–1944. *Bulletin of the Oxford University Institute of Statistics* **8**:14–21.
1951 Reproduction and replacement. *Population Studies* **4**:421–431.
Institute for Social Sciences, Stockholm University.
1941 "Population Movements and Industrialization: Swedish Counties, 1895–1930." London: P. S. King and Son.
Keyfitz, N.
1977 "Introduction to the Mathematics of Population," rev. ed. Reading, Massachusetts: Addison-Wesley.
Knodel, J. E.
1974 "The Decline of Fertility in Germany, 1871–1939." Princeton, New Jersey: Princeton, Univ. Press.
Lax, D. A.
1975 "An Interim Report of a Monte Carlo Study of Robust Estimators of Width." Department of Statistics, Princeton University, Princeton, New Jersey, Technical report no. 93, series 2.
Lee, R. D.
1975 Natural fertility, population cycles and the spectral analysis of births and marriages. *Journal of the American Statistical Association* **70**:295–304.
1977 Methods and models for analyzing historical series of births, deaths, and marriages. *In* "Population Patterns in the Past" (R. D. Lee, ed.), pp. 337–370. New York: Academic Press.
Leridon, H.
1977 "Human Fertility." Chicago: Univ. of Chicago Press.
Lesthaeghe, R.
1977 "The Decline of Belgian Fertility, 1800–1970." Princeton, New Jersey: Princeton Univ. Press.
Livi-Bacci, M.
1971 "A Century of Portuguese Fertility." Princeton, New Jersey: Princeton Univ. Press.

1977 "A History of Italian Fertility During the Last Two Centuries." Princeton, New Jersey: Princeton Univ. Press.

McCarthy, J. F.
1977 Patterns of marriage dissolution in the United States. Ph.D. Dissertation, Department of Sociology, Princeton University, Princeton, New Jersey.

McNeil, D. R.
1977 "Interactive Data Analysis." New York: Wiley.

McNeil, D. R., and Tukey, J. W.
1975 Higher-order diagnosis of two-way tables, illustrated on two sets of demographic empirical distributions. *Biometrics* **31**:487–510.

Menken, J. A.
1979 Seasonal migration and seasonal variation in fecundability: effects on birth rates and birth intervals. *Demography* **16**:103–119.

Mosher, W. D.
1980 Demographic responses and demographic transitions: a case study of Sweden. *Demography* **17**:395–412.

Mosteller, F., and Tukey, J. W.
1977 "Data Analysis and Regression." Reading, Massachusetts: Addison-Wesley.

Orav, E. J.
1977 An expanded exploratory data analysis study of age-specific fertility. Senior thesis, Department of Mathematics, Princeton University, Princeton, New Jersey.

Page, H. J.
1977 Patterns underlying fertility schedules: a decomposition by both age and marriage duration. *Population Studies* **30**:85–106.

Page, H. J., and Lesthaeghe, R., eds.
1981 "Child-Spacing in Tropical Africa." New York: Academic Press.

Rindfuss, R. R., and Sweet, J. A.
1977 "Postwar Fertility Trends and Differentials in the United States." New York: Academic Press.

Ryder, N. B.
1951 The cohort approach: essays in the measurement of temporal variations in demographic behavior. Ph.D. Dissertation, Department of Sociology, Princeton University, Princeton, New Jersey. (Reprinted 1980, New York: Arno Press.)
1955 The influence of declining mortality on Swedish reproductivity. *In* "Current Research in Human Fertility. Papers Presented at the 1954 Annual Conference of the Milbank Memorial Fund," pp. 65–81. New York: Milbank Memorial Fund.
1980 Components of temporal variations in American fertility. *In* "Demographic Patterns in Developed Societies" (R. W. Hiorns, ed.), pp. 11–54. London: Taylor and Francis.

Shryock, H. S., Siegel, J. S., and Associates
1976 "The Methods and Materials of Demography." New York: Academic Press.

Smith, D. S.
1972 The demographic history of colonial New England. *Journal of Economic History* **32**:165–183.

Stoto, M. A.
1982 Advances in mathematical models for population projections. *In* "International Population Conference, Manila 1981," vol. 3, pp. 417–434. Liège: International Union for the Scientific Study of Population.
1983a The accuracy of population projections. *Journal of the American Statistical Association* **78**.

1983b Estimating distribution functions for small groups: postoperative hospital stay. *In* "What Role for Government? Lessons from Policy Research." (R. F. Zeckhauser, and D. Leebaert, eds.), Durham, North Carolina: Duke Univ. Press.

Sundbärg, G.
1907 "Bevölkerungstatistik Schwedens 1750–1900." Stockholm: National Central Bureau of Statistics (reissued, 1970).

Sweden
1878 "Grunddrag af Sveriges Befolknings-Statistik for åren 1748–1875." Stockholm: National Central Bureau of Statistics.
1875–1910 "Sveriges Officiella Statistik: Befolknings-Statistik." Stockholm: National Central Bureau of Statistics.
1911–1959 "Sveriges Officiella Statistik: Befolkningsrörelsen." Stockholm: National Central Bureau of Statistics.
1960–1976 "Sveriges Officiella Statistik: Folkmängdens Förändringar." Stockholm: National Central Bureau of Statistics.
1976 Fertility for cohorts of Swedish women born in 1870–1960. *In* "Sveriges Officiella Statistik: Statistiska Meddelanden," Serie Be 1976 (8). Stockholm: National Central Bureau of Statistics.

Teitelbaum, M. S.
1972 Fertility effects of the abolition of legal abortion in Romania. *Population Studies* **26**:405–417.
1973 U.S. population growth in international perspective. *In* "Toward the End of Growth: Population in America" (C. F. Westoff, ed.), pp. 69–83. Englewood Cliffs, New Jersey: Prentice-Hall.

Thomas, D. S.
1941 "Social and Economic Aspects of Swedish Population Movements, 1750–1933." New York: Macmillan.

Trussell, T. J.
1974 Selected applications of model fertility schedules. Ph.D. Dissertation, Department of Economics, Princeton University, Princeton, New Jersey.
1979 Natural fertility: measurement and use in fertility models. *In* "Natural Fertility" (H. Leridon and J. Menken, eds.), pp. 29–64. Liège: Ordina Editions.

Tukey, J. W.
1949 One degree of freedom for non-additivity. *Biometrics* **5**:232–242.
1962 The future of data analysis. *Annals of Mathematical Statistics* **33**:1–67, 812.
1972 Some graphic and semigraphic displays. *In* "Statistical Papers in Honor of George W. Snedecor" (T. A. Bancroft, ed.), pp. 293–316. Ames: Iowa State Univ. Press.
1976 Transfactorial fits. 1. The linear geometry in the two-way case. Manuscript, Department of Statistics, Princeton University, Princeton, New Jersey.
1977 "Exploratory Data Analysis." Reading, Massachusetts: Addison-Wesley.

United Nations
1967 "Methods of Estimating Demographic Measures from Incomplete Data." Manual IV of Manuals on Methods of Estimating Population, Series A, Population Studies, no. 42. New York: United Nations.

United Nations, Department of Economic and Social Affairs
1966 "Demographic Yearbook 1965." New York: United Nations.
1976 "Demographic Yearbook 1975." New York: United Nations.

Utterstrom, G.
1954 Some population problems in pre-industrial Sweden. *Scandinavian Economic History Review* **2**:103–165.

1962 Labour policy and population thought in eighteenth century Sweden. *Scandinavian Economic History Review* **10**:262–279.

Van de Geer, J. P.

1971 "Introduction to Multivariate Analysis for the Social Sciences." San Francisco: Freeman.

Van de Walle, E.

1974 "The Female Population of France in the Nineteenth Century." Princeton, New Jersey: Princeton Univ. Press.

Van de Walle, F.

1975 Migration and fertility in Ticino. *Population Studies* **29**:447–462.

Winsborough, H. H.

1978 Organization of demographic research: problems of the next decade. *In* "Social Demography" (K. E. Taeuber, L. L. Bumpass, and J. A. Sweet, eds.), pp. 315–330. New York: Academic Press.

Index

A

$\alpha_i^* A_j^*$ component, *see also* Standard-form components of fertility distributions, function of
  marital fertility distribution implied by, 188, 192, 199–200, 212
  overall fertility distribution implied by, 109–111, 201
  relation to age pattern of natural fertility, 186–192
  shape for marital fertility, 104–105
  shape for overall fertility, 101
  for two- and three-component fits, comparison of, 112
Additive fit, relations to multiplicative fit, 34–35, 277
Age cut, definition, 20
Age-cut effect, 21, 24–25; *see also* EHR age parameters
Age grouping, effect on age pattern of fertility, 42
Age misreporting
  correction for, on basis of EHR parameters, 228–229
  effect on age-specific marital fertility schedules, 208
  in Swedish birth data, 11, 208
Age parameters, *see* EHR age parameters
Age pattern in demographic data, precedents for modeling, 46–47
Age pattern of entry into childbearing
  EHR-parameter evidence of change in, 136–138, 149, 151–155, 223–226

  relation to age pattern of marriage, Sweden, 137, 180
  relation of indices of cohort pace of childbearing to, 132
Age pattern of fertility, *see also* Cohort age pattern of marital fertility; Cohort age pattern of overall fertility; Cross-sectional age pattern of marital fertility; Cross-sectional age pattern of overall fertility; Normalized rates
  approaches to modeling, 1–3
  change in, importance of relating to change in total rate, 47–48
  expression in terms of EHR age standards, procedure, 239–240
  need for time sequence model of, xxi, 16, 161
  normalized rates as expression of, 21, 45–46
  time-sequence compensation of, for fertility level, 132–135
Age-specific fertility rates, *see also* Time sequences of age-specific fertility
  for marital fertility, overview for Sweden, 197
  for overall fertility, overview for Sweden, 13
Age-specific proportion married, approximation from EHR fertility parameters, 209–215
Age-truncated sequences, 44;
  see also C20 sequence; MX20 sequence; X20 sequence; XX20 sequence

STUDIES IN POPULATION

Under the Editorship of: H. H. Winsborough

Department of Sociology
University of Wisconsin
Madison, Wisconsin

Doreen S. Goyer. International Population Census Bibliography: *Revision and Update,* 1945-1977.

David L. Brown and John M. Wardwell (Eds.). New Directions in Urban–Rural Migration: *The Population Turnaround in Rural America.*

A. J. Jaffe, Ruth M. Cullen, and Thomas D. Boswell. The Changing Demography of Spanish Americans.

Robert Alan Johnson. Religious Assortative Marriage in the United States.

Hilary J. Page and Ron Lesthaeghe. Child-Spacing in Tropical Africa.

Dennis P. Hogan. Transitions and Social Change: *The Early Lives of American Men.*

F. Thomas Juster and Kenneth C. Land (Eds.). Social Accounting Systems: *Essays on the State of the Art.*

M. Sivamurthy. Growth and Structure of Human Population in the Presence of Migration.

Robert M. Hauser, David Mechanic, Archibald O. Haller, and Taissa O. Hauser (Eds.). Social Structure and Behavior: *Essays in Honor of William Hamilton Sewell.*

Valerie Kincade Oppenheimer. Work and the Family: *A Study in Social Demography.*

Kenneth C. Land and Andrei Rogers (Eds.). Multidimensional Mathematical Demography.

John Bongaarts and Robert G. Potter. Fertility, Biology, and Behavior: *An Analysis of the Proximate Determinants.*

Randy Hodson. Workers' Earnings and Corporate Economic Structure.

Ansley J. Coale and Paul Demeny. Regional Model Life Tables and Stable Populations, Second Edition.

Mary B. Breckenridge. Age, Time, and Fertility: *Applications of Exploratory Data Analysis.*

In preparation

Neil G. Bennett (Ed.). Sex Selection of Children.